Super Healing
FOODS

◆ Frances Sheridan Goulart ◆

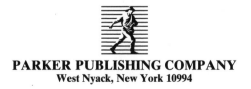

PARKER PUBLISHING COMPANY
West Nyack, New York 10994

This book is a reference work based on research by the author. The opinions expressed herein are not necessarily those of or endorsed by the publisher. The directions stated in this book are in no way to be considered as a substitute for consultation with a duly licensed doctor.

10 9 8 7 6 5 4 3 2 1

Illustrations by Juan DeGuzman

Interior design by Emily Adler

Library of Congress Cataloging-in-Publication Data

Goulart, Frances Sheridan.
    Super healing foods / Frances Sheridan Goulart.
        p.   cm.
    Includes index.
    ISBN 0-13-108820-3 (cloth).—ISBN 0-13-108838-6 (paper)
    1. Nutrition. 2. Diet therapy—Popular works. I. Title.
RA784.G68   1995   95-13636
613.2—dc20   CIP

ISBN 0-13-108820-3
      0-13-108838-6 (pbk.)

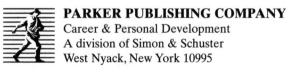

PARKER PUBLISHING COMPANY
Career & Personal Development
A division of Simon & Schuster
West Nyack, New York 10995

Printed in the United States of America

Dedication

To Liz McRory,
for her super healing support every page of the way
and to Doug Corcoran for his affirmative presence and patience

CONTENTS

PART ONE

The ABC's of Super Healing Nutrition ◆ *1*

PART TWO

Common Health Problems
and Their Food "Cures" ◆ *231*

PART THREE

Super Healing Nutrition in Action ◆ *337*

Index ◆ *382*

INTRODUCTION

If you've got a lemon, as they say, make lemonade. But why stop there? Lemons aren't the only super healing foods that alleviate a cold,* that satisfy one quarter of your daily requirement for cholesterol-lowering, immunity-boosting vitamin C, or that energize you as effectively as coffee while cleansing. and stimulating—rather than irritating—your gallbladder.

Consider ginger root. According to USDA medicinal herb authority Dr. James Duke, it's a better-than-Dramamine™ remedy for travel sickness** and a side-effect-free way to prevent nausea.

Or how about super healing chicken soup—that four-star remedy for the common cold? According to a Mount Sinai Medical Center Research study headed by Dr. Marvin Sackner, it provides better-than-Contac relief for upper respiratory infections and better yet, you can access all those benefits *without* the chicken.†

Is it any surprise? Herbs, vegetables, fruits, and nuts provided our first super healing medicines and still do. Virtually every major breakthrough in the development of pharmacology has come from plants, says the Herb Research Foundation. Plant remedies are still the major medicinal source of healing for 80% of the world's population, and botanicals—not chemicals—are the key players in the development of more than half the pharmaceuticals the rest of us rely on.

A TREASURE CHEST OF REMEDIES
Both Ancient and Modern

Five thousand years ago plants were used as medicine by the ancient Sumerians, who recorded the use of 250 medicinal plants on clay tablets. The ancient Egyptians, too, used plant medicines such as gum benzoin, elderberries, wild lettuce, and cinnamon. And in Pliny the Elder's 47 volumes on natural history, there is information on roughly 1,000 plants. In the second century, a Greek pharmacist-physician, Galen, authored 20 books containing numerous food-based healing formulas.

---

* See details, p. 121.

** See details, p. 90.

† See details, p. 265.

Food is often your best remedy and your safest. According to a Johns Hopkins University study, over 125,000 of us die annually as a result of drugs prescribed by medical doctors. Virtually no one has ever succumbed to an overdose of parsley, garlic, or chamomile tea. On the other hand, many plant-based folk remedies are about just that. The hair of the dog is *not* what any reputable medical doctor ordered for a hangover. (Originally, the expression described the folk medicine practice of applying a few hairs of a rabid dog that bit you to speed healing. That didn't work either.) So what's hooey and what's not?

Let's consider a few old chestnuts.

◆ *An apple a day keeps the doctor away.* *Your* doctor might say no, but in a recent three-year study at the University of Michigan, two-a-day apple eaters had fewer headaches along with fewer colds and fewer skin and arthritic complaints. One reason: Apples contain lots of pectin, a fiber which prevents constipation, a leading cause of headaches. Regular apple munching also helps lower LDL (low-density lipoprotein) cholesterol by up to 16%.

◆ *Egg white gives you smoother skin.* Reason? Egg white is composed of water and albumin proteins. When you apply egg white to your face, the water evaporates and the proteins dry, taking loose dead cells on the skin's surface with them, says Page Blankinship, a spokeswoman for the Cosmetic Toiletry and Fragrance Association.

◆ *Drinking milk or beer will cool your mouth after a spicy meal.* It's a chemical reaction, say sensory evaluation experts. The chemicals in hot, peppery foods are dissolved in both fat (milk) and alcohol (beer).

◆ *When you eat Chinese food, you feel hungry an hour later.* Not necessarily. If you are, blame the vegetables, says the gastroenterology department at New York University Medical Center. "Water-chestnuts, Chinese cabbage, bamboo shoots, and sprouts are high in fiber and distend the stomach. When your stomach empties out an hour later, there's such a change you feel hungry even though you ate enough. Solution: Eat more slowly and be sure the meal is balanced with protein and fat.

◆ *Chewing green olives helps prevent motion sickness.* True, says Dr. Cecil Hart of the American Academy of Otolaryngology and Northwestern University Medical School in Chicago. Green olives contain tannins, which dry the mouth and reduce the saliva that drains into the stomach when it's upset, interfering with the contraction of stomach muscles.

◆ *Putting cereal in your socks prevents foot odors.* Hooey, says Dr. Edgar B. Smith, chairman of the department of dermatology at the University of Texas Medical Branch in Galveston. But cereal bran alone does absorb sweat almost as well as talc.

◆ *Honey on a cut speeds healing.* True to an extent, says Richard Knutson, M.D., of the Delta Medical Center of Greenville, Mississippi. The ancient Egyptians used a poultice of grease and honey on wounds, and all sugars appear to absorb moisture and reduce swelling. Sugars are thought to contain a natural antibacterial agent, but this remains to be proven clinically.

◆ *Gargling with salt water will cure a sore throat.* Believe it or not, a saline solution is more effective than cough drops and commercial gargles. Salt's antiseptic properties work best in a ratio of one-quarter teaspoon salt to eight ounces warm water.

◆ *A cold teabag on your eyelids will reduce puffiness.* True, but it's the coldness, not the tea leaves, that constricts blood vessels. A chilled teaspoon works equally well.

◆ *Carrot soup will cure diarrhea.* True, says Dr. Jan Soule, pediatrician in Portland, Oregon. Carrot soup supplies balanced amounts of sodium and potassium, two electrolytes that a dehydrated stomach needs. No time to do it from scratch? Make a shortcut carrot soup by mixing equal amounts of water and a jar of puréed baby carrots.

THE HEALING POWERS IN YOUR KITCHEN

Ready to explore the safe super healing powers of ordinary fruits and vegetables? There's no time like the present. Statistics from the American Dietetic Association tell us that more than four out of five (82%) Americans recognize the importance of good nutrition, but only 39% do anything about it, and barely one third of us consciously shop with the healthiest choices in mind. When we do the right thing, for 52% of us it's simply eating more vegetables, and for 36% of us it's eating more fruit. And the younger you are (under 35), the less likely you are to do even that. Worse, less than a third of us know what recommended daily guidelines we aren't living up to. (Seventy percent of us, for example, believe that one or two servings of fruits and vegetables daily does the trick. The recommended minimum is five.) And only 23% of those of us who know the goal meet it on a regular basis.

You don't have to be among the soon-to-be-sick-or-sicker if you keep reading this book.

HOW TO USE THIS BOOK FOR SUPER HEALING HEALTH

1. Nature's 50 top super healing foods are individually profiled in Part I with recipes and remedial formulas so you can incorporate super healing nutrition into every meal and snack.

2. The 50 common ailments that these foods can help prevent, alleviate, or reverse are profiled in Part II with one or more recipes or formulas and references to other helpful foods and formulas found throughout the book.

3. The Super Healing Master Plan diet in Part III is a lean, green, high-fiber low-fat meatless regimen that even nonvegetarians can follow for high-level wellness for a week, a month, a year, or a lifetime. There are four variations to accommodate all your nutritional needs no matter what super healing path you're on or what your progress.

4. In addition to the recipes in Parts I and II, there are recipes, menus, and meal plans, each with variations, in Part III which show you how to put super healing nutrition into action every day.*

5. What's where? It's as easy as ABC to find any food or any disorder because the Super Healing Plan has been organized alphabetically. And you'll find cross-referenced cues at the end of each entry to lead you to even more super healing help elsewhere in the book.

6. Beyond food and nutrition? You'll find nutrition-supportive exercises, tips for bad habit control, affirmative spiritual action, and

---

* The body has ten health support systems—The Dermal, Cardiovascular, Respiratory, Skeletal, Digestive, Endocrinal, Neuro-muscular, Audiovisual, Reproductive and the Immune System There are certain illnesses and food remedies that pertain to those systems which have been identified, numbered, and will be referred to throughout this book as "Target Healing Zones."

more in Part III plus a guide to mail order sources for hard-to-find foods and health aids.

Ready to start healing? Here's how to use your knife and fork as tools to access the uncommon healing benefits in common everyday fruits, vegetables, nuts, legumes, and grains. (A super healing food is defined here as one that favorably affects at least one or more of the body's 10 healing zones in one or more more-than-marginal ways.) See "Ten Mind/Body Healing Zones chart on pp. 339.

Let the next bite you take be the beginning of the rest of your super healing life.

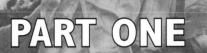

PART ONE

The ABC's of Super Healing Nutrition

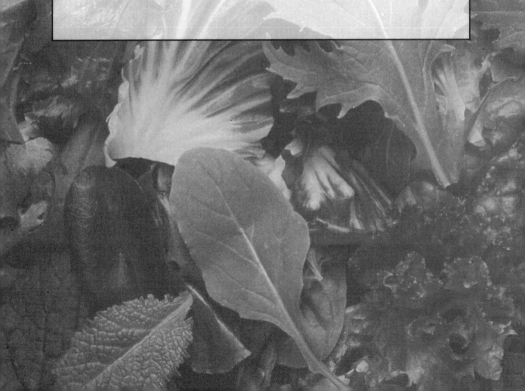

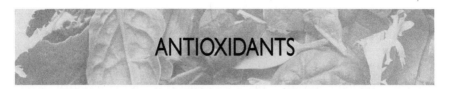

ANTIOXIDANTS

Is your diet rich in health-friendly carotene, genistein, tocopherols, and flavonoids? It should be if you're out for super healing because these are the nutrients known as antioxidants found in carrots, red peppers, broccoli, and other red, yellow, and green vegetables as well as nuts, beans, and whole grains. According to the National Council for Responsible Nutrition, U.S. health care costs could be reduced by $7 billion if we increased our collective consumption of antioxidant carotene-carrier foods alone.

ANTIOXIDANTS FOR HEALTH DAMAGE CONTROL
Only an Onion or an Apple Away

There are more than 1,500 recognized antioxidants and related phytochemicals in everyday common foods that do an uncommonly good job of combating free radicals in the body—those substances released internally during the process of oxidation and formed externally by environmental forces such as radiation, X-rays, drugs, pesticides, air and water pollutants, hydrocarbons, food additives, alcohol, smoking—you name it. Free radicals damage living cells and contribute to a continuing roll call of complaints, including interference with DNA programming, premature aging, heart disease, AIDS, arthritis, cancer, cataracts, allergies, and diabetes. Here's how the antioxidant force can be with you when you eat.

Perhaps the most celebrated of the free radical foes are the carotenoids (named for the carrots in which they were first isolated), of which there are approximately 40, including alpha and beta-carotene (found in carrots, apricots, and sweet potatoes) and lutein (found in spinach, celery, and kale). The carotenoids are especially potent in blocking cancer, fighting allergies, and slowing the aging process.

The most powerful members of the antioxidant family are probably the pycnogenols (a.k.a. flavonoids), which are 20 times more potent than vitamin C and 50 times more active than vitamin E. Pycnogenols protect against capillary damage, bruising, and improve your overall immunity to heart disease and cancer. Best sources: onions, green peppers, red wine, green tea, and selected herbs.

Beyond what it does for the common cold and the flu, the vitamin-antioxidant ascorbic acid (vitamin C) can slow the onset of Parkinson's disease, reduce the risk of hardening of the arteries by increasing the amount of protective high-density lipoprotein (HDL) cholesterol in your bloodstream, help prevent cataracts by guarding the eyes against oxidation, help lower blood pressure, and protect against a wide spectrum of cancers.

Vitamin E (tocopherol) is a fat-soluble vitamin-antioxidant and important immune system stimulant that helps alleviate fatigue and provides tissue oxygen to accelerate the healing of wounds, burns and skin disorders such as acne and eczema. In partnership with the mineral selenium, it neutralizes free radicals that accelerate cellular and cerebral aging and raise the risk of cancer.

20 ANTIOXIDANTS/40 FOOD SOURCES

Of the 20 nutrients critical in the prevention of cancer, says John Bertram, Ph.D., professor of genetics and molecular biology at the University of Hawaii Cancer Research Center, half are antioxidants. And what's true for cancer is true for heart disease and most other degenerative diseases. If your health's on hold, your body's not equipped to fight back because it's inadequately supplied with these food-based free radical scavengers. What do you need on a meal-to-meal basis to protect yourself? Take a look.

Antioxidant	Selected Food Sources
Carotenoids/Vitamin A	Carrots, squash, apricots, red peppers, sweet potatoes, celery, spinach, tomatoes, oranges*
Vitamin C	Parsley, citrus fruits, kiwi fruit, red and green peppers, cabbage, leafy greens, green tea
Vitamin E	Nuts and seeds, nut oils, wheat germ, soy foods

---

* Carotenoids are not well absorbed without fat. To maximize uptake, combine nuts and oils with vegetables and fruits.

Indoles	Broccoli, cauliflower, cabbage, mustard greens, radishes
Amino acid Proteins	Dairy foods, soy foods, nutritional yeast, high-protein cereal grains
Genisteins	Soy foods, tofu, tempeh, miso
Ellagic acid	Apples, berries, tea
Protease inhibitors	Nuts, seeds, grains, soybeans
Selenium and Zinc	Nuts, seeds, whole grains, nutritional yeast

Note: Other important free radical fighters and fighter helpers found in the aforementioned foods include B complex (especially pantothenic acid, vitamins B_1 and B_6), sulphur compounds, quercetin, pangamic acid (vitamin B_{15}) and Coenzyme Q_{10}.

Your Herbal Antioxidant Arsenal

Good herbal antioxidants to sip, sniff, or cook with include alfalfa, rosehips, peppermint, nettles, hawthorn, goldenseal and fenugreek, cumin, capsicum (red pepper), cinnamon, and basil (all available as teas and tinctures).

FOUR ANTIOXIDANT EATERS' TIPS

◆ Your best source for all the antioxidants known and unknown are whole foods—five or six servings a day of fruits and vegetables at the top of the list, says the National Institutes of Health. Supplements cannot provide the unknown protective factors which work in synergy with recognized free radical fighters.

◆ Fresh raw fruits and vegetables are a more potent source of antioxidants than frozen. If you must cook, short and fast does minimal damage, and always steam (don't boil), bake, or broil—don't fry. Long-cooking, noninstant whole grains and dried beans deliver more antioxidants than instant or fast-cooking types.

◆ The deeper the color (orange, red or purple, yellow, green), the higher the antioxidant level in any food or drink.

Note: In the following recipe, any natural whole grain may be substituted for amaranth (i.e., brown rice, whole wheat, or rye berries).

RDA Ratatouille

This recipe provides your recommended daily allowance (RDA)* for at least six antioxidants, including C, E, and beta-carotene.

> *1 tablespoon sesame or sunflower oil*
>
> *4 cups cooked amaranth (or other whole grain high-protein cereal such as quinoa or kamut)*
>
> *2 cups (1 medium) diced zucchini or yellow squash*
>
> *1½ cups coarsely shredded carrots*
>
> *2 green or red peppers, seeded and diced*
>
> *3 cloves garlic, crushed and minced*
>
> *2–3 medium tomatoes, coarsely chopped*
>
> *¼ teaspoon basil*
>
> *pinch cayenne pepper*
>
> *½ bunch minced fresh parsley or cilantro*

Heat oil in a heavy skillet. Add grains and sauté for 5 minutes. Remove grain from skillet and add zucchini and sauté (adding a few spoonfuls of water if the mixture sticks). Return grains to skillet.

In second skillet, steam-cook carrots and peppers in a few spoonfuls of water until tender (but not browned). Add garlic.

Place tomatoes over carrots, peppers, and garlic in the skillet, sprinkle with basil and cayenne, and cover. Steam over low heat for 5 minutes. Uncover, stir vegetables over medium-high heat for 30 seconds. Sprinkle with parsley or cilantro and remove skillet from heat.

In casserole dish, layer alternating tomato mixture with the grain-zucchini mixture, beginning and ending with tomatoes.

Cover casserole and bake at 350 degrees for 15–20 minutes. Garnish with orange or kiwi slices.

TIP: May be prepared in advance and chilled before baking.

Makes six generous servings.

Benefits healing zones: All

Also see: Beta-carotene, Cruciferous Vegetables, Broccoli, Carrots, Vitamin C, Vitamin B, Vitamin E, Coronary Heart Disease

Call the American Institute for Cancer Research hotline at 1-800-843-8114 for more information.

---

* Also known as Daily Quota.

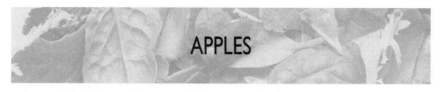

APPLES

Did you know that the United States produces 8 billion pounds of apples annually and that the average American polishes off 18.1 pounds of them a year?

Here are a few more health and healing historical facts for apple polishers.

♦ The apple that almost wasn't: All of America's harvest of McIntoshes (number 3 on America's bushel-and-a-peck Hit Parade) owe their heritage to the single tree that survived transplanting by Ontario farmer John McIntosh at the turn of the century.

♦ The most perfectly red apple—Ida Red, a cross between the Jonathan and Wagener varieties—was hybrid in Idaho in 1942.

♦ America's newest apple, Paula Red, is named for Paula Arend, wife of a Sparta, Michigan, apple aficionado and grower.

♦ Big byte: The name *Apple* was chosen by health-conscious computer whiz Stephen Wozniak in 1976 because he felt the fruit epitomized naturalness and good health.

♦ There are more than 500 apple varieties in the United States. But only 14 favorites account for 90% of the crop harvested.

♦ Not like father, like son: Every apple seed produces a slightly different variety than its parent.

♦ The Rome apple, the baker's first choice and America's number 4 favorite, actually originated in southern Ohio.

♦ America's first homegrown apples came from the "Pippins," which Massachusetts colony's Governor John Winthrop planted in Boston in 1639.

♦ New York City's nickname, the "Big Apple" (i.e., the Mecca), was coined by jazz musicians in Harlem speakeasies of the 1920s and 1930s.

♦ One of America's earliest golf courses was created on a 3-acre apple orchard in Yonkers in 1892 by a group of Scottish golfers who called themselves the Apple Tree Gang.

◆ The world's biggest big apple is an Oregon red weighing 17½ pounds.

◆ Celebrity apple polishers: The longest single unbroken apple peel on record was 172 feet, 4 inches long, peeled in 11½ hours by a Big Apple New Yorker. Paul McCartney named the Beatles' company Apple Corp. and their record company Apple Records. All Beatles recordings featured photos of a shiny green Granny Smith apple.

◆ The expression "apple of one's eye" arose from the superstition in ancient times that the pupil of the eye was an apple-like globe (the Anglo-Saxon word *aeppel* referred to both the seeing eye and to the edible fruit).

SIX REASONS FOR AN APPLE A DAY

As for the old chestnut that an apple a day keeps the doctor away: There are plenty of super healing reasons why that's so. Apples are rich in natural fruit sugars, low in calories (about 80 each), high in water, and rich

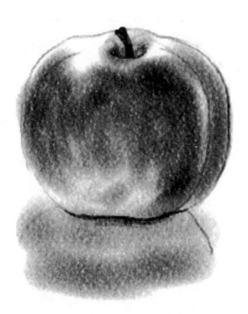

in carbohydrate food fibers, including cellulose, hemicellulose, and pectin plus the noncarbohydrate fiber lignin in the apple peel, which lowers cholesterol, normalizes blood pressure, and prevents digestive disorders. (The homeopathic remedy for diarrhea is podophyllum, compounded from the May apple.) Another cardiovascular bonus: Apples have little sodium, no fat or cholesterol, and provide 70% more potassium—the mineral that enhances heart muscle function—than fresh oranges.

THREE APPLE ANTIOXIDANTS FOR 20 TO 50 TIMES MORE HEART PROTECTION

The flavonoid-antioxidants in apples may even keep the pacemaker away and prevent bypass surgery. Flavonoids are antioxidant compounds 20 times more potent than vitamin C and 50 times more potent than vitamin E, according to the British Heart Foundation. A five-year study of 805 Dutch men from 65 to 84 years old led by Dr. Michael Hertog, an epidemiologist at the National Institute of Public Health in Bilthoven, The Netherlands, found that men who consumed the greatest amounts of this widely dispersed antioxidant suffered half as many fatal heart attacks as men who consumed the least. (High consumption of flavonoids is the equivalent of one large apple a day, or four cups of regular tea.) Flavonoids appear to protect the heart by preventing the formation of plaque that clogs arteries and by lowering blood pressure and cholesterol.

PECTIN
A Bushel and a Peck of Benefits

In typical studies, the equivalent of two large apples a day causes a 16% drop in cholesterol levels, attributed to the fruit's high pectin levels as well as its flavonoids. Pectin appears to form a gel in the stomach that prevents total absorption of the fats in food.

Pectin also helps regulate blood sugar in diabetics and is a natural antidiarrheal aid (purified pectin is an ingredient in many over-the-counter [OTC] correctives such as Kaopectate). Apples are one more of the few fruits to supply the potent compound ellagic acid which blocks the cancer-causing action of many pollutants and protects you from the toxic effect of carcenogenic benzene compounds.

A BIG MAC A DAY FOR MENTAL CLARITY

Apples also contain the trace mineral boron, which improves mental alertness. According to a 1993 USDA study, brainwave levels fell in response to reductions of boron from 3 mg (the super-minimal amount most of us consume) to 250 µg a day but rose when the dose was adjusted. Boron also appears to curb calcium losses that lead to osteoporosis.

SIPPING APPLE CIDER TO RELIEVE INSOMNIA, SUNBURN AND AGING SKIN, AND MORE

According to French folklore, insomnia is cured by applesauce or stewed apples, and a grated apple applied topically is said to have a germicidal effect on sores and sunburns. Thin apple slices or puréed apples also make good skin toners and antiwrinkle masks, says food historian Ruth Ward, because of their alphahydroxy complex acids (try a nightly splash of fresh apple juice as a rejuvenating astringent). Studies indicate that apples' acids remove damaged aged cells, soften skin, and slow aging (for antistress relief, apply a poultice of grated apples to the eyelids) by stimulating dermal collagen production.

ENERGIZE WITH AN APPLE'S FRUIT SUGARS AND VITAMINS

Carbohydrate loading? An 8 ounce glass of apple juice or cider supplies more sugar (22 g) in a healthier ratio of fructose to glucose to sucrose than a glass of cola (18 g) or milk (8 g). A standard-sized apple supplies small amounts of vitamin A and B Complex and 6 mg of vitamin C.* Apples are also one of the few fruit sources (along with mangos, blueberries, and currants) of vitamin E (two large apples supply 20% of your RDA).

---

* Some varieties have a higher than average vitamin C content per 100 g—for example, Ribston Pippin (30 mg), King of the Pippins (18 mg), Northern Spy (16 mg), Blenheim Orange (13 mg), Cox's Orange Pippin (10 mg), Golden Delicious (8 mg). Best of the culinary varieties: Golden Noble (29 mg), Reinette du Canada (17 mg), and Bramley's Seedling (16 mg). Overall, botanists number 3,000 varieties of applies.

Buying, Storing, and Using

Look for firm, clear-skinned apples, but avoid bruised ones, which (in apples) may signal an enzyme that accelerates oxidation of phenols and produces brownish pigments. Surface brown spots called russeting are safe and edible.

If you're an avid apple eater, look for certified organic produce (apples and pears are heavily sprayed crops, and peels are often colored artificially as well). Or use a good-quality produce pesticide wash (see Mail Order Sources in Part III).

Apples should be refrigerated to preserve natural flavor and prevent inner browning (near the core). Out of the refrigerator, apples spoil 10 times faster.

Don't peel or slice an apple until you're ready to eat. Dipping raw slices and/or peeled apples into a lemon and water solution will retard browning. Keep a saucer of lemony apple slices and pear wedges in the fridge for postmeal damage control. They counteract the fat consumed in meats, desserts, sweets, and other rich foods.

To get twice as many nutrients (with the exception of vitamin C, which is lost in dehydration), snack on dried apple rings as a chip or candy substitute.

Eat your macs with iron-rich foods such as nuts, seeds, or grains to up your intake of vitamin C (the two nutrients potentiate one another).

Best juice partners: carrot, lemon, camomile, grape.

TIP: For a catalog of 124 grow-your-own apple varieties, including heirloom and hard-to-find apples, write St. Lawrence Nurseries, Box 324, Potsdam, NY 13676.

Apple Whip and Chill

Whip two egg whites with ½ teaspoon cream of tartar until stiff. Put 1 cup of lukewarm water in blender with one package of plain gelatin and process until frothy and milky colored.

Combine the two mixtures. Fold in ¾ cup of coarsely grated raw apple (squeezed of extra juices) and 1 tablespoon honey, ½ teaspoon cinnamon, and ½ cup plain yogurt.

Spoon into two parfait glasses, sprinkle with crushed raw nuts or granola.

Chill until firm.

Variation: Substitute a Bosc pear for apple or the apple-flavored apple banana. Substitute lemon yogurt for plain.

Benefits healing zones: 2, 7, 8

Also see: Coronary Heart Disease, Fatigue, Indigestion, Antioxidants

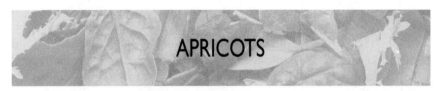

APRICOTS

What's low in calories, high in beta-carotene, and a legacy of the Garden of Eden? Ordinary apricots. Three fresh apricots provide over 50% of your daily quota (RDA) for beta-carotene and only 50 calories. According to a counter legend, it was apricots, not apples, which grew in the Garden of Eden, and this is the same super healing fruit (known as the Khubani) which keeps the Hunza octogenarians in the Himalayas young.

ANTICANCER SNACKING

Studies indicate that diets rich in beta-carotene-rich fruits, such as apricots, lower the incidence of cancer dramatically—especially of the larynx, lungs, and pancreas, And apricots offer super healing to ex-smokers since they have the ability to defuse the latent effects of nicotine. Beta-carotene also helps prevent the build-up of plaque in the arteries that triggers coronary heart disease.

FOUR BIG MINERAL BOOSTS IN EACH LITTLE FRUIT

Apricots also supply potassium for healthy cardiovascular function; boron, which promotes estrogen in postmenopausal women; iron for the prevention of fatigue and infection; plus silica for healthy skin, hair, and nails.

Buying, Storing, and Using

Look for unsulphured dried fruits free of the sulphur additives, which can trigger asthma in the sensitive. For super healing, use dried apricots, which have more than triple the fresh fruit's concentration of beta-carotene and fiber.

Benefits healing zones: 2, 3, 7

Also see: Beta-carotene, Cancer, Coronary Heart Disease

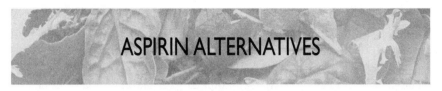

ASPIRIN ALTERNATIVES

According to the International Association for the Study of Pain, Americans take 30 billion aspirin a year to put pain—everything from migraine and lower back ache to menstrual cramps—in its place. The pain-pain-go-away impulse has reached such proportions that since 1960, hundreds of pain centers* have opened to treat the phenomenon of *chronic pain* (the kind that persists after the original cause is gone or when all else fails) as a disease all its own. With this new approach, new therapies—including biofeedback, low-energy lasers, and acupuncture and hypnosis—have appeared. But in-clinic relief comes at a price—usually hundreds of dollars a month—and may take many months to work.

ASPIRIN
The Good News

Aspirin, acetaminophen, and other analgesics have their virtues. Aspirin improves the efficiency of thymosin, a substance secreted by the thymus gland that prevents suppression of immunity by internal or external forces and even appears to promote longevity, says the American Academy of Orthopedic Surgeons. When taken regularly by heart patients, it reduces cardiovascular deaths by almost 25% and nonfatal strokes by nearly 50%.

Aspirin even appears to stimulate production of two cancer-fighting components of the immune system: gamma interferon and interleukin-2, says the National Cancer Society.

TEN REASONS TO AVOID ASPIRIN

Unfortunately, you pay the price for aspirin's benefits. Aspirin reduces pain by suppressing the body's natural inflammatory reaction, says

---

* For a referral to a center in your area, write the American Association for the Study of Headache, P.O. Box 5136, San Clemente, CA 92672, or call the National Headache Foundation, 800-843-2256.

Michael J. Shkrum, M.D., of the Victoria Hospital in London, Ontario, Canada. "Salicylate has widespread metabolic effects, too, that can mimic other medical conditions, leading to delayed diagnosis of salicylate intoxication." According to researchers at the Oregon Health Sciences University in Portland, 6,000 aspirin taken over a long period of time (three tablets a day for three years) can cause permanent kidney damage. Make that a more potent OTC painkiller like Naproxen and you may have double trouble because its effectiveness is twice as long lasting.

Aspirin also increases bleeding tendencies and can cause stomach bleeding (especially beyond the conservative preventive aspirin therapeutical dose of one every other day) and is contraindicated for anyone with diabetes, kidney or liver disfunction, or ulcers.

Aspirin also alters the effects of other medications, including anticoagulants, diabetic drops, insulin, and cortisone, and it triples your body's excretion of vitamin C. Aspirin substitutes such as acetaminophen aren't much better. Taken twice daily for a year, acetaminophen can triple your risk of serious kidney damage, admits John T. Walden of the Nonprescription Drug Manufacturers Association.

15 SAFE ALTERNATIVES

So what's the safe do-it-yourself solution? Here are 15 solutions that use nutrition and natural therapies:

1. *Beef up your diet with B, C, and carrots, not beef.* The least headache-prone group in the country? The largely vegetarian Seventh Day Adventists. A diet rich in vitamins C and B complex and calcium-rich foods can headache-proof your diet. Another deficiency pain maker? Vitamin A (found in carrots, eggs, liver, and leafy greens).

2. *Beat the pain with botanicals.* The best plant painkiller is *feverfew,* says the London Migraine Clinic. Used in fever, migraine, and arthritis control for over 2,500 years, the active ingredients which produce even stronger-than-aspirin relief are sesquiterpene lactones and parthenolide. Fifty to 100 mg daily is the usual dose level. Or try kudzu, a staple in the Chinese pharmacopeia for 1,800 years, available as an herbal powder. The pain-suppressant effect, which is migraine-specific, is produced by flavonoids, an antioxidant also found in tea, apples, and red wine.

3. *Consider niacin, not Advil.* And consider the cause. Headaches can be caused by chronic poor posture and/or poor diet, says the National Headache Foundation. Try 50 mg of niacin (vitamin B₃) at the first sign of pain, not aspirin, whose enzyme-inhibiting side-effects can include indigestion.

4. *Ban the bar, and say no to nitrates (and keep a cap on caffeine).* Health food stores carry a variety of preservative-free alternatives to chocolate bars, cocoa, chocolate desserts, etc., which contain tyramine, another common headache-maker, plus caffeine. Too much caffeine can also be a mini-migraine maker, warns the New England Headache Treatment Program in Stamford, Connecticut, by causing dilation of blood vessels in the cranial cavity. If chocolate fasting doesn't fix it, have your doctor check your sensitivity to MSG—a headache-provoking seasoning used by many restaurants and food processors.

5. *Empirin-Plus.* Activate your body's natural painkilling endorphins with DLPA (DL-phenylalanine) supplements—a combination of natural and synthetic amino acids more effective than OTC aspirin and Valium that is especially useful in whiplash, cramps, neuralgia, and arthritis. You can get a handle on what hurts with two 375-mg tablets. Best natural DLPA sources: dairy foods, lean meat, and poultry.

6. *Take it lying down.* Minor persistent back pain often responds to a simple change in position that takes the stress off your spine and relaxes key back muscles. Try the 90/90 solution: Lie on the floor, legs on a chair, with thighs at a 90-degree angle to hips and calves at a 90-degree angle to thighs. Variation: Lie on your side in same position. If that doesn't do the trick, ask your neighborhood naturopath about oxygen therapy.

7. *Rub it in.* Let your fingers do the healing with a painkilling herbal oil: ½ teaspoon eucalyptus and 1 tablespoon pure olive oil, or equal parts of fresh ginger juice with sesame oil. Another variation is this botanical capsaicin liniment: Simmer 1 tablespoon of cayenne pepper (capsaicin) in 1 pint of cider vinegar gently for 10 minutes. Bottle hot and unstrained. Apply freely and massage gently for 15 to 20 minutes three to four times a day. This even beats the pain of black and blue spots—capsaicin is a healing compound that raises your pain threshold by neutralizing substance P, a neuropain transmitter.

8. *Head off athletic aches and pains,* advises Dana Ullman, MPH, in
   Everybody's Guide to Homeopathic Medicines (Tarcher), with pre-
   workout homeopathic formulas which speed healing and restore
   the immune system to a state of balance without drugs. Health
   food stores also carry homeopathic ointments for soreness, stiffness, and bruising. The best all-purpose bets to prevent postexer-
   cise lactic acid build-up: arnica montana, sarcolacticum acidum,
   and rhododendron.

9. *The AC/DC aspirin alternative.* Can't decide whether to soothe the
   pain with an ice pack or a heating pad? Use both—alternating for
   30-minute periods—advises the National Headache Foundation,
   until you feel better.

10. *Wear a migraine-bandit headband:* an elastic band with two small
    discs that apply pressure over areas of maximum pain. Provides
    relief by putting pressure on important acupressure points.

11. *Try P.M. relief for A.M. pain.* A nightly rub with a muscle relaxant
    cream at bedtime helps reduce chronic stiffness associated with
    arthritis and rheumatism. Another reliever is a weekly aquacise-in-
    water fitness program.

12. *Use your imagination.* According to Dennis Turk, Ph.D., director
    of the Pain Evaluation and Treatment Institute at the University of
    Pittsburgh School of Medicine, creative visualization can distract
    your senses from the distraction of pain. One favorite: "Close your
    eyes and imagine a lemon on a white china plate. See a knife next
    to it. See yourself pick it up and slice the lemon. Hear the sound it
    makes cutting through. Smell the aroma. Bring the lemon up to
    your face and imagine its taste." TIP: The more detailed the image,
    the more rapid the pain distraction.

13. *Check your stress levels.* Stress can lead to pain anywhere in your
    body if it provokes tensing, slouching, hunching, clutching, tooth
    grinding, nail biting, etc. Check out your stress levels twice a day
    and have an M.D. do it annually.

14. *Last but not least,* if you must take aspirin, you can offset its
    potential ill effects by alternating with an aspirin alternative that
    normalizes activity of the body's anti-inflammatory agents
    (prostaglandin, serotonin, and leukotrienes). A good one from the
    garden patch: Feverfew (*Tanacetum parthenium*)—a centuries-old
    garden patch painkiller and second cousin to the common garden

mum that can be taken daily as a tea or in tablet form without side-effects. Even better, grow your own. Write to Companion Plants, 724 N. Coolnette Ridge, Athens, OH 45701 for information.

15. For an analgesic education in a nutshell, dial 1-800-253-8394 for a copy of the Long Beach Medical Center's brochure "Pain Talk," or call 1-800-756-PAIN.

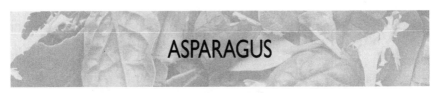

ASPARAGUS

Asparagus? Think Easter, onion, and antiquity. A Mediterranean member of the lily family and first cousin to the orchid, lily of the valley, and yellow onion, asparagus is grown in 100 varieties worldwide, and many nations claim it as their own. Of the several varieties native to France, for example, the most notable if not the most nutritious is the celebrated Argenteuil variety, prized for its tenderness and delicate flavor. Originally cultivated for Louis XIV, it is raised underground to abort "greening" and is not widely available outside France.

There is also a unique purple German asparagus; a white Belgian; and a white German type plus small and large continental green spears. America produces several varieties, both white and green.

A SPEAR TO SAFEGUARD WHOLE BODY HEALING
Five Factors

This slinky root vegetable, known in England as "sparrow grass" until the eighteenth century, was known as a healing food as far back as the second century B.C. Chinese herbalists also used "asphargos" (a name meaning "wind pipe" applied by Greeks of Aristotle's day) to cure everything from arthritis to infertility. In the fifteenth, sixteenth, and seventeenth centuries, asparagus was a remedy of choice for toothaches, heart disorders, dropsy, and bee stings.

In Japan, asparagus juice tonics have been a time-honored botanical treatment for cardiovascular disorders. There are five nutritional reasons for this: Our favorite first-of-spring vegetable satisfies 200% of your RDA for blood-pressure-regulating, electrolyte-balancing potassium, plus 49% of your need for antioxidant vitamin C (including the bioflavonoid rutin, which protects the capillaries and prevents varicose veins). Heart-healthy factors four and five? Pectin, the cholesterol-lowering fiber that also regulates bowel functions, and vitamin K for normal blood clotting.

GOOD ASPARAGUS
Better Sex and Reproductive System Health

Asparagus contains substantial amounts of aspartic acid, an amino acid that neutralizes the excess amounts of ammonia in the body that cause fatigue and sexual lassitude. "Experiments with potassium and magnesium salts of aspartic acid," observes food historian Robert Hendrickson, "have overcome cases of chronic exhaustion and increased sexual responsiveness."

Asparagus is also the sole source of the alkaloid asparagine, an essential for prostate gland health. (A good way to benefit, according to the Bastyr College Health Information Project is to juice asparagus with carrots and cucumbers and drink daily.) And 1 cup of cooked asparagus

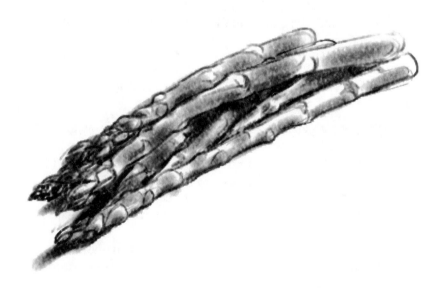

spears supplies 66% of your 400-µg RDA for folate, which helps lower the risk of birth defects, and colon and cervical cancer.

Diuretic and Detoxifier

An asparagus aperitif is a good once-a-week way to detoxify all 10 of your healing zones—especially the bladder, kidneys, and urinary tract—since asparagus's highly alkaline salts and the trace elements silicon and molybdenum are all essential for the health of all the glands and major organs and for prevention of gout, acne, eczema, and other skin disorders, says the American Botanical Council.

Asparagus's vitamin B_6 makes it one of nature's four top diuretics (along with watermelon, cantaloupe, and artichokes) for relief of premenstrual bloating and edema. (The characteristic odor that asparagus leaves behind in the urine is a sign of kidney-bladder cleaning.)

Raising Immunity, Lowering Weight

Asparagus can increase your immunity while you decrease your weight: 1 cup cooked supplies 1,300 IU (international units)* of beta-carotene and only 30 calories, with only a trace of sodium. Asparagus is the ideal food for dieters.

Buying, Storing, and Using

The tip of asparagus is your tip-off. Fresh tips are firm, dry, compact, and end in a sharp point and should smell clean and green. (Tips that are open rather than compact or feathery are past their prime.) The greener the spear, the more tender the texture. (Before you cook it, taste the raw pea flavor of the spear.) *Note:* No asparagus spear is 100% tender tip to butt. As much as 75% or more of a mostly white spear will be tough and woody. Use asparagus as soon as purchased or wrap in damp paper towels and store in a vegetable crisper.

Commonest cooking method: Place loosely string tied bundles of whole spears in boiling salted water (salting keeps stalks firm) and simmer uncovered for 12 minutes. Or prepare diagonally sliced spears in a

---

* IU or international units is the form of measurement used for oil soluble vitamins such as vitamins A and D. IUs are five times greater (in number) than REs a newer unit of measurement for oil soluble vitamins. 5,000 IU = equals 1,000 RE (Retinol equivalent)

steamer (if you have a three-tiered version, steam rice or noodles and vegetarian dumplings while you're at it). To sweeten stalks, add 1 tablespoon sugar to a pot of water. Add standing bunch of asparagus and steam until tender.

Try the following uses:

Toss cooked spears in grated cheese and fine whole wheat bread crumbs which have been sautéed in oil.

Sprinkle cooked spears with cheese and oil, and broil for 60 seconds.

Top warm or cold asparagus with healthy mayonnaise blended with the juice of one blood orange and grated lemon peel.

Add tips to spring salads.

Steamed stalks/spears may be pureed for healing soups and sauces or juiced to supplement other juices or store-bought soups. Best asparagus partners: parsley, green pepper, celery, spinach.

Sparrow Grass Dills (No-Cuke Pickles)

> *3 wide-mouthed pint canning jars*
>
> *4 cups vinegar*
>
> *1 cup natural sugar*
>
> *2 teaspoons whole allspice*
>
> *12 whole cloves*
>
> *6-inch stick cinnamon*
>
> *4 pounds asparagus, washed and ends trimmed to fit jars*

Heat jars in a 250-degree oven to sterilize. Place vinegar, 2 cups of water, and sugar in medium pot. Tie allspice, cloves, and cinnamon in a cheesecloth bag and add to pickling liquid; simmer for 15 minutes.

Boil 4 cups of water. Add asparagus, cook for three minutes, and drain. Return boiling water to pot and return to a boil.

When cool, pack spears in sterile jars, cover with pickling liquid, leaving ½-inch headspace, and seal. Process jars in boiling water for 10 minutes.

Makes 3 pints.

Benefits healing zones: 2, 6, 7, 9

Also see: Basic Dieting Facts and Advice, Coronary Heart Disease, Prostate, Cystitis

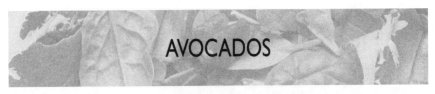

AVOCADOS

The avocado (a.k.a. the "alligator pear,"* although it is kin to neither)—the fruit we treat and eat like a vegetable—is in fact the product of the *Persea americana* tree (a relative of the laurel), which now thrives on semitropic turf throughout the Western Hemisphere.

Originally native to Mexico and Central America, there are over 400 wild and cultivated varieties today of this buttery-textured, hazelnut-redolent plant maverick, which is classified as a "neutral" fruit because it is compatible with (and can be eaten with or as) either fruits or vegetables.

The modified English spelling of the Spanish word for avocado resembles the Spanish *bocado,* meaning "delicacy."

THE NUTRITION OF A FRUIT, VEGETABLE, AND NUT
All in One

A prolific producer like the banana bush, or an average avocado tree can produce 500 to 2,000 fruits in its lifetime. The avocado is considered the most highly nutritionally evolved of all food plants, according to the Natural Food and Farming Associates. With the biochemical profile of a nut rather than a fruit, the average avocado provides enough protein to replace the meat or cheese in a light meal. (In parts of Mexico and South America, where avocados often appear as dessert and are even transformed into ice cream, avocado, tortilla, and coffee may constitute a square meal.)

THE GREEN BUTTER FOR CARDIOVASCULAR FITNESS

Avocado is a source of 13 essential minerals, including iron, copper, and magnesium, which work as a team to build and repair red blood cells and prevent nutritional anemia. A serving of guacamole also gives you monounsaturated fats (including oleic and linoleic acids) for maintenance of normal cholesterol levels and provides a more potent source of heart-rhythm-regulating potassium than such potassium-source standards as peaches, potatoes, and prune juice. In fact, studies suggest that

---

* Another name for the black, pebbly skinned California *fuerta* variety.

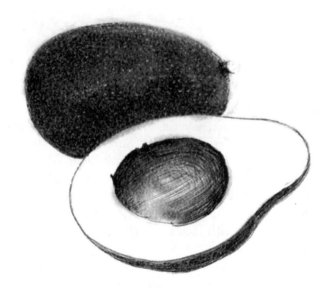

half an avocado a day not only satisfies your "fat tooth" a lot better than butter but lowers cholesterol by 8% to 42%. As a bonus, avocados are low in sodium and cholesterol free.

ANTIAGING BENEFITS

A spoonful of avocado oil a day (internally or externally) provides vitamin A for smooth, age-resistant skin and vitamin E, which prevents premature aging. In addition, avodaco promotes youthful neurological function and enhances the uptake of vitamin A.

An avocado smoothie or green vichyssoise is a good defense against malnutrition and essential fatty acid deficiencies, a common side-effect of dieting, which rob skin of oil needed by the sebaceous glands.

Avocados are a top-rated source of three important B vitamins: folate (if you don't care for other source foods such as figs or oatmeal) as well as pyrodoxine(B_6) and pantothenic (B_5), the two nerve-stabilizing B vitamins.

BODY BUILDING AND HEALING FROM THE WAIST DOWN

Getting a little guacamole in your meals may be the only fast-acting food laxative you need, according to medical anthropologist John

Heinerman (mash two avocados with 1 teaspoon cider vinegar or lemon juice; take a spoonful at a time as needed). The creamy, nonirritating consistency of the avocado makes it prescriptive for colitis, ulcers, and bowel disorders, says the American Nutritional Medical Society.

The Avocado: Face Value

Puréed avocado also makes a healing moisturizing mask for dry skin (mix with a bit of ground oats to bind and apply to clean skin for 20 to 30 minutes, or simply massage your just washed face and neck with the inside of the avocado skin). Give rough knees, feet and elbows the same oily massage.

Buying, Storing, and Using

Buy avocados hard (but avoid bruised ones, which can affect quality) and allow to ripen at room temperature (to quick-ripen, brown-bag your avocado a day or two; the paper retains natural ripening qualities). Avocados are at their peak when semisoft. If not completely eaten, sprinkle exposed avocado with lemon juice to prevent discoloration, and refrigerate.

TIP: An avocado is one of those it's-not-over-till-it's-over vegetables. Save the skins to massage your face and neck for wrinkle relief or soothe rough elbows, knees, and pads of feet. Then bury the pit (flat end down) in potting soil and watch it sprout leaves.

Try these uses as well:

Slice or dice and float in soups and sprinkle on salads.

Stuff halves and serve as appetizers, or combine ½ avocado and blend with soups and sauces.

Use as a no-sodium, no-cholesterol vegetable sandwich or crepe filling or cracker butter.

Add cubed meat to fruit and vegetable cocktails.

Add avocado oil (not to be heated) to vinaigrettes to boost nutrients.

Super Healing Guacamole

1 large ripe avocado, mashed (1½ cups), reserve pit

1 tablespoon lemon juice

3 tablespoons minced green onions

2 tablespoons minced fresh coriander

⅛ teaspoon pepper

Dash of hot-pepper sauce

Mix all ingredients in a medium-size bowl. Place reserved pit in center to prevent darkening. Cover and chill for flavors to blend.

Tasty over roasted peppers and rice.

60-Second Avocado Coulis

1 peeled, chopped avocado

½ cup vegetable stock

2 tablespoons lemon juice

2 cloves garlic, minced

2 teaspoons dried basil

In a food processor, purée avocado, stock, lemon juice, garlic, and basil until smooth.

Note: A coulis is a thick purée. Use as a cold or warm sauce or dip.

Benefits healing zones: 1, 2, 7, 6

Also see: Coronary Heart Disease, Indigestion, Fatigue

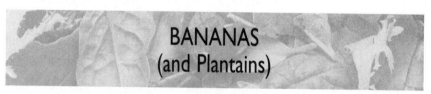

BANANAS
(and Plantains)

Plum crazy about bananas? Keep peeling—there is hardly a more fruitful way to protect yourself from ulcers, indigestion, high cholesterol, chronic fatigue, you name it.

The sages of India, according to legend, refreshed themselves by resting in the shade of lush banana-bearing bushes, which, when transported to the Canary Islands by adventurers, became known by the African name *banana*. (*Banana* is also Aussie slang for a one-pound note.)

The banana was known in medieval times as the original forbidden fruit and was identified in the *Koran* as "the paradise tree" (a misnomer since bananas grow on a bush).

Our favorite mellow yellow fruit did not appear in America until the sixteenth century but by the late 1800s was being hawked like hot dogs on street corners as a 10-cent snack. Today the typical American consumes 27 lbs a year.

Botanically classified as the world's largest herb, there are 200 varieties of bananas worldwide (30 grown in Asia just for the local market), including an East Indian variety grown solely for the purpose of making beer.

The banana bush, like the avocado, is one of nature's most prolific food plants, producing up to 300 "fingers" (fruits) in a single "hand" (bunch), perhaps to compensate for the fact that the bush bears fruit only once.*

The most popular commercial banana, the Cavendish, is also the largest, most compact, and easiest type to ship. Other varieties include the Gros Michel, the stubby Claret or red banana, which has a slightly glutinous flesh; the Lady Finger, which is the smallest and most delicate; the slightly tart Apple Banana, the green and white Hawaiian, and a new plantain-like hybrid from Brazil and Southeast Asia called the Gold Finger which doesn't turn brown when cut.

NATURE'S BEST FRUIT SOURCE OF MINERALS

Nutritionally, the banana is richer in minerals than any other soft fruit, with the exception of strawberries. Bananas provide calcium and phosphorus for healthy skin, teeth, and bones. Bananas also provide more potassium than yogurt—for stabilization of blood pressure, and as much pectin fiber as an apple—which both prevents and alleviates constipation and dysentery and helps block absorption of fats that elevate blood cholesterol.

CHROMIUM SOURCE FOR DIABETICS, DIETERS, AND ATHLETES

Better yet, bananas are one of the few fruit sources of chromium, the micromineral responsible for the synthesis of fatty acids and cholesterol. Chromium is also critical for diabetics because it stimulates the metabolism of glucose for energy. Chromium speeds weight loss and fat loss and promotes an increase of lean muscle. As a bonus, bananas are

---

* See Mail Order Sources

low in calories (80 to 100 apiece) but high in satiety value. As a bonus, a warm, ripe banana can help curb your "fat tooth," providing the same "mouth feel" as a pat of butter or a cube of cheese, with fewer calories and no fat. Bananas are among the most digestible of all fruits when ripe. (Central African pygmies are said to polish off up to 60 a day.)

The banana is starchy or sugary depending on the stage of ripeness it has reached. Color is the tip-off: When the peel is yellow-green, a banana is 40% starch; when fully yellow, it's fully ripe, and 91% of those carbohydrates have broken down into the three sugars—glucose, fructose, and sucrose—that make bananas such high-energy eating.

Bananas: Preventing Deficiency

Bananas help prevent or pay back nutrient deficiencies of B complex vitamins potassium, and vitamin C created by regular use of aspirin, laxatives, contraceptives, caffeinated drinks, and alcohol. And bananas are one of the two known reliable fruit sources of infection-fighting vitamin B_6 (the other is prune juice), which is essential for the synthesis of hemoglobin.

Buying, Storing, and Using

◆ Bananas can be bought green since they sweeten as they ripen. (The brown spots on an overripe peel are called "sugar spots.") And the riper it is, the sweeter a banana tastes. But bananas should not be eaten green* because unripened they harbor compounds that inhibit amylase, an enzyme that facilitates the digestion of complex carbohydrates.

◆ Bananas will keep three to four days longer if refrigerated than at room temperature. They also freeze well (but thaw in the refrigerator, to preserve color, and use immediately).

◆ To slow the browning of peeled bananas, dip them into a solution of lemon juice and water or toss sliced bananas in a fruit salad.

---

* However, there is a good reason to get your bananas green. Green bananas grown and harvested in environmentally responsible ways, says the Rainforest Alliance, are healthier and safer, while banana growers in Central and South America use vast quantities of chemicals and pesticide-impregnated plastic bags on banana bunches that are often discarded near rivers and carried out to sea. Environmental activists also claim that banana cartels have demolished vast areas of rainforest acreage. Responsibly grown bananas wear a green "smart banana" seal (for more information contact Rainforest Alliance, 270 Lafayette St., Ste. 512, New York, NY 10012; Mercantile Food Co., 4 Old Mill Road, P.O. Box 1140, Georgetown, CT 06829, phone 203-544-9891).

Overripe, discolored bananas can be used in baking or in blender drinks, where their intense sweetness allows you to reduce sugar by one third or more.

◆ Got the banana blahs? Try the Polynesian "Ice Cream Banana," so named because of its frothy, extra-rich tasting pulp. The silvery blue-green skin is yellow when ripe. Eat raw or prepare like plantains.

◆ Bananas (and plantains) are not, strictly speaking, for juicing, but you can purée them and then combine the purée with other juiced fruits for super healing smoothies and thick shakes. (Or try a frozen, slightly thawed, puréed banana as an ice cream alternative.)

◆ Have a dried banana for triple the bone building calcium, boron, and energizing potassium.

PLANTAINS FOR THE HEALTH OF YOUR BOWELS AND INTESTINAL TRACT

As for plantains, if you're prone to ulcers or irritable bowel syndrome, forget Tagamet™ and bunch up on plantains—the economy-sized "cooking banana" second cousin of our everyday "dessert" or "fruit" banana.

Plantains, which are larger than bananas and don't grow in bunches, are never eaten raw but are cooked when green, greenish-yellow, yellow, or even black. Like bananas, plantains begin life as high-starch fruits and sweeten during the ripening process but unlike bananas, they retain their firm texture. Mild-flavored when green and sweet when yellow, plantains are similar to potatoes and cooked in much the same way (a popular Dominican breakfast is mashed boiled green plantains with sautéed onions).

Plantains are valuable for their antipeptic and duodenal ulcer properties as well as their gastritis/flatulence- and dyspepsia-fighting ability. (A plantain flour gruel mixed with milk and plantain-flour chapattis is East Indian's Rx for digestive upset.) The healing substance in plantains is an ulcerogenic enzyme that mimics the action of the antiulcer drug Corben Oxolene, triggering a release of a protective substance that prevents hydrochloric acid damage to the stomach. Like bananas, plantains feed the natural acidophilus bacteria of the bowel.

Two Plantain Fibers—for Inner and Outer Health

The hemicellulose and high pectin fiber content of green, unripe plantains (and, to a lesser extent, bananas) help lower the bad LDL and elevate the good HDL cholesterol levels. Plantains also supply calcium, iron, and vitamin A (the yellower the fruit, the higher the content). Another bonus for acne and cellulite relief: Plantains are classified as "depuratines," herbs that provide a system-purifying acid for clarifying the complexion.

TIP: What's your plantain pleasure? To find out, buy several green plantains, cook half when green, and cook the remainder when riper. If the taste of green plantains appeals, refrigerate and use within 10 days. Ripening can be slowed with no loss of quality.

Blue Bananas

Purée in blender 1 cup fresh or frozen drained blueberries plus one very ripe banana. Add one drop vanilla extract.

Serve as a pudding-type dessert sprinkled with wheat germ or lecithin.

Makes two servings, about 100 calories each.

Variations: Black-and-blue bananas: Use ½ cup each blackberries and blueberries in place of 1 cup blueberries. Or add ½ teaspoon dried mint or garnish with a fresh sprig of mint.

Banana First Aid

For bruises (to reduce discoloration and pain): Peel a ripe banana, apply the peel inner side to bruise, and bind in place with dampened gauze.

Wrinkle Roll-Back Masque

Mash one or two very ripe bananas and add 2 teaspoons nut oil (peanut, sesame, walnut, etc.). Pat onto damp face and neck and let "set" for 30 minutes or more. Remove with tepid water. Apply twice a week. (Have a rejuvenating banana smoothie while you wait.)

Plantain Soup

> *2 teaspoons extra-virgin olive oil*
>
> *1 small onion, peeled and finely chopped*
>
> *1 carrot, peeled and finely chopped*
>
> *2 ribs celery, finely chopped*
>
> *2 cloves garlic, peeled and minced*
>
> *5 cups broth, homemade or low-sodium canned*
>
> *2 green plantains, peeled and diced (see Mail Order Sources)*
>
> *1 bay leaf*
>
> *1 teaspoon ground cumin, plus more to taste*

Heat olive oil in a large, heavy saucepan over medium heat. Add onion, carrot, celery, and garlic and cook until soft (about three to four minutes).

Add the broth and bring to a boil. Add plantains, bay leaf, cumin, and pepper. Return the soup to a boil, reduce heat, and simmer, uncovered, until tender (about 40 minutes).

Remove and discard bay leaf. Place half of the soup in a blender or food processor and purée into the remaining soup.

Before serving, reheat and correct seasoning.

Makes four servings. Leftovers may be frozen.

Variations:

◆ Substitute canola or safflower oil.

◆ Use parsnips in place of carrots.

◆ Use celery root in place of stalk celery.

Benefits healing zones: 1, 6, 7

Also see: Indigestion, Fatigue, Low Blood Pressure

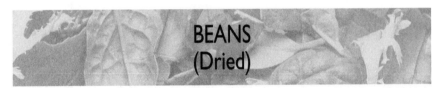

BEANS
(Dried)

What's the best food to take to a desert island? Bag the ham and rye and pack beans and grains.*

BEAN PROTEIN FOR FAT-FREE ENERGY

Dried beans,** available in 1,000 varieties, are nutritionally neck and neck with beef or cheese as a high-quality protein source. Kidney beans,

---

* The protein patterns of beans and grains become complete when combined for example: rice and kidney beans, corn and lima beans, to supply the 8 essential amino acids which the body cannot manufacture and which are essential for life, (a ninth amino acid *histidine* is essential for infants and children only).

** Beans come under the broad terms of *legumes, pulses,* or *grams* (Indian), referring to field varieties of beans or peas. Beans are a link between vegetables grown under and above the ground and are treated in symbolism as a transitory form between life and death: It is said that the Pythagoreans believed that upon leaving the body, certain souls became beans, and thus because the bean was half-human, it should not be eaten.

lentils, pintos, limas, and their like are also near zero in sodium, fat, and cholesterol and low in calories, 25% of which they derive from protein. As a bean bonus, an average serving of cooked kidney beans supplies just one third the calories and twice the satiety value of a serving of lasagna.

THE BEANS
Strong Bones Connection

Using your bean provides you with bone-building, nonheme iron (a nonorganic form that becomes more available and more readily digestible when eaten in combination with a vitamin C-rich food), magnesium, and the critical mineral that's missing in meat—calcium—for cardiovascular health and osteoporosis prevention. One cup of navy beans supplies as much calcium as a serving of broccoli or a dish of ice cream, says the National Osteoporosis Foundation, while two servings of beans daily—boiled, baked, sprouted, or puréed into soup or sandwich spread—lower cholesterol as effectively as oat bran (7 to 27%), according to Dr. David A. Jenkins, nutritional science professor at the University of Toronto.

FIGHTING DIGESTIVE DISORDERS WITH BEANS

Beans also provide more soluble fiber per serving than most cereals or whole grain pastas, accounting for 10 of the top 25 best food sources for the dietary fiber that normalizes digestion and cardiovascular functions. Because of their fiber, beans are just what the doctor ordered for hemorrhoid/constipation relief and prevention and normal colon functions.

The six best classic bean dishes for soluble fiber (2.5 g per serving) are bean soup; vegetarian chile (with pinto beans); three-bean salad (kidney beans, chick peas, and green beans); lentil soup; and minestrone soup (kidney beans).

BEAN CUISINE FOR DIABETICS AND DIETERS

A one-a-day cup of beans in the form of soup, mock meatloaf, bean "butter," or salad sprouts often helps regulate insulin levels better than drugs. Type I diabetics often cut their insulin needs by 30% or more on a bean regime, according to Dr. James Anderson, University of Kentucky, while Type II diabetics, whose bodies produce some insulin, reduce their insulin replacement needs by up to 90%.

Even better, the complex carbohydrates in beans are digested slowly, which makes them ideal for both diabetics and dieters. A longer transit time also, as a byproduct, suppresses the appetite.

THE ANTISTRESS FACTOR PLUS

Beans are rich in the antistress B-vitamin complex, especially B_6, and B_3. And of the 25 best sources for the vitamin folate—which the body uses to manufacture new blood cells and boost immunity—12 are legumes. Studies by the American Institute for Cancer Research indicate that folate improves the body's resistance to carcinogens and its ability to repair their damage.

Beans also benefit your heart by providing more blood pressure-stabilizing potassium in ½ cup than one serving of yogurt, one banana, or 1 cup of orange juice.

ANTIAGING/ANTICANCER BENEFITS

Beans in general are a rich source of the antiaging substance, CQ-10 (a co-enzyme that occurs naturally in the body), while chick peas specifically provide stamina-building DMG (dimethylglycine), which the American Association of Nutritional Consultants describes as "a metabolic reactive food factor that enhances immune system function, acts as an inflammatory agent, and improves sugar and fat metabolism."

Beans are one of the best ways to reduce your risk of cancer, concludes a recent Australian study. The diet of 88 patients with melanoma (skin cancer) differed from that of 88 cancer-free people in one way: It was significantly lower in beans.

FLATULENCE
Cause and Cure

What's *not* so good about this good-hot-or-cold near-ideal food? Beans are moderately high in purines (thus off the menu for gout sufferers), can trigger migraines or rashes for some people, and cause flatulence (some beans more than others; see the list in the following TIPS section) for almost all of us—unless you take a few flatulence-defensive steps.

Beans cause flatulence because of the three sugars they contain—raffinose, stachyose, and verbacose—which the body cannot break down or absorb as is. Instead of being digested and absorbed in the small intestine like other sugars, these sugars are passed along to the large intestine. There, bacteria break down and ferment these sugars, producing carbon dioxide, hydrogen, and a few other gases as byproducts. Carbon dioxide and hydrogen comprise over 95% of the gas. The distention these gases cause can lead to bloating, cramps, and even diarrhea.

Like bean sugars, bean starch ends up in the large intestine, where friendly bacteria take over, fermenting the carbohydrates they contain as one byproduct and producing, as a second, a social problem—flatulence.

TIPS:

1. Soak beans four to five hours. For best results, add 9 cups of water for every cup of beans. (Soaking in cold water removes 2% of the sugars.)

2. Switch beans. Some beans are less gassy than others. The 22% protein adzuki bean provides a reduced flatulence alternative to pinto beans—with a similar flavor and nutritional value—but 75% fewer of the pinto's gaseous sugars, says Joseph Maga, Ph.D., director of food research at Colorado State University. It's a good, safe, company's-coming bean (available at health food stores or from Adobe Milling, P.O. Box 596, Dove Creek, Co 81324).

3. Get the quick cookers. Freshly harvested beans cook faster, don't need overnight soaking, taste better, and provide more nutrition than supermarket dried types.

And what about our old-fashioned favorites? Food study researchers at the Nutritional Sciences Department of Chapman College in Southern California rated beans on a scale of 1 to 10, with 1 being the most gassy and 10 the least.

(1) Soybeans

(2) Pink, navy beans

(3) Black beans

(4) Pinto beans

(5) California small white beans

(6) Great Northern beans, white cannellini

(7) Lima beans, small

(8) Garbanzos (chick peas)

(9) Lima beans, large

(10) Blackeyed peas

4. Add rice. Cooking beans with an equal measure of rice eliminates up to 60% of their flatulence, says Dr. Louis Rockland at the USDA's Western Regional Research Laboratories. In the process, it increases usable protein by 2 to 8 g per cup by completing the amino acid pattern and creating a complete protein. Other whole grains, such as buckwheat, millet, barley, or the new high-protein quinoa seed, can be substituted for rice.

5. Cook beans longer. Beans are not food for the fast-track chef unless he or she has fast-track equipment. High-speed bean steamers and pressure cookers qualify. Even better are the overnight simmer-while-you-snooze, plug-in crock pots.

According to Bonnie Liebman, nutritionist for the Center for Science in the Public Interest, your body can't digest beans when the starch is not broken down by the appropriate amount of cooking. Beans require soaking—often one to three hours (unless the label says otherwise)*—and then gentle simmering for a minimum of one hour to prevent toughening of the protein. (Adding a bit of dried seaweed, such as kombu or dulse, also tenderizes bean protein.)

6. Season beans. Various university studies indicate that adding a generous pinch of summer savory or 1 teaspoon of ground ginger (per each pound of beans) at the start of cooking counteracts legume gassiness and adds flavor. Or for each cup of dry beans, add 1 teaspoon of castor oil to the cooking water (you won't taste it after cooking). But skip the salt; added during the cooking process, it draws moisture out of the beans and reduces chewiness. So does baking soda, but it also leaches out B vitamins.

7. Build up your tolerance. According to the Connecticut Agricultural Extension Service, eating smaller amounts of the more digestible beans—such as lentils, limas, and split peas—and gradually upping your intake improves your bean tolerance. The more often a food appears in your system, experts advise, the better your chances of developing the appropriate digestive enzymes your body needs to digest it.

---

*Look for the Frieda's Finest label—four field-ripened beans (blackeyed peas, garbanzo beans, green peas, and lima beans)—in supermarket produce departments. These beans are rehydrated for quick cooking (25 to 35 minutes).

Chewing thoroughly also aids digestion and minimizes problems. Or check the antiacid aisle for Beano™—an enzyme supplement that breaks down beans' sugars before your digestion deals with them.

   8. Sprout beans. According to the Vegetarian Information Service, sprouting dried beans destroys their ability to generate gas. In the case of the soybean, sprouting performs the same biochemical transformation as heating at 140 degrees for 2½ hours—unlocking protein and increasing vitamins B, C, and A. But sprout beans long enough to be on the safe side, and steam briefly before serving. As few as five or six raw beans can cause intestinal problems. According to bean researchers, the problem-causing compound is lectin, which attaches to the intestinal lining once consumed. In England, packages of kidney beans carry a warning that kidney beans should be placed in boiling water for at least 10 minutes before eating.

   Once they are pot ready, the best way to prepare beans is under pressure—a method that cuts cooking time by two thirds. Two of the best and most energy-efficient pressure cookers are the Innora and Magefesa Rapid 2 (about $100 each).

Buying, Storing, and Using

Look for smooth skins, uniform shapes and even color. Vitamin B_6 is destroyed by air and light, so to prevent loss, store beans in air- and moisture-proof containers.

Wash and sort beans before using.

Dried, untreated beans are higher in B-complex vitamins than canned or presoaked varieties.

GETTING BEANS' GOODNESS INTO EVERY MEAL
Eight Tips

   1. Beans on the QT whenever you have a taste for them? Here's how: Soak beans overnight according to directions (see the accompanying Cooking Timetable). Pour off soak water, and spread beans in a single layer on a cookie sheet. Freeze. Then pour into a plastic bag (they don't clump up) and use directly from the freezer.

   2. Keep an open jar of cooked or sprouted and/or marinated beans (one or more varieties) in the fridge for quick snacks or to use in salads with cottage cheese or yogurt.

COOKING TIMETABLE

Note: Presoak beans one to three hours or overnight unless package directs otherwise.

Bean	Cooking Time Regular (hrs.)	Pressure (mins.)	Cooking Water	Dry Beans	Cooked Beans
Blackeyed peas	1	20–25	3 cups	1 cup	2 cups
Pinto beans	2.5	20–25	3 cups	1 cup	2 cups
Kidney beans	1.5	20–25	3 cups	1 cup	2 cups
Soybeans	3 or more	20–25	3 cups	1 cup	2 cups
Garbanzos	3	40–45	4 cups	1 cup	4 cups
Lentils and split peas	1	10–15	3 cups	1 cup	2.5 c.
Great Northern beans	2	20–25	3.5 cups	1 cup	2 cups
Navy beans, white beans	1.5	20–25	3 cups	1 cup	2 cups
Lima beans	1.5	20–25	2 cups	1 cup	1.5 cups

Note: Any two beans with the same cooking time can be prepared together (e.g., navy and limas).

3. Use cooked beans in place of potatoes or noodles.

4. Use cooked, puréed beans in place of butter, peanut butter, and mayonnaise.

5. Toss white beans with chunks of tuna and with tofu in pesto. Add white beans to pasta sauces. Stir white beans into simple bouillon, consommé, and broths, and sprinkle with cheese for quick whole-meal soups.

6. Mash any dried bean with nutmeg-scented mayonnaise, yogurt, or pot cheese to make vitamin-rich spreads for bread and whole grain crackers.

7. Toss dried red beans and fresh green beans with quartered, hard-cooked eggs and chopped scallions and spinach; add vinaigrette for on-the-spot, whole-meal salad.

8. Why stop after blackeyes and Great Northerns? Forty more varieties—not including such "heirloom" specialties as Jacob's cattle

and yelloweye or "New Age" varieties like the black scarlet runner—are available from Le Marche Seeds International, P.O. Box 566, Dixon, CA 95620 (catalog $2.00).

TIP: For 1,000 varieties of organic dried beans, write to Salt Spring Seeds, Box 33, Barger, BC, Canada VOS 1EO.

Benefits healing zones: **2, 3, 5, 6**

Also see: **Basic Dieting Facts and Advice, Indigestion, Osteoporosis, Vitamin B**

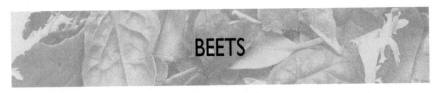

BEETS

Does your daily diet pass the test for building better blood pressure, a stronger immune system, and an ailment-proof liver, gallbladder, and bowel? It may not if beets are persona non grata on your weekly menus.

TWO HEALING VEGETABLES IN ONE

The beet, whose roots and leaves are both edible (like carrots and turnips—but unlike rhubarb, whose greens are toxic), is that rarity among plant foods—a root vegetable with a second super healing leafy green vegetable attached.

Common table beetroot is closely related to the sugar beet,* to Swiss chard, and to a type of wild beet, martima, which still grows in the Mediterranean. The edible garden beet can be dark purple, bright

---

* The beginning of the nineteenth century marked the discovery that certain yellow-white types of beets contained large amounts of natural sugar, from which a commercial sweetener could be produced. Production boomed during Napoleon's blockade of Europe, which halted the importation of cane sugar, and the new industry flourished because of the efficiency and economy with which the beet could be produced. Sugar beet pollen is wind borne, and fertilization of plants of the species occurs even over long distances. (GREEN THUMB TIP: Garden and sugar beets are not good garden bedfellows; cross-pollination occurs readily and ruins both crops.)

vermillion, or even white (see Mail Order Sources for heirloom and endangered and specialty plant sources and the yellow beet, which is sweeter—rarely pickled—and more common outside the United States).

FIVE B.C. BENEFITS OF BEETS

Beets were used medicinally to relieve toothaches and headaches and for spring rejuvenation tonics long before they were pickled, juiced, or puréed into borscht. Theoprastus of Dyplylos (371–287 B.C.), the Greek philosopher and naturalist, praised beets for their diuretic effects.

In the first century A.D., Celsus recommended beets as the perfect laxative and applauded their anti-inflammatory properties. A century later, Greek physician Galen recommended beets for problems of the liver and spleen. German healer Sebastian Kneipp advised that beets aided digestive disorders.

By 4 B.C., beetroots had become a staple in the Roman diet but were not cultivated widely in Europe until the beginning of the seventeenth century. They did not appear in the United States until the early 1800s. Today, we know why beets—no matter how you slice, juice, or soup them—are whole body super healers.

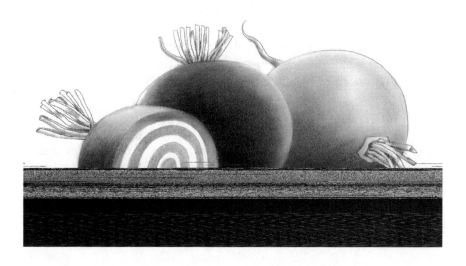

THERAPY IN DEEP PURPLE FOR THE WHOLE BODY

Beets are a rejuvenative food for every organ in the body—especially the gallbladder, liver, bowels, and digestive and lymphatic systems, say researchers at the American College of Clinical Nutrition—and an effective healing agent for the disorders that afflict these organs, including low blood pressure, alcoholism, cirrhosis, hepatitis, and indigestion. (TIP: Bran intolerant? Get your fiber from beets, which rarely cause flatulence. The natural red color is a good tipoff that the pigments are not digested but pass straight through the system to be eliminated.) Thanks to the beetroot's rich supply of beta-carotene (22,700 IU) and organic mineral salts that speed tissue repair, detoxify the bloodstream, and nourish the circulation that feeds every living cell in the body, beets are also a good brain and antifatigue food. In addition, they are high in two amino acids (glutamine and asparagine), betaine (a vitamin-like substance that aids brain function), and B-complex vitamins, especially folate, the antidepression B vitamin.

BEATING CANCER WITH BEETS

In 1919, the German pharmacologist Hugo Schulz reported that beet extracts slowed cancerous growths, and further German studies from 1951 through 1964 substantiated these findings. In 1983, German cancer specialist professor H. O. Kleine, M.D., reported that a liter of unsweetened red beet juice taken daily was both a preventive measure against cancer and the best natural remedy for improving blood chemistry.

The antitumor effect of beetroot juice is attributed to beetroots' rich supply of iron plus the antioxidants, the flavonoids, the beta-carotene, and ascorbic acid, all of which oxygenate cancer cells and improve cell respiration, according to Nobel Prize winning researcher Dr. A. Ferenczi.

TURN AN ANTIAGING LEAF WITH BEET GREENS

Even better than a beet's roots are its greens, because they rank among the five top-rated sources of three antiaging pigment antioxidants: (1) the flavonoids, which produce "vitamin P" activity for strengthening the immune system (which becomes more vulnerable with age) as well as the joint structures and vascular system; (2) the alpha and beta anticancer carotenes; and (3) chlorophyll, the fat soluble substance that stimulates hemoglobin and red blood cell production (and is useful in relieving heavy menstrual flow) and provides protection from free radical threats to the immune system.

Because beet greens also contain calcium, potassium, iron, and vitamins A and C, they are an essential addition to any healthy-heart program.

Buying, Storing, and Using

Good-quality beets should have fresh-looking greens (slightly flabby greens can be restored to freshness if refrigerated in water). Roots should be firm, smooth, and vibrant red-purple. Remember, the younger the root, the richer the nutritional rewards. A bad-buy beet can be identified by its short neck and the circles of leaf scars around the beet top. Smaller beets are best for juicing, larger ones for steaming, baking, pickling, etc. Beets can be stored three to 5 days in the refrigerator or, with greens removed, two to four weeks.

BEEF UP YOUR BEET INTAKE
Seven Tips

Incorporate beets and greens into any meal by doing the following:

◆ Freshly grate into salads or soups.

◆ Serve sliced and pickled as a near-zero-calories snack (50 calories a cup).

◆ Enjoy beets puréed as a cold borscht (soup) in summer or roasted as a spud substitute in winter (see the following recipe).

◆ Juice first, sauté later: Remember, juicing liberates more nutritional compounds in beets than any other method of preparation. (Making apple cider? For a more golden color, add a beet.)

◆ To benefit from as broad a range of carotenoids as possible, juice both the root and the leaves and combine with other carotene-source foods—carrots, squash, collards, spinach.

◆ For a wrinkle-reducer mask (and for crow's feet and under-eye puffiness), try mixing grated raw beets with whipped cream. Apply to clean, slightly damp skin, and rinse off after 20 to 30 minutes. (*Variation:* Combine raw grated potato and grated beet for a half-and-half mask.)

Big Red:
The Baked Apple/Baked Potato Alternative

Preheat oven to 375 degrees. Scrub two large fresh beets. Cut off leaves and stems about 1 inch above beet top. Pat dry. Rub each beet with a little olive or canola oil and sprinkle with a few drops of water. Place in a baking dish and cover with baking parchment or foil. Roast 45 minutes or until tender. Serve as you would a baked apple or a baked spud with a dab of yogurt (instead of sour cream) and a sprinkle of Super Healing Salt (p. 276). Makes two servings.

Variation: Stuffed Beet: Bake 20 minutes. Remove from heat, cool, hollow out, and stuff with stir-fried sprouts or puréed carrots and replace top half. Bake for 15 minutes longer. Makes two servings.

Note: Baking is the best flavor-savor way to cook a beet.

A Beet Split

Prepare as in the Big Red recipe, then chill, slice, top with fruit yogurt, or serve with a spoonful of Two-Root Coulis (p. 69) in place of yogurt.

Roast a few extra beets to eat cold as diet snacks; reheat for a baked potato alternative.

Spiced Beet Purée with Walnut Oil

> *6 medium-sized beets (about 2 pounds), with 1 inch of stem attached*
>
> *2 large cloves garlic, unpeeled*
>
> *2 bay leaves*
>
> *4 cloves*
>
> *1 teaspoon walnut (or other nut) oil*

Preheat oven to 400 degrees. on a large double sheet of baking parchment or foil, place beets with the garlic, bay leaves, and cloves. Wrap up and roast until beets are tender (about 2 hours).

Open package, cut stems, peel, and place beets in a food processor until smooth. Stir in oil and serve warm.

Makes four servings.

Benefits healing zones: 2, 6, 7, 9

Also see: Antioxidants, Leafy Greens, Juices, Low Blood Pressure, Mail Order Sources

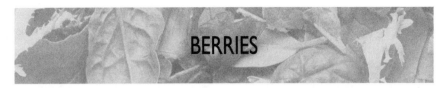

BERRIES

For super health and healing, berries are terrific. Cranberries,* blueberries, raspberries, gooseberries, currants, or wild blackberries all are rich in vitamin C and pectin (the soluble fiber that lowers cholesterol and normalizes colon and bowel function), plus boron, the bone builder, and a number of antioxidants.

SIX WAYS TO STAY HEALTHY WITH STRAWBERRIES**

Strawberries provide twice the vitamin C and half the calories and fiber of raspberries. Like celery, strawberries are a good source of 20 different antiaging trace minerals, including chromium, zinc, and selenium. More importantly, they are a top source of the cancer-deactivating compound ellagic acid, which also occurs in Brazil nuts, cherries, and grapes and in lesser amounts in raspberries. Strawberries also contain flavonoids, the miracle phytochemical that fights cancer and heart disease and prevents certain carcinogens from damaging DNA, according to 1993 studies by the National Cancer Institute.

Raspberries, whose varieties range from whites to pink, to purple, and orange, but for most of us are represented by the red or black varieties—have twice the fiber of strawberries and more immunity-boosting folate and blood-building iron than strawberries and are a good tonic for the respiratory system. Rich in the vitamin-antioxidant combination A and C, they make an excellent first-rate, alcohol-free, appetite-stimulating aperitif when juiced alone or in combination with other berries.

---

* Pilgrims who saw the head of cranes in the shapely pink blossoms of the bush named the bitter fruit "crane berries."

** Strawberries are so called because they were once cushioned between layers of straw for winter storage and speared on pokers of straw to be carried uncrushed to the marketplace. Incidentally, strawberry hives are usually provoked by the outer fuzz, not the fruit on non-vine-ripened berries. Rinsing the berries in hot and then cold water usually neutralizes the allergen.

Raspberries are a time-honored remedy for reversing mucous and catarrhal conditions, says the Office of Alternative Medicine at the National Institutes of Health.

A HANDFUL OF BLUEBERRIES
Four-Way Defense against Diabetes, Diarrhea, and Urinary Tract Infections

One cup of blueberries or huckleberries (the wild variety which is more delicately flavored) supplies one third of your RDA for ascorbic acid plus heart-healthy potassium and silica, the trace mineral that rejuvenates the pancreas and helps prevent bone disorders and diabetes. Blueberries are also a source of myrtillin, another phytochemical that regulates blood sugar. Like blackberries, blueberries are antidotal for diarrhea because of their flavonoid content. (Flavonoids are the phytochemicals that make blueberries blue, blackberries black, grapes purple, etc.) Blueberries and the huckleberries are also potent bacteria fighters and defend against infections of the urinary tract and kidneys, according to studies by the Weizmann Institute of Science and Tel Aviv University.

Blackberries, blueberries or brambleberries (a highly perishable relative of the raspberry and loganberry) are the most fibrous of the berry family and supply half your daily vitamin C requirement and four major minerals: potassium, iron, calcium, and phosphorus. Blackberries have been used therapeutically for centuries to build blood and put the damper on dysentery.

According to herbal healers, a blackberry cordial or two should be on every woman's weekly menu. These slow excessive menstruation, help reverse "tired blood," and thanks to their boron content, help prevent bone disorders such as osteoporosis. Blackberries also provide a good, safe, sweet sipping remedy for acid indigestion, heartburn, and colitis.

RED AND BLACK ALL OVER
Cranberries and Blackberry Cocktails for Healthy Heart and Kidney Function

Cranberries (one of the three fruits native to America, along with the Concord grape and blueberries) were, along with limes, the first anti-scurvy fruits used in Colonial New England and are still highly regarded as a pantry corrective for hemorrhoids, kidney stones, and rectal disturbances. Like blueberries, cranberries fight urinary tract infections. In addition, their iodine content makes them a good medicine for an underactive thyroid.

RED CURRANTS

The red currant (the anchor ingredient in the jelly of the same name) in berry or juice form is good medicine for yeast infections. It is also helpful for inducing a "healing sweat" to relieve respiratory tract infections. The high bioflavonoid content of red currants accounts for their healing in conditions of bruising, periodontal bleeding, hemorrhoids, and capillary damage. They are used as an internal antiseptic by naturopathic herbalists and to counteract jaundice, food poisoning, and acidic blood conditions.

THREE BERRY BONUSES

All berries are first-rate cool-down foods. Any kind of berry juice, says medical anthropologist John Heinerman, helps the body readjust its internal thermostat to a more comfortable setting in hot weather. All berries are nutrient dense, and their fewer than 100 calories a cupful makes them a must for dieters, who need to prevent nutritional deficiencies while cutting back on calories. In addition, all berries supply the antioxidant catechin (also in green tea) and are an oil-free source of heart-protective vitamin E.

Buying, Storing, and Using

Buy berries, which are highly perishable, at peak freshness for the most nutrition. Second choice: frozen. Avoid overprocessed, sugary, canned berries. Buy in quantity and freeze what you can't use immediately for future meals. Store fresh berries in the refrigerator in a single layer to prevent mold and spoilage. Avoid cooking, which destroys 50% of the nutrients. (Frozen berries retain about 80% of their vitamin C stored at 0 degrees Fahrenheit.)

Try the following uses:

- ◆ Strawberry juice will soothe a sunburn, and mashed and mixed with plain yogurt and lemon it makes an antiwrinkle skin toner. Or add puréed peaches and oatmeal and you have an effective creamy cleanser (spread on damp skin and rinse off after 10 minutes.)

◆ Try growing firm strawberries and make kebob combinations.

◆ Substitute strawberries for half the beets in standard borscht recipes or for the tomatoes in barbecue recipes.

◆ Make "cherry popcorn": As a high-fiber diet snack, spread sweet, ripe cherries on a large cookie sheet. Freeze. Store frozen in a large sack. For snacks, thaw a handful and eat while slightly icy.

◆ Make "melted berries" syrup: Put ½ cup fresh berries in a small saucepan. Sprinkle lightly with sugar, and mash. Add 1 tablespoon of water and heat until sugar dissolves.

◆ Make a no-sugar cranberry cocktail alternative. Put whole, fresh cranberries in a blender with nonfat yogurt and 1 tablespoon of honey.

How about a cranberry houseplant that produces berries every year? Verdean Berry Farm's got them. For details, write to Verdean Berry Farm, P.O. Box 3395, Wareham, MA 02571.

Raspberry Antiplaque Paste

Wash and gently blot dry ½ pint each of fresh strawberries and fresh raspberries. Gently crush berries by hand (don't purée) and combine with enough baking soda to make a paste. Add warm water if needed.

Use to scrub teeth as you would using powder or paste. According to the American Holistic Medical Association (AHMA), brushing the teeth with a thick paste of strawberries or raspberries helps combat tartar buildup and gingivitis.

For a good postscrub cocktail, combine juices of both the berries to help cleanse the bloodstream of toxins, suggests the AHMA.

Very Berry Beauty Mask

Combine 2 cups of puréed fresh strawberries or raspberries with 1 cup whipped cream (for dry skin) or egg yolks (for oily skin).

Variation: Mix the fruit purée with Fuller's earth in place of the yolk or cream (appropriate for either skin type).

Super Healing Fruit Soup

3 cups of fresh raspberries, blueberries, or strawberries

¼ cup of natural sugar (optional)

½ cup of alcohol-free red wine or grape juice

2 teaspoons of fresh lemon juice

1 cup of soft tofu

Fresh mint or lemon curls for a garnish

In the blender or food processor, combine the berries with ½ cup of water. Purée. Strain and discard seeds, if any.

In a medium saucepan, combine berry purée with the sweetener. Bring to a gentle boil, reduce heat, and simmer for five minutes. Remove from heat. Add wine or juice and lemon. Stir and allow to cool.

In a blender or food processor, whip the tofu until smooth. Add the berry mixture and blend until thoroughly combined.

Chill and serve. Garnish with whole berries and fresh mint or lemon curls.

Benefits healing zones: 1, 3, 4, 6, 7

Also see: Antioxidants, Indigestion, Cystitis, Basic Dieting Facts and Advice, Vitamin C, Juices, PMS

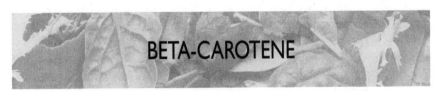

BETA-CAROTENE

What's the best way to turn the corner on healing? Put more carrots, squash, broccoli, and dandelion greens on the menu. All four are top-rated sources of beta-carotene, the pro-vitamin-A antioxidant that, says Michiaki Murakoshi of Japan's Kyoto Prefectural University of Medicine, protects your DNA by inactivating the gene that promotes tumor growth and blocking the growth of malignant cells.

FREE RADICALS' BIGGEST FOE

Along with other major antioxidants such as vitamins A and C, selenium, and vitamin E (see Antioxidants), beta-carotene snuffs out free radicals, which cause the cellular changes that lead to degenerative diseases such as rheumatoid arthritis, diabetes, cardiovascular ailments, and cancer.

Beta-carotene is the most celebrated and certainly the most visible (it's the plant pigment that makes pink grapefruit pink and oranges orange) of all the antioxidants, but it is only one of the 30 to 50 of the carotene complex,* including alphacarotene, gammacarotene, lycopene, lutein, and capsanthin, known to contain vitamin A.

While all of the carotenes have the ability to partially convert on command into vitamin A (depending on the health of your thyroid and the presence of zinc and protein in your system) none are as readily found in common foods as beta-carotene.

In 1972, researchers compared 220 Japanese stomach cancer patients in Hawaii with 440 Japanese Hawaiians who didn't have cancer. Vegetable eaters had half the rate of stomach cancer as those who didn't eat vegetables.

When Singapore researchers compared 233 Chinese immigrants who had lung cancer with 300 who didn't, those who ate the most beta-carotene-rich foods had less than 50% of the lung cancer as those who didn't each such foods.

Beta-carotene-rich foods may be your best defense against coronary artery disease as well, since this vitamin A precursor appears to help prevent the oxidative damage of lipids believed to promote plaque. In a 1991 Boston study, middle-aged men who suffered from angina reduced their risk of heart attack and stroke by 50% after adding beta-carotene to their diets. What's a healing dose? Since beta-carotene is converted to vitamin A, 12 to 15 mg a day—three times the level suggested by the U.S. Department of Agriculture (USDA) and the National Cancer Institute—may be a good idea, especially since beta-carotene, unlike other forms of vitamin A, is nontoxic at any dose. Only about 16% of all beta-carotene ingested is translated into vitamin A in the body. The rest circulates unchanged in the bloodstream and is readily absorbed by the cells.

---

* Beta-carotenes should not be confused with carotenes. For example, spinach contains the carotenes lutein and xanthin, which are not found in carrots, the largest source of beta-carotene.

SHOPPING TIP: The more intense the color of the vegetable or fruit (usually red, yellow, orange, or green), the greater the concentration of beta-carotene. And beta-carotene in food beats beta-carotene from supplements.

SOURCES OF BETA-CAROTENE

Sources of this healer are at your fingertips in the familiar and not so familiar. Mangoes, for instance, supply 20% more beta-carotene than cantaloupe and 50% more than apricots (they also have twice the vitamin C of oranges). But you've got to eat up. The richest sources of beta-carotene in terms of milligrams per 3.5-ounce portions—a typical serving size—are dandelion greens (8.4); carrots (6.6); sweet potato (5.9); watercress (5.6); kale (5.3); spinach (4.9); mango (2.9); winter squash (2.4); cantaloupe (2.0); apricots (1.6); and broccoli (1.3).

VITAMIN A

Don't forget about your need for the vitamin A that doesn't become carotene—retinol (the nonplant form of A), which has been useful in treating acne, wrinkles, and other internally and externally atopic troubles.

Vitamin A also has potency as a cancer inhibitor (see Beta-carotene) and a cholesterol lowerer and protects your body's vitamin C stores from oxidation. In the form of Retin-A cream, vitamin A helps remove age spots and heal impetigo, boils, and open ulcers. To benefit to the max, concentrate on vitamin A foods that are also rich in E and zinc (additional A increases your tocopherol requirement, and zinc, is needed to activate the A you eat and store).

TIPS:

◆ Your need for A is increased if you consume alcohol and/or take antacids, aspirin, laxatives, contraceptives, and many other OTC and non-OTC drugs, especially cholesterol-reducing medications.

◆ Your vitamin A needs are satisfied by beta-carotene source foods.

12 WAYS TO PUT VITAMIN A ON THE MENU

Food	Portion	% RDA
Carrot, raw	1	203
Pumpkin	½ cup	269
Sweet potato, baked	1 (approx. 4 oz.)	249
Lamb's quarters, chopped, boiled (wild green)	½ cup	87
Spinach, boiled	½ cup	74
Butternut squash, baked cubes	½ cup	71
Hubbard squash, baked cubes	½ cup	62
Dandelion greens, chopped, boiled	½ cup	61
Cantaloupe, cubed	1 cup	52
Mango	½ (approx. 3½ oz.)	40
Turnip greens, or beet greens, cooked	½ cup	40
Persimmon	1 (6 oz.)	36

Beta-carotene Frappé

Put ½ cup fresh carrot juice in blender with 1/2 peeled mango. Add three crushed ice cubes. Blend until frothy. A good can't-break-for-breakfast snack.

Benefits healing zones: All

Also see: **Antioxidants, Carrots, Squash, Leafy Greens, Acne, Vision, Cancer, Vitamin E**

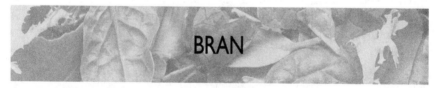

BRAN

If you want to be independently healthy, pick bran and take your pick.

RICE BRAN, WHEAT BRAN, CORN BRAN, AND OAT BRAN

Rice bran is the outer shell of a grain of rice, medium brown, the texture of fine cornmeal, with a sweet, nutty taste. It provides a high percentage of the RDA for blood-pressure-modulating magnesium, healthy amounts of B vitamins for healthy nerves and proper energy production, and almost as much fiber as wheat bran. It lowers cholesterol levels as much as oat bran. One downside: Almost 60% of rice bran's calories are from fat.

In an airtight, moisture-free container, refrigerated or frozen, rice bran keeps for months. Use it to replace up to half of the flour in quick bread and muffin recipes and in place of bread crumbs or oats and to fortify nut loaf and casseroles.

Wheat bran, the nutritious fibrous covering of the wheat berry, is yellow to russet brown and, depending on milling method, flaky or powdery fine. With 3 grams of fiber per 2-tablespoon serving, wheat bran is rich in magnesium for normalizing blood pressure, with a modest amount of blood-boosting iron.

Store in the refrigerator or freezer in a moisture-proof container. Use in hot cereals, quick breads, atop casseroles, or as crumb alternative in battering fritters and croquettes.

TIP: To improve flavor, toast in a medium hot skillet until amber.

For maximum fiber, fill your sugar bowl with corn bran. With almost 8 grams of fiber per 2 tablespoons for cancer protection and cholesterol reduction, corn bran is coarse, tan or white, with the aroma and consistency of corn meal. Use as you would other brans and in place of cornmeal in recipes. Mix with natural dry sugar and butter to top muffins and cakes.

Oat bran offers other health benefits—more soluble fiber than oatmeal, plus thiamine and iron for energy and magnesium for the conversion of vitamin D. Use as a hot cereal or cereal fortifier, add to soups and stews, use to thicken sauces in place of bread crumbs, and replace part of the flour or meal in baked goods, batters, and doughs. Toasting enhances flavor.

ANTICANCER ROUGHAGE

Pentose, a fiber sugar found only in cereal brans, appears to be twice as effective as other fibrous foods in reducing the incidence and risk of cancers of the colon and bowel, says the American Health Foundation. One reason is that it increases stool transit times. In addition, oats are one of the seed foods that supply protease inhibitors, antioxidants that prevent activation of viruses and cancerous chemicals in the intestines.

ANTI-INFLAMMATORY/ANTIVIRAL/ANTICHOLESTEROL

Oat bran has the ability to inhibit biosynthesis of prostaglandins, which are linked to inflammatory disorders—especially of the skin, as in psoriasis and eczema. Oat bran also provides anti-infectious capabilities, especially against intestinal disorders. Oat bran has been shown to lower serum cholesterol. Oats' cholesterol-lowering effect works best when eaten at intervals throughout the day.

BRAN PLAN MULTIPLE HEATH BENEFITS

Bran is nature's most effective prevention and cure for constipation (wheat beats other grains; (½ ounce a day does the trick), reducing your risk in the process of hemorrhoids, varicose veins, and various types of cancer and high cholesterol. How much is enough? As a laxative, a mere 3 tablespoons of bran or ⅓ cup of 100% bran cereal is usually enough.

Remember, the coarser the bran, the more remedial the results. CAUTION: Intake of more than 40 grams a day can lead to gastrointestinal distress and may interfere with your body's ability to absorb nutrients, such as iron, zinc, and calcium. So vary fiber sources and space intake throughout the day to maximize beneficial effects.

Benefits healing zones: 1, 2, 3, 7

Also see: **Indigestion, Cancer, Coronary Heart Disease, Hemorrhoids, Whole Grains, Antioxidants**

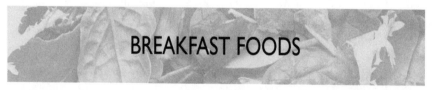

BREAKFAST FOODS

On any given morning, 50% of us go without breakfast, and in fact 12% of all soft drinks are consumed at breakfast time (*Berkeley Wellness Letter*, Palm Coast, Florida, May 1993). Does it matter whether you cut a croissant and pour an orange juice to start the day or just leave the house on an empty stomach? It not only matters, it's a matter of life or slow death.

According to a recent study by University of California researchers, devoting an extra 5 or 10 minutes—especially if you have 5 to 10 pounds to lose—to the first meal of the day (ideally, one you've prethought) beats going without for two primary reasons.

◆ First, it provides mood-boostering energy that fuels the brain and actually promotes weight loss. (Skippers generally make up for early-in-the-day deficits by overeating in the evening.) Furthermore, A.M. calories are more rapidly burned off than P.M. excesses.

◆ Breakfast eaters live longer. Death rates are typically 40% higher for men and 28% higher for women who only rarely or sometimes eat breakfast, compared to those who do it daily.

WHY YOU SHOULD PAMPER YOUR PANCREAS WITH PANCAKES
Three Payoffs

Another study at the University of Iowa Medical College concluded that starting the day with breakfast is associated with better mental performance, too. Breakfast eaters are generally more productive during the early part of the day, with faster reaction times and less muscular fatigue than do-withouters. Breakfast eating may protect you from diabetes and other blood-sugar disorders. According to a study by F. John Service, M.D., and colleagues at the Mayo Clinic in Rochester, Minnesota, "The pancreas can't keep up with the demand for insulin later in the day, and insulin has less effect on the tissues, later than in the morning. From a standpoint of blood sugar, it's best to have your big meal of the day at breakfast."

DO YOU SUFFER FROM BREAKFAST SKIPPER'S DEFICIENCY SYNDROME?

Missing the first meal of the day means you're missing out on super healing nutrients such as vitamin C, riboflavin, and calcium, and if you miss out you might not make good those losses in the two meals that remain, a deficit that can lead to osteoporosis, periodontal disease, chronic fatigue syndromes, and worse. According to Dr. Helen A. Guthrie, professor of nutrition at Pennsylvania State University, breakfast skippers consume 40% less calcium and vitamin C during the day and 10% less iron and thiamine. Even worse, you cheat your heart of good health. According to *Nutrition and the MD,* Vol. II pp. 83-85, March, 1988, cereal fiber eaten on a regular basis (especially oat and wheat bran) can reduce cholesterol by up to 15 to 20%. This is a significant reduction when you consider the fact that a 1% drop in cholesterol reduces the risk of heart disease by 2%.

How to Rate a First-Rate First Meal of the Day

A bad breakfast may be worse than none at all. Many dry cereals, for example, are 60% sugar, almost three times sweeter than a sugar cookie, while convenience and microwave meals and fast-food breakfasts typically derive up to 80 calories from fat and supply almost your whole day's RDA for sodium in one serving but only one tenth of your need for fiber—to say nothing of the toxic potential of the chemicals added for flavor and color.

So how does a model breakfast shape up? Here are three menus (to go or to stay) that provide the basics: one third of your mandatory RDA for vitamins and minerals; one quarter to one third of your daily carbohydrate and protein and fat needs; and one third of your fiber requirement (10 grams). Last but not least, both benefit two or more of your body's 10 healing zones.

Note: If you must have sugar, use a minimally processed, unbleached organic cane sugar, maple granules, or sparing amounts of raw organic honey (see Mail Order Sources).

#1 SUPER HEALING NUTRITION IN A BOWL (HOT)

Mush, porridge, hot cereal—it can be as appealing as it is healing. Here's how to benefit the most.

1. Stock up on a good selection of healing whole grains (instant and regular), including amaranth, quinoa, oats, rye, barley, brown rice, wild rice, cornmeal or riz-cous (the rice-couscous hybrid), polenta, bulgur, kamut, cream of wheat and rice, couscous, and millet from your health food store, co-op, or mail order food supplier (see Mail Order Sources).

2. To prepare, put ½ cup grains in a saucepan with 1½ cups water. Bring to boil. Lower heat, cover, and simmer according to direc-

tions. Stir in fruit, sweetener, milk, or cream substitute (such as nut or soy milks fortified with calcium and beta-carotene).

Super Healing Nutrition to Go (Variation)

²/₃ cup any whole grain

¹/₈ teaspoon salt

Boiling water, thermos

Topping: Yogurt, maple syrup, nut butter, skim or soy milk

The night before (or an hour ahead), put cereal and salt into a preheated, wide-mouth, 1-pint thermos. Fill thermos to within 1 inch of threading with boiling water; screw on lid. Before eating in the morning, thin cooked cereal with milk substitute. Stir in sweetener.

Optional: Add raisins, dried fruit, or raw nuts before capping; or carry and add.

Note: Use "To Go" method for a fast-as-flakes at-home breakfast. Just spoon thermos cereal into bowl.

#2 SUPER HEALING NUTRITION IN A BOWL (COLD)

Cold cereal is a just-as-healthy alternative if you choose the right ingredients. Best bets: sugar free, low or no sodium, minimally processed, additive-free flaked, puffed, nuggeted, or shredded biscuits from single or multigrain flakes (sold in health food stores and better supermarkets). Top with a low-fat skim milk or a nondairy substitute milk. Add fruit, nuts, or seeds.

#3 SUPER HEALING NUTRITION IN A SINGLE BITE

This multipurpose, sweetener-free formula for a 15-minute, six-ingredient breakfast makes muffins, waffles/hotcakes, or big cookies, depending on how you vary, beat, and bake the batter. The dry ingredients provide fiber and carbohydrates; liquid ingredients supply protein; oil and eggs supply fats. Add your own natural sweetener to taste.

Basic Mix Plus

2 cups whole grain flour plus ¹/₂ cup meal (corn, grits, oats, etc.)

1 teaspoon low-sodium baking powder

1 cup dairy or soy milk, yogurt, or substitute*

1 egg or substitute*

2 tablespoons nut or vegetable oil

Combine dry ingredients and liquids separately, then combine. Don't overmix.

For a week's worth of muffins today/waffles or muffins tomorrow, refrigerate batter in a covered container.

Variations: Sweeten (to taste) with berry or carrot purée or other natural sugar. To increase protein and minerals, add 1 to 2 tablespoons each skim milk powder, wheat germ, bran, or nutritional yeast.

Use the Basic Mix formula to make these breakfast treats:

◆ *Muffins:* Fold in ¼ additional cup meal, flakes, or nuts. Or for "lite bite" muffins, fold in one slightly beaten egg white. Fill greased muffin pans or paper cups half full of batter and bake for 10 to 12 minutes in 375-degree oven. For crunch, add 2 to 4 tablespoons seeds or chopped raw nuts. *Variation:* Instead of 12 regular 2-ouncers, make 24 bite-sized muffins.

◆ *Pancakes/waffles:* Pour batter from measuring cup onto preheated griddle or waffle iron. Brown, flip, and brown.

◆ *Big breakfast cookies:* Add additional meal, flour, or dry cereal flakes and/or nuts or unsweetened coconut until cookie-batter consistency is reached. For a flavor spike, add grated citrus peel, dried raisins, or dried tea herbs such as lemon, mint, or chamomile. Use tablespoon or soup spoon to drop batter onto lightly oiled cookie sheet. Bake 7 minutes in preheated, 400-degree oven.

13 BETTER-BREAKFAST TIPS

Morning super healing nutrition doesn't have to be eaten out of a bowl or a muffin cup. Here are 13 ways to have a better super healing breakfast in no time flat.

1. Have a bakeoff Sunday morning and make breakfasts for a month. Mix a double batch of Basic Mix and make muffins first, waffles

---

*See Substitutes and Dairy Substitutes for other alternatives.

next, and cookies last. Cool, freeze individually, and then pop into large freezer bags for easy, one-serving meals (brunch, coffee breaks, brown-bag lunches, and kids' snacks).

2. *Breakfast in a single scoop:* Fill a large cup-style ice cream cone (whole wheat sugar-free brands are sold at health food stores) half full of low- or nonfat frozen yogurt. Add sliced fresh fruit and wheat germ or crushed nuts. Top with more yogurt and sprinkle with crushed toasted sunflower or poppy seeds or grape nuts flakes.

   Express breakfast variations: In advance, fill four to six cones with alternate layers of puréed banana, persimmon, or mango or papaya and flavored yogurt, cottage cheese, or whipped tofu. Cover with eco-safe freezer nonplastic paper* and freeze until needed. Thaw for five minutes. Eat on the run.

3. *Milk-free Breakfast in a Single Gulp.* Combine half a ripe peeled avocado, half a peeled medium orange or one kiwi, ½ cup sprouts (optional), and 1 teaspoon honey (optional), and 1 or more table- spoons wheat germ, bran, or protein powder. Purée in blender. Makes two servings.

4. Make your own no-fat fruit or vegetable "bacon." Put 1 cup unsul- phured apricots (or other unsulphured dried fruit or dried vegeta- bles, such as tomatoes, peppers, etc.) through a food grinder, alter- nating with one slice dry, whole wheat bread or ½ cup coarse bran or wheat germ. Sweeten if desired. Add pinch of dried grated lemon peel. Press into a greased square dish, smooth, and score into bacon-sized strips. Cover with eco-safe nonplastic wrap. Chill 1 hour or dry in dehydrator according to directions. Break into strips.

5. Think locally but eat globally. If you're bored with breakfast, plan a week's worth of worldly menus worth getting up for.

   In Egypt, breakfast means a cooked bean dish called *Fuul Mudammas;* in Japan, it's rice, grilled fish, salad, and a fermented soybean soup (miso); Isreal breakfasts on yogurt, fish, vegetables, eggs, and cheese; in Nigeria, it's gari, a hot and spicy soup made from fried cassava rich in vegetables; in the former Soviet Union

---

*See Mail Order Sources.

it's kashka porridge, cold meat, smoked fish, cheese, potatoes, salad, and tea; eye openers in England include eggs, cereal, and kippers; and in Norway, people breakfast on assorted breads, smoked fish, goat cheese, and boiled eggs. Or try this fresh fruit and grain ambrosia from Finland:

Breakfast Whole Grain Ambrosia

> 1 cup wheat berries
>
> 1 teaspoon fresh ginger, grated
>
> $\frac{1}{2}$ teaspoon lemon rind, grated
>
> $\frac{1}{8}$ teaspoon ground allspice
>
> $\frac{1}{8}$ teaspoon ground cinnamon
>
> $\frac{1}{8}$ teaspoon ground cloves
>
> $\frac{1}{4}$ cup nonfat plain yogurt
>
> 1 tablespoon honey
>
> 2 green onions, chopped
>
> 2 tablespoons fresh parsley, minced
>
> 2 tablespoons fresh mint, minced
>
> 1 tablespoon toasted pecans, chopped
>
> 1 fresh peach, sliced
>
> 1 cup fresh blueberries

Place berries in a medium-sized bowl, cover generously with water, and soak overnight. Drain, transfer grains to medium saucepan, and cover with fresh water. Bring to a boil, reduce heat, cover, and cook for 30 minutes until tender and all water is absorbed. Place in a large bowl, and refrigerate.

Combine ginger, lemon rind, allspice, cinnamon, cloves, yogurt, and honey. Stir mixture into chilled grains.

Add green onions, parsley, mint, toasted pecans, sliced peaches, and blueberries and toss gently. Serve cold or at room temperature.

Makes four servings, 2 grams of fat each.

Variation: Substitute brown rice or kamut for wheat berries. Use blackberries or raspberries in place of blueberries.

May be served as a lunch or dinner salad or side dish.

6. As long as you keep fat, sodium, and sugar down, anything goes. Tried retro-eating? Have a light dinner at 8 A.M., a hearty breakfast

at 8 P.M. Or start the day with a luncheon salad and have a sit-down 6 P.M. raw foods smorgasbord brunch.

7. The cinnamon toast alternative: Spread your toast with calcium-rich sesame butter (tahini), sprinkle with potassium-rich maple syrup granules. For a better breakfast PB&J, pair sugar-free jelly with cashew, almond, or macadamia nut butter.

8. The no-cholesterol scrambled egg alternative: Heat 2 tablespoons of oil in a heavy skillet. Combine ½ cup lowfat plain or flavored tofu and 2 tablespoons yogurt, 1 teaspoon oil or melted butter, and 1 teaspoon dried salad herbs or fresh chives or parsley. Scramble over medium heat until dry.

   Variation: Substitute dry curd cottage or farmer's cheese for tofu.

9. Who needs the added fats and cholesterol of cereal cream? To get half the calories and twice the protein, make Super-Healing Half-and-Half. Combine one 6-ounce square of tofu with 3 ounces of water or calcium and beta-carotene-fortified soy milk (or mild herb tea). Sweeten to taste. Purée until smooth. Spoon on hot or cold cereal as a presweetened cream. To thin, add water. To thicken, increase tofu. For fruit flavored half-and-half, blend in 2 to 4 tablespoons fresh berries or melons.

10. Sprout a meal. Add one cup of sprouted wheat, rye, alfalfa (or ¼ cup of each) to one cup of cooked hot cereal for Porridge Plus, and top with Healing Half-and-Half or skim milk.

11. Breakfast on a Stick: Alternate chunks of raw, fresh, firm fruit—bananas, pineapple, melon, oranges, apples, grapes, pears—on 6- to 8-inch bamboo skewers. Brush lightly with oil or honey. Broil for three minutes 6 inches from heat. Rotate and broil for three more minutes. Roll immediately in crushed cereal flakes and/or skim milk powder or lecithin granules.

12. Try apple, pineapple, grape, or orange juice concentrate as a tasty calorie-trimmed fruit pancake syrup or cereal cream substitute. Just thaw, dilute slightly, heat gently, and pour.

13. For more vitamin C and minerals, make Tutti-Frutti Breakfast Punch: Combine 1 cup cranberry or cranapple juice, 1 cup fresh orange juice, and 1 cup freshly squeezed pineapple juice. For Breakfast Punch Plus, add one teaspoon vitamin C (1000 mg) or

1 tablespoon healing aloe vera* to the pitcher. Makes three servings.

TIP: No time to squeeze fresh orange juice? Add the juice of one fresh lemon to a container of store-bought juice. It improves flavor and adds bioflavonoids. (To keep breakfast citrus fresher longer, put whole lemons and limes and oranges in sterilized canning jars, cover with water, cap tightly. They keep for months.)

GETTING BACK TO BREAKFAST
Four Tips for Motivating Yourself

1. Start a cereal shelf. Stock it with a dozen grains (try a different one every hot-cereal day): for example, polenta, cornmeal (white and yellow), grits, buckwheat groats, millet, barley, amaranth, brown rice, quinoa, wild rice.

2. A ready-when-you-are kitchen is often all you need to get started. Stock up on alternatives (see Stocking Up) to sugar and cereal creams—like kefir, goat's milk, acidophilus milk, fruit juices, soy milk, and homemade half-and-half—and all the extras that make cereal a complete meal. Make a list of what you've got, what you can do with it, and how long the recipe takes, and post the list on the fridge or the bathroom mirror (or both!).

3. To make sure you have 15 minutes to eat before you run, set the alarm 15 minutes early and start tomorrow's breakfast tonight by setting the table and assembling all ingredients on the top shelf of the fridge or counter.

4. Take time to bone up on breakfast-out options. If you eat on the go, ask for nutritional analysis sheets of menu items at all fast-food restaurants you frequent and check out the fat, calories, sodium, and nutritional information on the labels of your favorite microwave, frozen, packaged, and convenience breakfasts. Make a "do-eat/don't-eat" list and keep a copy in your kitchen and wallet/briefcase/backpack/shopping bag.

---

* Available as a clear gel or liquid at natural health food stores and health pharmacies.

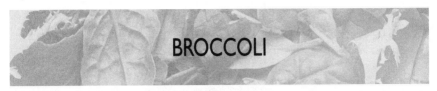

Broccoli is the most popular member of the *Brassica* or cruciferous cabbage patch family of vegetables originally cultivated by the Romans and later-day Italians and now eaten worldwide. The name is actually an acronym blending of the scientific name, *Brassica oleracea italica*, meaning "sprout or shoot" (the broccoli head is actually a flower shoot, botanically speaking).

Among the foods richest in life-extending, health-enhancing phytochemicals that protect all 10 of the body's healing zones from cancer, cardiovascular disorders, and premature aging, broccoli is the undisputed star of the vegetable crisper and number one on the National Cancer Institute's list of nutritional all-stars. (Consumption of broccoli has increased 800% in the United States within the last two decades alone.)

ANTICANCER INSURANCE

One half cup of broccoli a day provides protection from several forms of cancer, including cancer of the esophagus, stomach, colon, lung, larynx, prostate, mouth, and pharynx. The chief reason? Sulforaphane (an antioxidant found in other cruciferous vegetables, such as Brussels sprouts, carrots, and kale) which, concluded a recent study* by Paul Talalay, Ph.D., and colleagues at Johns Hopkins University in Baltimore, "work by bonding with toxins encountered, preventing the chemicals from reaching the cell's genetic material and instead flushing the noxious substance from the body."

A second reason is the antioxidants, which, among other protective good deeds, inactivate estrogens called 16-alphahydroxyestrone that promote cancer of the ovaries, breast, and cervix. Last but not least, broccoli contains both the beta- and alphacarotenes (two spears provide your RDA for beta-carotene), which accounts for broccoli's ability to resist and help reverse lung cancer and slow the growth rate of other tumors, say researchers at the Johns Hopkins School of Hygiene and

---

* *New England Journal of Medicine,* January 17, 1991

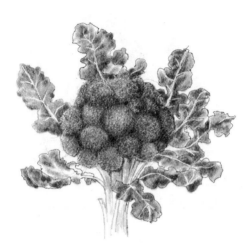

Public Health. Broccoli also has a high chlorophyll content, which effectively blocks precancerous cell mutations and also stimulates hemoglobin and red blood cell production, say researchers at the Organic Food Council.

The amino-sulphurous compounds in broccoli help detoxify excess cobalt, nickel, and copper in the body as well as normalize blood sugar levels that are too high (hyperglycemia) or too low (hypoglycemia).

WHITTLE YOUR WAISTLINE

Another reason to fill the snack bowl with raw broccoli rather than cheese nachos? A cupful of buds sets you back only 45 calories—all derived from energy-intensive carbohydrates (your body uses only 1 calorie to turn 50 calories of fat into energy but 12 to use the same 50 calories of carbohydrate). Broccoli also gives you 20% of your daily value for appetite-appeasing, bowel-regulating fiber in a form that's better assimilated than bran (broccoli has as much bran as cabbage and more than carrots).

STALKING VITAMINS AND MINERALS

One serving of broccoli also provides 125% more vitamin C than a cup of orange juice for infection protection, which, together with the anticancer antioxidant beta-carotene, reduces your risk of gastrointestinal and respiratory tract tumors.

Ounce for ounce, broccoli supplies as much calcium as cow's milk and in a form that's more easily assimilated than from most green plant sources. And it's one of the few plant foods rich in amino acid protein. One cup provides as much amino acid protein as a cup of corn or rice— for only one third the calories.

BROCCOLI JUICE FOR BETTER BRAIN FUNCTION AND VITAMIN UPTAKE

But that's not the end of broccoli's goodness. One serving of steamed, raw, or juiced broccoli also supplies 6% of your niacin, 12% of your phosphorus, and 10% of your RDA for iron, the mineral which improves mental alertness as well as the absorption of vitamin C. (For more brain perks, have a bowl of cream of broccoli soup; the combination of protein and iron sends amino acids to the brain.)

Broccoli is good eating. As John Randolph of Williamsburg noted in his food treatise in 1775, "The stems will eat like asparagus and the heads like cauliflower." It pairs well with hot or cold pasta, improves quiches, omelets, and flans; and adds an autumnal root vegetable flavor to juices and soups.

Growing Tips

- ◆ Plant in a 6.2 pH soil for best results. Broccoli needs plenty of phosphorus.

- ◆ You can start broccoli seeds indoors and set out the transplants when they are four weeks old, or sow seeds right in the garden. But transplants are easier to keep weeded.

- ◆ Buy transplants with fewer than six true leaves and no woody patches on the main stems.

- ◆ Best beginner's broccoli—Packman (see sources).

Buying, Storing, and Using

- ◆ Look for brightly colored broccoli with tightly closed buds (the smaller the head, the better the flavor).

- ◆ Keep broccoli in the vegetable crisper to protect vitamin C (at 32 degrees Fahrenheit, it retains vitamin C levels for two weeks).

◆   To use, rinse well, cut away leaves and woody section of stalks, and divide head into florets and stalk into thin slices.

◆   During cooking, the shorter the cooking time, the less breakdown of broccoli's mustard oils into odorous sulphur compounds. The best method for vitamin retention and odor and color control is blanching 2 cups of cut broccoli in 3 tablespoons water for three minutes at 600 watts. Second-best method: Quick steaming with very little water.

◆   Broccoli bored? Save a row in your garden for some *gaailaan* (see sources), the nutrient-dense Chinese broccoli.

Broccoli Butter

> *1 1-inch slice dry bread, crust removed*
>
> *1 medium onion, peeled and quartered*
>
> *2 garlic cloves, peeled*
>
> *½ teaspoon minced fresh chili pepper*
>
> *2 cups broccoli buds*
>
> *2 tablespoons fresh lemon juice*
>
> *⅓ cup olive oil*
>
> *2 teaspoons vinegar*

Soak bread in water for five minutes. Squeeze to remove excess water. Place half in food processor with the onion, garlic, chili pepper, and broccoli. Process until pasty. Add remaining parsley, bread, lemon juice, and half of the olive oil. With machine running, slowly add the remaining olive oil and vinegar. Taste and adjust seasoning if needed. Scrape, spread into bowl.

Makes 1½ cups.

Broccoli Gazpacho

Put in blender: Six broccoli flowerets; 1 fresh tomato, chopped; one quarter diced small cucumber; 1 tablespoon minced bell pepper; 1 tablespoon chopped onion; 2 teaspoons lemon juice; 1/4 teaspoon dried oregano; dash of hot pepper sauce. Blend to a slightly chunky consistency. Chill and serve sprinkled generously with fresh parsley or avocado slices. Serves two.

Variation: For Beta-carotene, add two chopped carrots and one handful spinach leaves.

Benefits healing zones: 3, 5, 6

Also see: Basic Dieting Facts and Advice, Antioxidants, Cancer

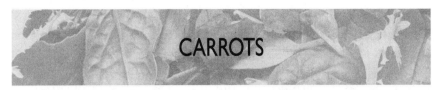

CARROTS

The carrot, a member of the 3,000-year-old *umbelliferous* family (celery, parsnips, caraway, fennel, dill, and chervil), is a root vegetable to root for. Therapeutic as it is for a wide range of ills—from the common cold to chronic fatigue, asthma, cancers, and a whole lot more—of the 25 vegetables the USDA rates tops, carrots provide the most protein, calcium, iron, and vitamins A, C, and B—finishing ahead of squash, green beans, and cauliflower and just behind broccoli, tomatoes, and corn.

Did you know that carrots were originally purple? Europeans developed the familiar carrot-orange varieties in the early seventeenth century. During World War II, the British developed the high-beta-carotene Mediterranean carrot most of us eat today. Carrots, however, are grown worldwide in a variety of shapes, sizes, and colors.

CARROT-A-DAY WAY TO BEAT CANCER
AND CORONARY HEART DISEASE

Like asparagus and artichokes, carrots were first a taproot pharmaceutical and only later an edible. The ancient Greeks called carrots *philons,* from the root word for *loving,* reflecting the belief that the root had aphrodisiacal powers. The English word derives from the Latin *carota,* meaning "to burn." Greek physicians used carrots before cooks did, prescribing carrot root and juice tonics to treat cancer, indigestion, snakebite, and skin ulcers. And they weren't far off the mark. A carrot a day today (or 1/2 cup of grated or sliced or juiced carrots), indicate recent studies by Regina G. Zegler, a National Cancer Institute epidemiologist, appears to reduce the risk of lung cancer by half. At twice that dose, carrots lower cholesterol levels by an average of 11%. Carrots, like other all-star carotene-rich foods (spinach, broccoli, etc.), effectively block the progressive cellular damage characteristic of cancers of the larynx, esophagus, prostate, bladder, cervix, and liver as well as premature aging and cataracts, says the American Institute for Cancer Research. Carrots are the fifth best source of the carotene complex after collard greens, kale, spinach, and butternut squash. One large raw carrot supplies 13,500 units of pro-vitamin A beta-carotene (a source second only to beef liver).

Carrots, in fact, are the top-rated source of alphacarotene, too, along with the other phytochemicals—p-coumaric and chlorogenic acids—which 1994 studies by epidemiologists at the University of Minnesota indicate effectively interrupt the formation of carcinogens in their early stages. Carrots' cancer-fighting flavonoid antioxidants, concludes a five-year study in The Netherlands, also protect your heart by reducing the formation of oxidized LDLs, a major factor in hardening of the arteries.

HOW ONE CARROT A DAY PREVENTS TWO DEFICIENCY DISORDERS

Carrots provide vitamin C and folate, says James G. Penland, Ph.D., a research psychologist at the Nutrition Research Center—a combination that makes carrots potent as a nutritional defense against respiratory ills from the common cold to the killer flu (regular carrot juice therapy makes breathing easier for asthmatics, too, reflecting the ancient Greeks' practice of feeding carrots to horses to improve their respiration). This combination also fights against periodontal disease (in which there is typically a deficiency of these two vitamins) and even birth defects triggered by folic acid deficiency. The phosphorus in the feathery carrot tops (a waste-not-want-not parsley substitute) is a good source of energy for the nerves.

Another source of energy in carrots is iron (the C and iron in carrots work together, making each other more available than when found singly). Juiced carrots are also a first-rate source of easily absorbed pure, phosphorus-free vegetable calcium and important digestive enzymes.

CARROT COCKTAILS FOR SEX, SPORTS, AND ARTHRITIS CONTROL

A dose of *Daucus carota* (carrots) is even libido liberating since carrots supply an estrogen-like compound which stimulates the sexual appetite, and ancient Greeks used them as an aphrodisiac. Carrot juice (or soup) is also the best fluid food going for travelers' diarrhea, sports fatigue, or flu-induced intestinal dehydration because (unlike soft drinks or sport "ades" or plain water), it supplies balanced amounts of sodium and potassium, two important metabolic electrolytes (this is one reason carrots juiced with endive are a time-honored aid to heal arthritis, a disorder in which these minerals are in short supply).

FIBER FOR HEART, HIPS, AND HEMORRHOIDS

Other studies indicate that the calcium pectate fiber in carrots fights elevated blood fats. Healthy volunteers given two medium carrots a day for three weeks had a blood cholesterol reduction of 11%. Calcium pectate in carrots bonds bile acids to block the formation of cholesterol in the liver. Pectate does double duty as a constipation- and hemorrhoid-battling bulking agent.

That same carrot fiber, which retains 30 times its weight in water, works as a safe appetite suppressant, satisfying the appetite without excess calories (one carrot contains about 42 calories). There are even studies that suggest that the noise created when eating crunchy carrots is stress reductive.

Carrots, are also free of the saturated fat found in other vitamin A rich foods such as in liver, egg yolks, and butter. Last but not least, eating carrots before sunbathing is said to prevent sunburn.

Beta-carotene Carrot Paté (Mock Salmon)

> *2¹/₂ cups carrots, diced*
>
> *2¹/₂ stalks celery, diced*
>
> *3 tablespoons natural peanut butter*
>
> *2 tablespoons onion powder plus dash cayenne or cajun seasoning*
>
> *2 tablespoons chopped parsley*
>
> *2 tablespoons tahini or mayonnaise*
>
> *¹/₃ cup almonds, ground in blender or processor until mealy*

Purée carrots and celery in food processor, juicer, or food grinder. Blend in other ingredients, mix well. Add more almond meal if needed to shape.

Press into lightly oiled terrine, casserole dish, or loaf pan.

Chill, garnish with avocado or kiwi slices, and serve on a bed of greens with crackers and breadsticks.

Makes four to five servings.

Two-Way Carrot Slurpy

> *2 medium carrots, finely grated*
>
> *1¹/₂ cups orange juice*
>
> *¹/₂ apple, cored and cut in eighths*

Lemon juice, dash
1 teaspoon ground cinnamon (optional)

Place all ingredients in blender container. Blend until thick and smooth. Contains about 100 calories per cup; makes two servings.

Variation: One-Way Slurpy: Serve chilled as a "gazpacho" or as a thick slurpy with straws.

Benefits healing zones: 1, 2, 3, 4, 9, 10

Also see: **Antioxidants, Beta-carotene, Cancer, Coronary Heart Disease, Basic Dieting Facts and Advice, Juices**

CELERY AND CELERIAC

If your favorite super healing green is parsley, celery's not a bad pale-green runner-up. *Apium graveolens,* or common celery,* is celebrated for its near-zero calorie count (18 a diced cupful) and its crunch (in the words of Ogden Nash, "Celery raw develops the jaw, but celery stewed is more quietly chewed"); but its value as a super healing food extends well beyond these things. Historically, celery and celeriac have been intertwined with parsley, another member of the prolific umbelliferous family.

In classical times, the two (celery and celeriac) shared the same name and both were used medicinally. Wild celery (smallage) may be the plant *selinon* mentioned by Homer in the *Odyssey.* Celery was employed as a laxative, diuretic, gallstone nostrum, and antistress and antibacterial agent. Celery was even utilized by eighteenth-century Dutch healers, who believed that celery's acids excited the urinary tract in passage. Celery is the only vegetable which produces androsterone, a hormone produced by both sexes (but largely by men) that is released through perspiration. Celery was not cultivated and eaten as a vegetable until the seventeenth century, when the bitterness was bred out, and by the nineteenth century the first blanched varieties (from which the healing chlorophyll is removed) became available.

---

* From the French *céleri.*

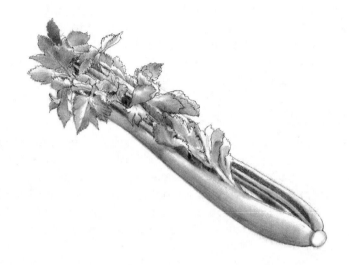

STALKING HYPERTENSION

Why do traditional oriental healers use celery whereas we use potent hypertension drugs? Celery contains the substance 3-butylphthalide, which researchers at the University of Chicago describe as a chemical that reduces blood pressure by relaxing the smooth muscle lining of blood vessels. A dose of phthalide equivalent to four stalks of celery a day prompts a decrease in blood pressure and cholesterol. Celery also provides three more healthy-heart nutrients: potassium, vitamin C, and more fiber (1.9 grams per ½ cup) than parsnips, cabbage, or squash. That fiber—cellulose, hemicellulose, and lignin—is what accounts for celery's crunch, which in itself has stress-reductive properties.

FIVE BODY CHEMISTRY BALANCING ACTS

Since it is 90% water and classified as a protective alkaline food, a celery cocktail or a few stuffed or plain stalks a day are a remedial way to deal with acidosis, halitosis, other acidic conditions of the body (including arthritis, which many naturopathic physicians classify as an acidic disorder), and imbalances due to overindulgence.

In the Roman Empire, celery was fed to livestock to improve (de-acidify) the flavor of their flesh, and it was eaten to counteract the morning-after effects of feasting.

Celery juice also helps support the integrity of the intestinal tract and muscular flexibility. Celery is sometimes juiced to extract the special healing oil *apiol* it contains, which helps purify the blood and clean the urinary tract, says the Nutritional Health Alliance. Celery juiced with endive and carrots often provides asthma relief.

HAVE AN ANTIAGING CUP OF *APIUM GRAVEOLENS*

Celery is a youth and beauty food. The compounds it contains called psoralens help prevent the chronic skin condition psoriasis. Along with B complex (especially folate) plus the electrolytic potassium, phosphorus, and sodium (which are essential for athletic stamina and antiaging and prevention of age-related calcium deposits), celery is an essential in any juice diet for inner cleansing and makes a healing electrolyte-rich sports drink.

Celeriac, common celery's cousin (a.k.a. celery root, knob celery, or turnip root celery) is a parsley-scented root vegetable rich in phosphorus and potassium for the health and healing of lymph, nervous, and urinary systems. It is low in calories (about 20 calories each serving); with half the vitamin C of regular celery but triple the calcium (42 mg per serving) and twice the fiber.

Buying, Storing, and Using

CELERY

◆ Look for crisp, medium-sized, pale green stalks with fresh leaves. Of the two varieties commonly sold—Pascal (green), which is stringless, and Golden (or yellow)—the former has the most pronounced flavor and the latter has the lowest beta-carotene levels.

◆ Avoid bruised stalks, which may harbor potential carcinogens, says the Natural Nutritional Foods Association.

◆ Celery should be washed and wrapped in damp paper towels before refrigerating.

◆ Keep up to seven days.

CELERIAC

◆ Select smaller roots to avoid woodiness.

◆ When ready to use, peel the tuber, removing leaves, roots, and buds, and then strip and slice and boil or steam (10 minutes), bake, or stew, or grate raw into salads or soups. (TIP: Blanching in salt water and lemon juice helps temper celeriac's slightly bitter aftertaste.)

◆ Wrap in paper towels and store, as for celery.

USES

◆ Celery is a good flavor booster (grated, diced, or shredded) in raw fruit and vegetable drinks as well as cooked soups, stews, and egg dishes. (It is a basic aromatic seasoning in French cuisine.)

◆ Diet snack: Fill stalks with puréed tofu, hummus, puréed avocado, or puréed root vegetable (carrots, turnips, beets, etc.).

◆ Celery may be braised (preferred ancient Roman style), steamed, sautéed, or even fried and served with mustard or a low-fat bechamel sauce.

◆ Celery leaves can be used as a cilantro or parsley substitute in salt-free salads and cold soups.

◆ Celery juice is compatible with almost all vegetables and fruits.

◆ Cooked celeriac purée adds body and a salt-free flavor spike to mashed potatoes, puréed carrots, and guacamole.

◆ Celery can be used as a cooked cauliflower substitute (whose taste it mimics). Or serve whole celeriac stuffed and baked like a bell pepper.

Thinny-Thin Celery Borscht

1 cup diced celery or celery root

1½ cups cooked beets

1 tablespoon fresh lemon juice

1 cup low- or no-fat yogurt

Blend all ingredients until thick and smooth. Serve cold, garnished with celery leaves or crushed celery seeds.

Two-Root Coulis

1 celery root (about 1 pound), peeled and chopped

2 large potatoes, peeled and chopped

3 carrots, peeled and chopped

2 cups vegetable broth

Place potatoes in medium saucepan, add cold water to cover. Bring to a boil, cook until tender (15 minutes). Drain and mash using a food mill, electric mixer, or hand-held masher.

In a second saucepan, combine celery root and carrots. Add cold water to cover. Bring to a boil and cook until tender (about 15 minutes). Drain. Combine the two mixtures. Pureé. Serve hot over steamed vegetables or pasta.

Variation: Substitute parsnips (a close relative) for carrots.

Note: A coulis is a thick purée.

Benefits healing zones: 1, 2, 5, 7

Also see: **Juices, Basic Dieting Facts and Advice, Coronary Heart Disease, Arthritis**

CRUCIFEROUS VEGETABLES

Beyond broccoli, what? Plenty, if you're-cancer-proofing your diet with cruciferous (or *Brassica*) vegetables, which increase protective enzymes that deactivate excess estrogen. You have, in fact, 3,189 more plants (both pungent and acrid) to go unless you limit your eating to what Dr. Thomas Kensler, associate professor of toxicology at Johns Hopkins School of Hygiene and Public Health, calls the "cruciferous anticancer 12" (cauliflower, cabbage, Brussels sprouts, kale, turnips, radish, cress, horseradish, rutabagas, broccoli, kohlrabi, mustard greens).* All are as good as, and sometimes better than, sources of the cancer-fighting phytochemicals.

Here are a few of the other super healing properties provided by three typical cabbage-family plants.

---

* Called cruciferous because of their four-petaled flowers, which resemble a cross (or crucifer).

CABBAGE

Cabbage provides more anticancer benefits than any other vegetable family. It is rich in the two antioxidants—sulforaphane and the flavonoids complex—that stimulates the body's production of cancer-fighting enzymes. According to Lee Wattenberg, M.D., professor of pathology at the University of Minnesota Medical School, one serving of cabbage a week could cut your chances of colon cancer by 66%.

FOUR CABBAGE BENEFITS BEYOND ANTICANCER PROTECTION

Cabbage is among the five top sources of vegetable fiber, supplying beta-carotene (red cabbage also contains the carotene lycopene), potassium, and 150% of your RDA for vitamin C (in ½ cup). This potassium-C combination reduces cholesterol, prevents blood clotting, and reduces your risk of coronary artery disease.

Cabbage juice is also helpful in healing cirrhosis of the liver, PMS, yeast infection, anemia, and peptic and duodinal ulcers (the secret healing ingredient is the vitamin U factor) says Dr. Garnett Cheney of Stanford University's School of Medicine. Fermented raw sauerkraut juice is notable for its nourishing effect on intestinal flora; stimulates the bowels; alleviates chronic constipation; and provides a gentle and natural laxative. According to researcher Dr. A. I. Vertanen of Finland, biologically active substances in cabbage inhibit the hyperfunction of the thyroid gland. And ½ cup of cabbage juice a day makes a good antacid. Because of its vitamin C and beta-carotene, cabbage juice is a good citrus substitute for those allergic to orange juice: Combine red cabbage with tomato or celery.

CAULIFLOWER POWER

"The test of a good gardener is revealed in his or her ability to grow cauliflower," it has been said. Indeed, this *Brassica* is the aristocrat of the cabbage family ("cabbage with a college education" was what Mark Twain called it).

Cauliflower predates Christ and was originally known as "colewort" or "the cabbage of Cyprus." What we call the head is actually a flower (ditto broccoli). There are two white- and purple-headed varieties grown.

Although cauliflower's pale color tells you it is not as nutrient dense as other cruciferous foods (it has less vitamin A than cabbage but more protein), it is a good source of four anticancer compounds: sulforaphane, fiber, vitamin C, and lutein, an anticancer carotene also found in spinach.

TURNIPS
Versatility Plus

Although classified as a starchy vegetable, turnips provide only one third the calories (14 per ½ cup) of an equal serving of potatoes (42 per ½ cup), plus healthy amounts of heart- and bowel-normalizing fiber (5 grams per ½ cup). Turnip is also a good source of complex carbohydrates for energy that keeps blood sugar levels stable—thus it's a food of choice for both diabetics and hypoglycemics. Turnip greens are a top-rated source of beta-carotene (1 cup of cooked greens contains more than 150% of the RDA and provides about two thirds of an adult's RDA for vitamin C). The turnip bulb has no beta-carotene and only half the vitamin C of the greens. A half-cup serving of cooked turnip has nearly 5 grams of dietary fiber, more than most dried beans.

Reach for a turnip when you have a pain in the foot (sore, burning, or aching). An old world formula directs you to boil (or roast) one large turnip and mash and spread one half on a cotton handkerchief and the other half on a second handkerchief. Apply turnip paste to the soles of feet, bandage in place, and wait for relief.

A second European folk nostrum, purported to relieve the discomfort of emphysema and pneumonia, goes like this: Juice ½ bunch watercress with one small turnip. Combine with goat's milk and warm, dark honey. Sip at two-hour intervals.

Buying, Storing, and Using

Look for dark green, crisp-looking leaves and tender, firm stalks and stems. All cruciferous vegetables can be steamed, stir fried, and shredded or grated for salads and soup fortifiers. Some can even be cooked and puréed as calorie-conservative mashed potato substitutes (or mash with equal amounts of cooked potato).

Cauliflower, broken into curds, is tasty simmered in milk or steamed whole for a dramatic side dish. Cabbage, kale, and mustard greens can be steamed, stuffed and baked, broiled, or sautéed.

Super Healing Six-Crucifer Slaw

1 cup shredded cabbage
1 cup shredded cauliflower buds
1 cup shredded rutabagas
½ cup tomatoes
Torn watercress
½ cup grated turnips
3 thinly sliced red or white radishes*
1 cup low-fat cottage cheese and ½ cup low-fat plain yogurt
2 tablespoons cider vinegar

Combine vegetables. In another bowl, mix cottage cheese and yogurt. Toss salad ingredients and cheese mixture together. Add vinegar.

TIP: A cinch-to-make sauerkraut? Wash a few good, mature heads of cabbage, and remove outside leaves. Use a kraut cutter (or a knife) to finely shred the cabbage, then mix 3½ tablespoons of salt for every 5 pounds of cabbage. Pack into clean canning jars. Fill with water to within a half inch of their tops, screwing bands on tightly. Let the kraut ferment for three days. After a week, wipe off bottles and store them in a cool place.

Turnip Purée Plus

8 medium-size carrots, peeled and cut into 2-inch lengths
6 medium-size turnips, peeled and quartered
½ cup hot broth, homemade or low-sodium canned
Salt substitute to taste (see p. 276)
Freshly ground pepper to taste

Preheat oven to 400 degrees. Place carrots and turnips in a roasting pan. Roast until vegetables are tender, about one hour.

Place in a food processor with the broth. Process until smooth. Season.

Makes four servings.

Cauliflower Croquettes

1 head cauliflower (about 1½ lbs.)
1 egg

---

* Also cruciferous, as is horseradish, and oriental radish types such as Daikon.

2 tablespoons parmesan cheese

½ cup whole grain bread crumbs

½ cup wheat germ

½ cup brown rice (or other whole grain) flour

1 cup grated cheddar cheese

1 tablespoon chopped fresh parsley

1 tablespoon chopped fresh chives

¼ teaspoon garlic powder

¼ teaspoon black pepper

Clean cauliflower, break into flowerets, and steam for seven minutes.

Purée until smooth (adding a little cooking liquid if necessary).

Place purée in large mixing bowl and combine well with remaining ingredients.

Preheat oven to 375 degrees and lightly oil a large baking sheet.

Shape mixture into 1½-inch patties or "cigars" place on baking sheet, and bake for 10 minutes on each side, until golden. Serve hot with a dipping sauce of equal parts mustard and light sour cream.

Yield: Three dozen.

Benefits healing zones: 2, 3, 6, 7, 9

Also see: **Antioxidants, Broccoli, Cancer, Indigestion, Ulcers**

DAIRY SUBSTITUTES

If you're eating for health and super healing, you're eating more low-fat beans, greens, grains, and berries. But if you're downing them doused with high-fat creams, milks, and sauces followed by cholesterol-rich frozen dairy desserts, you're losing more than you're gaining. A diet that derives more than 30% of its calories from fat endangers your heart, blood vessels, and arteries and raises your risk of cardiovascular disease by 30%, says the U.S. Department of Health and Human Services.

What's more, a high-fat, high-cholesterol diet can make you fat fast—not just because fattier foods are higher in calories, either. According to Canadian bariatric specialist Dr. David F. Horrobin, a substance called gammalinolenic acid (GLA) is a normal body constituent formed within the body from a substance in the diet called linolenic acid. Adequate amounts of GLA in the body help prevent obesity, says Horrobin, activating "brown fat," which burns up excess calories without exercise. GLA also activates a calorie-burning enzyme and seems to inhibit appetite. But people who add weight easily often have defective brown fat reserves. And a heavy hand with the butter and cream doesn't help because it raises cholesterol and saturated fats, which in turn block production of GLA.

A low-fat diet, by contrast, builds cardiovascular health, which, in turn, triggers high-level wellness of other body systems. According to a study at the University of New Hampshire by psychologist Jim Davis, the body's DIT (dietary-induced thermogenesis) is improved 30% when the heart is ticking the way it should.

How to reduce or eliminate your dairy consumption? Here are 20 low-fat, little-or-no-dairy solutions.

MILK/CREAM

Do you dream of cream? Try a do-it-yourself, salt-free, spoon-on dessert cream, (healthier than store bought) that has 37 calories and 113 mg of fat per 2 ounces—that's one tenth the calories and fat of the real stuff.

Dream Cream

> *1/2 cup instant (dry) nonfat skim 1% soy milk or rice milk*
>
> *1/4 cup ice-cold water*
>
> *1 teaspoon vanilla, almond, or lemon extract*

In a chilled metal bowl, combine milk powder and water. Beat three or four minutes with electric mixer. Add extract and continue beating until stiff peaks form. Makes *2/3* cup.

Variation: Substitute *1/3* cup low-fat coconut milk* (a good source of nonanimal calcium).

---

* At better supermarkets, or call Andre Prost at 800-243-0897.

TIP: To make whipped toppings that keep up to three hours in advance, place whipped cream in a strainer lined with cheesecloth and suspend over a bowl in the fridge. Water will drip through without collapsing cream.

Nondairy creamers add more saturated fat (20 grams per 3 ounces) to your diet than the small chocolate bars you're probably avoiding, along with plenty of sodium and preservatives. Lighten your coffee with a healthier counterfeit. Combine equal parts of dry powdered milk, dairy, soy or buttermilk, and powdered soy lecithin granules (a natural emulsifier) in a jar. Add just enough warm water to make a slurry mixture when shaken. Agitate until smooth. Refrigerate.

Are you one of the wholly cow crowd of Americans who drink four times more whole milk than skim? Motivate yourself to change your milky ways. Pouring skim, not regular, milk in your breakfast bowl cuts 10 pounds of fat from your diet in one year.

Don't say yes to yogurt too often. Regular whole dairy milk versions have as much as 8.3 grams of fat per serving. But don't do without. Switch to soy yogurts, or make this no-milk formula, which even puts fiber into your diet.

Un-Yogurt

Let ½ cup of hulled sunflower seeds soak for 24 hours in warm water to cover. This will produce 1 cup of soft, chewy seeds. Put seeds and liquid in blender and grind. Add ½ cup of water and blend. Add a second ½ cup of water, and blend again. Consistency should be similar to heavy cream. Cover cream and let it "culture" 8 to 24 hours at 70 or 80 degrees in a yogurt maker or in a bowl next to an electric light bulb. Un-Yogurt is ready when it's tasty and a "black cap" has formed (discard or eat).

Sweet on sour cream? Whip up your own tasty 10-calories-a-tablespoon-no-fat version:

Substitute Sour Cream

Follow directions for Un-Yogurt, but allow culturing to continue for an additional 12 to 18 hours. Let cheese "drip dry" through a fine sieve for one hour. Refrigerate. May be sweetened to taste with honey or a natural dry sugar.

Sugar-free, Milk-free Blintz

½ teaspoon plain gelatin powder (or vegetarian agar-agar flakes) dissolved in tablespoon warm water

¹/₄ teaspoon lemon juice and ¹/₄ teaspoon vanilla

Combine all ingredients. Beat with electric mixer at high speed until soft peaks form. Makes 1 cup.

If you're drinking coffee without caffeine and you'd like to do it without fat, skip the half-and-half and light cream. Both have twice as much saturated fat (2 grams per serving) as this healthy homemade:

Fat-Free Coffee (and Cereal) Cream

Put 1 cup of skim milk, soy, or rice milk powder, 1 cup of liquid skim milk, and 2 tablespoons of safflower or canola oil into a blender and liquefy. Add more water or more powder to correct creaminess. Makes 1 cup.

Like your milk-free oatmeal really piping hot on cold mornings? Instead of cold soy milk, stir in ¹/₃ cup of toasted soy powder per serving and a little extra water as you cook it. Result? Creamy, smooth cereal that stays hot to the bottom of the bowl.

How about a nondairy cereal cream with no fat or cholesterol? Try this:

Fat-Fighters' Creamer

Combine:

> *1 tablespoon honey*
>
> *3 tablespoons cashew meal*
>
> *1 tablespoon peanut meal*
>
> *3 tablespoons walnut meal*
>
> *1 tablespoon tahini or sesame meal*
>
> *¹/₂ cup nonfat dry dairy or nondairy milk*
>
> *1 cup water*

Combine all ingredients and process in blender. To thicken, add more nuts; to thin, increase liquids.

One cup of evaporated milk has almost 20 grams of fat, half of them the saturated, artery-clogging kind. Solution: Buy skimmed canned condensed or, better yet, make your own.

Homemade Evap

Liquefy 1¹/₂ cups powdered soy, rice, or dairy milk, ²/₃ cup fresh skim, low-fat or, 1% soy milk, and ¹/₄ cup rice syrup or maple syrup in the blender until smooth.

Or combine 2 cups low-fat coconut milk with ½ cup milk powder. Chill. Liquefy and use as substitute for cream. Only 3 to 4 grams of fat per cup.

What's the low-fat *creme fraiche* alternative? Try this:

No-Cholesterol Carrot and Chip Dip

Combine 1 cup of soft plain tofu, ¼ cup of nut or vegetable oil, 2 tablespoons dry cottage cheese, and 2 tablespoons fresh carrot juice. Purée until creamy. Chill. Makes 1 cup with 30% less fat than real *creme fraiche*.

What's the next best dairy-free thing to a creamsickle? Try this:

Fruit Pops

> *4 bananas*
>
> *¾ cup 1% light soy milk*
>
> *½ cup frozen raspberries, thawed and drained*
>
> *¼ cup unsweetened apple juice*

Peel and slice bananas and puree with remaining ingredients in a food processor or blender.

Freeze mixture in an ice cream maker according to manufacturer's instructions.

Contains only 0.6 grams of fat per ½-cup serving.

Also see: Coronary Heart Disease, Basic Dieting Facts and Advice, Foods, Allergies Vegetarian, Substitutes, Mail Order Sources

Sworn off dairy? Milk a 0% fat squash or papaya.

Zucchini Milk

Peel three fresh zucchinis (don't remove seeds or pulp). Cut into 1¼-inch chunks. Fill blender one quarter full. Liquefy and run until zucchini turns white and thick. Presto, zucchini milk. Sweeten or season to taste. To fortify with calcium, add 1 or 2 tablespoons milk powder or 1 teaspoon powdered calcium lactate. For papaya, substitute 1½ cups peeled, chopped, ripe papaya for zucchini (contains 2% fat per serving). Use in place of dairy milk in recipes.

There are 11 grams of fat in a milkshake, as much as a lean lamb chop. A better way to get your juices flowing without milk fat? Try this:

Milk-free Fruitshake

> *1 cup grapefruit juice*
> *1 cup fresh strawberries*
> *1 cup low-fat coconut milk, 1% soy milk, or rice milk*

Put all the ingredients in a blender. Process until smooth.

Use in recipes calling for whole milk.

The good egg can be bad for you. Two yolks have more cholesterol than 3 small hamburgers plus 9 grams of fat. Don't make eggnog. Make a no-fat, no-cholesterol Nut Nog instead:

Nut Nog

Mix in blender or a large cocktail shaker: 5 cups fresh skim dairy milk or soy or buttermilk, ½ cup finely ground almonds, 1 tablespoon of plain gelatin, 2 tablespoons carob powder, 1 tablespoon fresh nut oil, and 2 tablespoons of honey. Process or shake until thick and creamy. Sprinkle with nutmeg before serving.

Cheese is a high-fat dairy indulgence; but it doesn't have to be.

DAIRY CHEESE
Charting Fat and Calories

Food	Calories from fat	Total calories
I cup of:		
Skim milk	0	86
Low-fat milk (1%)	12	102
Low-fat milk (2%)	37	121
Whole milk	72	150
Buttermilk	20	90
Plain low-fat yogurt	36	150
I tablespoon of:		
Kefir cheese	27	33
Cream cheese	45	50
Sour cream	23	25
Half-and-half	15	20
Heavy cream	45	45

Make a cheater's cheddar, a tasty taste-alike for toast and sauces, with only 4 grams of fat per serving.

Imitation Shredded Cheddar

Soak one block of plain or preseasoned tofu in ½ cup of canned or fresh carrot juice. Freeze until almost solid. Thaw slightly until texture is similar to semi-hard cheese. Grate coarsely by hand. (TIP: Try the Parmesan and Romano cheese alternative sapsago (also called green cheese)—with only a fraction of the former's 7 grams of fat an ounce, plus less sodium and far fewer calories. Tastes great, and it's gratable.)

Want a fat-free party cheese? Switch to the creamy, 80-calories-a-scoop *di latte,* a low-fat fresh mozzarella with only 6 grams of fat. Did you know you get more fat (16 grams) from those 2 ounces of mozzarella in your pizza than you do from 3 ounces of sirloin steak? Top the sauce on your pizza with a Mock Mozzarella (use the recipe for Imitation Shredded Cheddar but omit carrot juice). Or switch to a garlicky-flavored, 2-grams-of-fat, 90-calorie spread that beats Boursin:

Counterfeit Boursin

2 packages (8 ounces each) fat-reduced cream cheese, softened

¼ cup thick dairy, soy or seed yogurt

2 teaspoons Dijon-style mustard

2 tablespoons each finely chopped fresh chives and dill

1 clove garlic, minced

Beat cheese, yogurt, mustard, chives, dill, and garlic with electric mixer in a large bowl. When thoroughly blended, spoon into a 2-cup mold lined with foil. Cover and refrigerate overnight. Transfer to a serving plate; peel off foil. Serve with whole grain crackers. Makes 10 servings.

To top tomorrow morning's low-fat bagels, try this:

Cashew Cheese

⅓ tablespoon pimento

Dash garlic

½ cup cold water

½ cup cashews

1 teaspoon vegetable salt or home-grown dried herb

Purée the ingredients in blender. Add ¼ cup cold pressed oil, 2 tablespoons lemon juice, and set aside.

Or place 4 tablespoons agar-agar or gelatin in 1 cup cold water for five minutes. Cook until clear, about five minutes. Blend in first mix. Pour into oiled bowl. Allow to set.

Save on Camembert's cost, calories, and fat. One ounce of Camembert has as much saturated fat (8 grams) as a serving of fast-food chili. Switch to tempeh (a fermented tofu). Health food stores carry several types, each with a unique flavor, texture, color, and aroma to use in casseroles, spreads, dressings and dips: wine fermented, brine fermented, red, and savory fermented.

What's the baked Brie alternative? deep-fried bean curd: The four popular types are cutlets, pouches, puffs, and burgers. All have a hearty flavor, brown color, and a firm, meaty texture similar to fried chicken. This type of tofu stays fresh even at room temperatures.

Here's the American Heart Association's recipe for an all-purpose, do-it-yourself, de-fatted cheese:

Instant Reduced-Fat Cheese

Cut 4 ounces of cheese (Swiss, mozzarella, jack, or Muenster) in half-inch cubes and place in a single layer in an oiled baking dish. Cover with water. Bake in microwave (high) for three minutes. Stir mixture during baking.

Remove from the oven, cool for 15 minutes, and then put through a fine sieve. Rinse. Press excess moisture out by hand, wrap, and refrigerate. The texture is not as smooth as the original cheese. Use in cooking, for melted cheeses, sandwiches, etc. Contains only one quarter the calories, fat, and cholesterol of regular cheese.

What's the Oreo® ice cream alternative? Here's a dairy dessert with little or no chocolate, milk, eggs, or cream that tastes finger-lickin' good with only 25% of ice cream's 20 grams of fat and half the calories.

Dairy-free Un-Chocolate Ice Cream

10 ripe, peeled, medium-sized bananas

½ pound dried unsulphured figs

1 cup carob powder or low-fat cocoa powder

Water, as needed, or mild herb tea

Blend bananas until creamy. Spoon into a freezer container and chill until almost frozen. Remove from freezer. Separately, blend figs, adding enough water to make a thin paste. Gradually blend in carob or cocoa powder. Combine carob-fig paste and banana mix. Spoon into freezer container or into popsickle molds (for fudgesicle). Freeze.

Variations: Substitute dates for figs. Use peeled mangos in place of bananas.

Benefits healing zones: 1, 5, 6, 7

Also see: Coronary Heart Disease, Basic Dieting Facts and Advice, Vegetarian Foods, Mail Order Sources, Substitutes

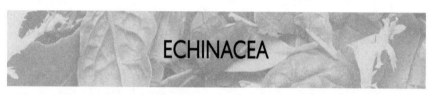

ECHINACEA

What's faster than a speeding antibiotic? Consider the herbal antibiotic and multispectrum healer *Echinacea,* the world's best-studied immune modulator, according to the Herb Research Foundation.

Various species of this purple coneflower, a wildflower native to the southeastern United States, are still used by Indian tribes of the plains. Native peoples call *Echinacea purpurea* "snakeroot," referring to its use for snakebites, and "toothache plant" because of the numbing effect it produces when chewed. As part of an ancient ritual, tribal medicine people mashed the fresh root and applied the juice to their hands, enabling them to handle fire without pain.

For over a century, this immunity-enhancing botanical has been used around the world to activate white blood cell production and fight infection and soothe inflamed mucous membranes caused by the flu and other infectious conditions, and without the side-effects caused by conventional antibiotics and even aspirin (which include immune function suppression, allergic reactions, and even minor liver damage).

According to hundreds of clinical tests, *Echinacea* also acts as a weak antibiotic, stimulates the adrenal glands, increases the production of bone marrow and new tissue, fights herpes, and counteracts immune suppression caused by cancer chemotherapy, and prevents tissue inflammation caused by allergies.

Echinacea in extract, tablet, capsule, or infusion (tea) form should be taken at the first signs of illness and repeated at two- to three-hour intervals for two to three days. For greater healing, *Echinacea* can be coupled with herbal preparations of goldenseal, artemisia, or astralagus.

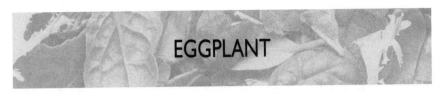

EGGPLANT

Eggplants (a.k.a. aubergines) are neither eggs (so named for the egglike shape of the elongated varieties) nor the "mad apples" they were alleged to be by sixteenth-century horticulturists; nor are they (as early Spanish settlers in America called them) "Guinea squash." The eggplant is, in reality, a member in good standing of the solanae or nightshade family (which makes them off limits for the arthritic, along with other nightshade foods such as tomatoes, green peppers, and tobacco). Although now associated largely with Eastern olive-producing cultures such as Greece, Italy, and Turkey, the eggplant is a native of Japan and India.

HEALTHY HEARTBEAT/HEALTHY BOWEL FUNCTION

Eggplant has the ability to bind up LDL ("bad") cholesterol and flush it from the body. It's also a good source of potassium, the healthy-heart mineral which normalizes sodium levels. As a juiced or puréed vegetable medicine, eggplant is useful as both a diuretic and a laxative because of its high soluble fiber content.

THE AUBERGINE ANTICANCER SOLUTION

According to the National Cancer Institute, the combination of soluble fiber and the antioxidant terpenes in eggplant may help prevent the steroidal hormonal effect which promotes certain types of cancer and help prevent the damage associated with this oxidative process.

COSMETIC AND REPRODUCTIVE BENEFITS

Eggplant supplies the healthy-pregnancy vitamin folate. Half a cupful provides a scant 13 calories (3 more than celery). And, according to tenth-century Hindu healers, eggplant is a vegetable medicine for sexual stamina.

Eggplant is a time-honored complexion clarifier as well. Here's a simple, two-ingredient formula for oily skin: Blend one entire small, diced eggplant with 1 cup plain yogurt. Apply to face and neck. Rinse off after 20 to 30 minutes. Fill a plant mister with herb tea and spray on as a finishing touch.

In addition, a compress of eggplant juice will help bleach freckles, and eggplant leaves can even be used as a poultice to soothe burns and cold sores.

Buying, Storing, and Using

There are 18 varieties of this satiny-skinned vegetable, which shines as both a meat accompaniment and a meat substitute. The commonest conformations of the eggplant are egg- or football-shaped, but there is also a white puffball variety, there are many elongated examples with thinner skins and fewer seeds, and there is a small Thai variety that can be eaten raw. There is even a bitter-orange-and-green bunchy variety sold in Oriental markets (in earlier times there were white, gray, green, brown, and striped varieties). The eggplant is one of the few U.S.-grown vegetables that thrive in the tropics as well. Some smaller "midget" varieties are grown as ornamentals, and all types of eggplants can be used for vegetable dyes.

Look for a satin-smooth, firm plant heavy for its size, of a uniform color with green cap intact.

Eggplant is highly perishable (keeps for one week) and is ethylene sensitive, so store away from fruits such as apples, which exude this gas as they ripen.

Do not peel until ready to use.

Eggplant will soak up to 10 tablespoons of oil when fried. To save calories and reduce fat, brush slices lightly with oil and broil until brown, turning once, or salt and drain before frying.*

TIP: To quick-cook a whole eggplant without peeling, puncture several times with a fork and microwave for 18 minutes.

Use eggplant as an appetizer, main course meat substitute (bread and bake as fake fishsteaks), a sandwich bread substitute, or bread spread. It is tasty cooked and tossed in cold grain and bean salads or breaded and baked. It is an anchor ingredient in mousaka, curry, parmegiana, and ratatouille dishes.

Try these super healing recipes:

Eggplant Oven Fries

Oven-sautéed eggplant: Cut in strips. Dip in eggs and fine bread crumbs or wheat germ and bran, and then bake at 450 degrees until tender (about 20 minutes). During the oven sautéeing, sprinkle several times with vegetable oil.

---

* The better the eggplant the less bitter it will be and the less need there is for salting, which leaches out water soluble vitamins.

These eggplant strips make delicious finger foods. Tasty when combined with tomatoes or simmered in a creole sauce.

Eggplant Caviar

> *2 two-pound eggplants*
> *2 large red peppers*
> *1 medium onion*
> *2 large cloves garlic, crushed*
> *⅓ cup olive oil*
> *Ground pepper to taste*

Puncture eggplants and microwave on high for 18 minutes, turning eggplants over once. Let cool. Meanwhile, wash, seed, and remove ribs from peppers. Dice. Peel onion and dice.

Peel eggplants, scraping pulp from skin. Combine eggplant, peppers, onion, and crushed garlic and grind to a coarse purée (or use a food processor or blender, working machine with an on-off motion).

Beat in oil and pepper, spoon into serving dish. Chill several hours. Correct seasoning. Serve cool, (but not cold,) as a first course or as a salad spooned over fresh greens with thin crackers or dark cocktail bread.

Serves six.

Benefits healing zones: 1, 2, 3, 7

Also see: Antioxidants, Coronary Heart Disease, Vegetarian Foods, Basic Dieting Facts and Advice

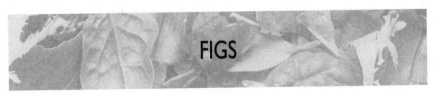

FIGS

According to legend, the shade of a fig tree is cooler than a tent, and to sit under one's own fig tree is a sign of peace and plenty. The first fruit mentioned by name in the Bible (Genesis 3:7, King James), figs were known as "provisions for the King's house" in the days of the Pharaohs. There were 150 words for fig in ancient Egypt, and figs were said to be Cleopatra's favorite true confection. Early Greek Olympians ate figs for strength and stamina and received them as recognition of athletic feats. Even today, in some southern European countries, figs are used in place

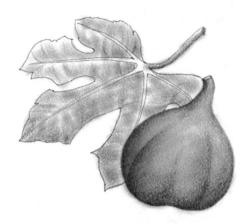

of rice at weddings, to symbolically shower newlyweds with health and longevity.

FIVE FIGGY HEALTH ENHANCEMENTS

Because of their mucin and pectin content, figs, like prunes, are natural laxatives (try juicing figs as an orange juice alternative or supplement). Swiss doctors used figs steamed in milk to treat abscesses, and black figs steamed in raw goat's milk is a time-honored European remedy for arthritis. Figs are an all-star pick-me-up energizer for kids and a valuable addition to the diets of osteoporosis sufferers because, pound for pound, they provide more calcium than milk, says the Alternative Health Foundation. They are fairly high in potassium and iron as well. A second pound-for-pound bonus: Even better, figs are higher in soluble fiber than most other fruits, vegetables, and nuts. There are 40 calories in one fresh or dried fig.

Buying, Storing, and Using

The two varieties of figs, yellow green or purple, offer similar super healing benefits. Look for unsulphured dried figs (the Kadota variety has the smallest seeds) and store them in a dry, cool place in a tightly closed container.

Try diced figs tossed with nuts, steamed grains, and vegetables and other subacid fruits (such as cherries and cranberries), or as an ingredient in fruit cocktails. Try fig juice as a calcium booster in breakfast drinks or combine with nut butter for a high-calcium PB&J. (*Note:* Diabetics and others with blood sugar disturbances should consult their physician before adding dried fruits to their diets.)

Dried Fruit Power Shake

> *½ cup chopped dates*
>
> *1½ cup milk (dairy, soy, or rice)*
>
> *Handful raw almonds or cashews (optional)*
>
> *1 tablespoon toasted wheat germ*
>
> *½ cup crushed ice*

Grind nuts and dates. Add milk and ice and blend until creamy. Strain and sip. Makes three small servings.

Variation: Use dates or prunes in place of figs.

Benefits healing zones: 5, 6, 7

Also see: Fatigue, Indigestion, Osteoporosis, Prunes

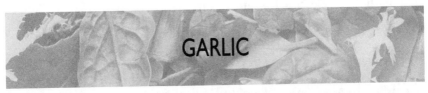

GARLIC

Garlic is nature's 100-watt bulb—its 100 or more healing ingredients are a boon to all 10 of the body's target healing zones. An important medicinal agent for the Chinese, Hebrews, Egyptians, Greeks, Romans, and Hindus, garlic was found in the tomb of Egyptian King Tutankhamen and was consumed by laborers who built the Great Pyramid. Muhammad used garlic to treat scorpion stings. Garlic is mentioned in clay tablets found in Nineveh (circa 668 to 626 B.C.) and cited in the Hebrews' Talmud for satiating hunger and improving circulation. Louis Pasteur, the bacteriologist, noted garlic's antibiotic effects. Albert Schweitzer used it to treat amoebic dysentery. During World Wars I and II, garlic was used by the British military to control infection and gangrene.

There are 500 or more benevolent bulbs (including onions) in the *allium* family, which is, in turn, ironically, a member of the *liliaceae* (lily) family.

SECRET INGREDIENTS

What makes garlic such good vegetable medicine? Its vitamin A, B, and C; its calcium, potassium, and iron; and the antioxidants, carotenes, germanium, and selenium plus the countless biologically active compound agents. But most important are garlic's 33 sulphurous compounds, especially the volatile amino acid allicin.* Allicin is released when the cell walls of the garlic clove are crushed or pressed. Allicin is what gives all *allium* family vegetables (including leeks, shallots, and chives) their characteristic pungency.

But vitamins and minerals aren't the only reason garlic helps reverse asthma and acne (using externally applied oil), treats ear drum disorders, and relieves bronchial congestion, gallbladder disorders, dyspepsia, and diarrhea. Like ginseng, it's in a class of so-called adaptogenic plants that restore metabolic equilibrium and block the free radicals that compromise the immune system. Or, as Dr. Gerhard Schrauzer, professor of chemistry at the University of California at San Diego, puts it, garlic is "a simple, nonprescription drug that helps detoxify the body and prevent disease." Indeed, naturopath-author Mildred Jackson claims that garlic can cleanse the entire circulatory system in less than an hour.

PREVENTING CANCER AND CARDIOVASCULAR DISEASE

According to New York University Medical Center professor of environmental medicine Sidney Belman and cell biologist Michael Wargovich at the University of Texas System Cancer Center in Houston, serious garlic eaters have a lower rate and risk of stomach and colon cancer. Studies by Dr. Wang Mei-ling, of the Shandong Medical Research Institute in Tianjin, China, indicate that cancer deaths in garlic-loving

---

* Short for allyl disulphide, this amino acid is also found in onions, a cousin vegetable.

countries are almost 10 times lower than elsewhere. (The dose that does it is seven cloves a day.)

Garlic is as good an earth medicine as you're likely to find to stay cardiovascular healthy. Reductions in LDL levels and increases in HDL of 20 to 40% are common. Garlic may even be better than aspirin at inhibiting the fibrogen that leads to blood platelet clumping, which causes stroke and atherosclerosis.

HYPERTENSION, DIABETES, AND ULCER CONTROL

Garlic therapy also has a healing effect on high blood pressure and eliminates angina pain, dizziness, and headaches without the frequently occurring side-effects of hypertension drugs. The magic ingredient appears to be garlic prostaglandin A. Garlic also inhibits the activity of liver enzymes and influences the way fats are metabolized, making it useful in treating gastric ulcers, and increasing blood insulin levels in diabetics, say USDA Human Nutrition Center researchers.

INFECTION PROTECTION

Known affectionately as "the stinking rose" and reverently as "Russian penicillin" by the legions of lovers whose admiration takes the form of newsletters and fan clubs, garlic's powers as an antibacterial and antifungal agent have been known and utilized since 1947. According to researchers at the Boston University School of Medicine, garlic has the effectiveness of 1% penicillin against strep, staph, fungus, and yeast infections as well as numerous strains of the flu. In fact, it not only kills existing bacteria but it inhibits further bacterial growth. And whereas penicillin inhibits only gram-positive bacteria, the allicin in garlic counteracts both gram-positive and gram-negative strains—and in smaller doses than most antibiotics.

Buying, Storing, and Using

Store your garlic heads in a net bag in a cool, dry room or soak cloves in vinegar overnight to increase acidity and eliminate the risk of botulism (which can occur with low-acid root vegetables), and then transfer the cloves to a jar of oil.

To prevent linger-longer odors, rub hands with parsley and lemon before handling raw garlic, or, if cooking, cut the garlic less and cook it longer (but at a lower heat).

To banish garlic breath, suck a lemon or chew parsley or fennel seed when eating garlicky food, or soak peeled cloves overnight in yogurt. An alternative is to switch to odorless bulbs, which are acid-aged and dried but taste and smell like the undoctored real thing.

Garlic Butter

Put garlic bulbs in steamer basket over boiling water and steam for 30 minutes. Separate and peel cloves, crush, and combine with olive oil. A ceramic garlic baker, which does the job with greater flavor retention, is a second option.*

Garlic butter/oil keeps up to two months refrigerated.

Benefits healing zones: All 10

Also see: Halitosis, Coronary Heart Disease, Indigestion, Cancer, Juices, Common Cold

Note: Baking reduces odor and mellows flavor, but it also reduces the medicinal benefits since allicin is heat sensitive.

Can't get your fill of garlic? Look for elephant garlic, four times the size of regular types with a milder flavor and an edible husk. Or grow your own garlic chives (a.k.a. gowchoy; see Mail Order Sources).

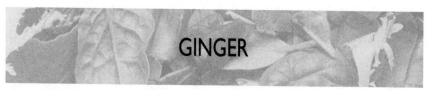

GINGER

Ginger (*Zingiber officinale***) is the root end (hand) of a tropical biennial herb indigenous to South Asia. one of the original spices which sent European explorers in search of a new sea route to Cathay, it was cultivated by the Greeks (the first people to use it as a Dramamine alternative), Romans, ancient Chinese (Confucius wrote that he never dined without ginger), and Hindus. It is commended frequently in the Greek

---

* Sold in cookware shops or large department stores and some health food stores.

** The Latin generic name *Zingiber* is derived from the Sanskrit *singabera* ("shaped like a horn"), so called because of the resemblance of the roots of the plant to a deer's antler.

De Materia Medica for its salutary effects on digestion and as a poison antidote, and it is cited in the Koran as one of the drinks of the righteous. In England before the Norman Conquest, it was, after pepper, the most common spice.

Ginger was successfully transplanted to the West Indies early in the sixteenth century by the Spanish. In the Middle Ages, ginger was so treasured a spice that the street in Basel where Swiss traders sold it was named Imbergasse ("Ginger Alley"). In sixteenth-century England, ginger was recommended by Henry VIII as a remedy against the Plague. Fancy gingerbread became popular during the reign of Queen Elizabeth I. Ginger even enjoyed a reputation as an aphrodisiac until it was outlawed during the Puritan era. Nineteenth-century English tavern keepers used ground ginger to sprinkle on top of beer or ale stirred with a hot poker.

HANDS-ON HEALTH

Slivered, dried, powdered, and preserved ginger root (ginger root is even steamed and roasted in the Orient) and ginger juice are obtained from the knobs of the roots called "hands," which are surprisingly nutritious and provide more protein than green beans, as much vitamin A and calcium as cauliflower, as well as iron, phosphorus, potassium, and riboflavin.

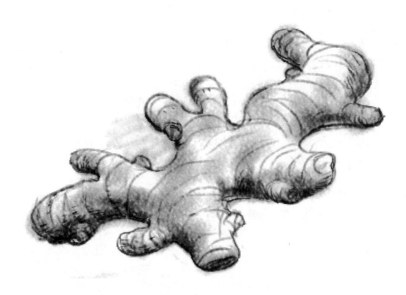

NATURE'S DRAMAMINE

For royalty and the very rich in ancient Greece, ginger was used as an antinausea drug (as it is even today). Ginger counteracts both vertigo and motion sickness better than OTC drugs, according to plant pharmacologists. A ½ teaspoon dose of powdered ginger outperformed 100 mg of Dramamine in controlled studies. (Ginger appears to work by increasing stomach acidity and ascorbic acids and acting on the inner ear canal, balancing that mechanism.) Stir 1 teaspoon of ginger juice (half an hour before traveling) into any drink or tea as prevention.

ANTICANCER/ANTIAGING

According to botanist and medicinal herbalist James Dake, studies show that ginger extract is effective in killing salmonella and inhibiting the fungi that produce aflatoxin, a potent carcinogen. Ginger contains two phenolic compounds, shogaol and zingerone, that protect fats from being damaged by highly destructive free radicals, which trigger cancer and accelerate the aging process.

HAVE A GINGERBREAD HEART

According to Danish researchers and Cornell University Medical College investigations, ginger is a better blood clot blocker than garlic or onion, working to inhibit blood cell synthesis of thromboxane, which triggers dangerous aortic coagulation. The chemical structure of the active ingredient *gingerol* resembles that of aspirin, another well-known blood thinner.

Indian research with test animals indicates that ginger in fresh and powdered form lowers blood cholesterol levels and helps offset the lipid-elevating effects of a high-fat diet. Other studies suggest ginger's usefulness in reducing blood pressure as well.

Research also indicates that ginger decreases the heart rate and increases the force of contractions in the upper (atrial) chamber of the heart, similar to Digitalis.

FOUR MORE BENEFITS

Ginger in your A.M. juice and your P.M. tea works as a drug-free painkiller, especially in relief of menstrual discomfort, and antacid and appears, say Japanese biochemists, to help block mutational cell changes that trigger cancer. Ginger also reduces fever and speeds recovery from respiratory ailments. (In India, children are administered ginger tea to counteract whooping cough.)

Buying, Storing, and Using

◆ For maximum effectiveness, use the juice or the grated pulp of the fresh ginger root. Use a garlic press to extract juice then mince the remaining pulp.

◆ Ginger root has an affinity for root vegetables such as beets and carrots and is tasty in nut dishes and stock-based soups. Use no more than ½ teaspoon of fresh minced grated or juiced root per serving. (To reinforce, add more just before serving.)

◆ Caution for cooks. Simmering mutes ginger's bite; but burned, ginger becomes acrid.

◆ Take a ginger break once a day: Enjoy it as tea, as juice, or salad dressing supplement, or added to a healing tub.

For treating hoarseness or speaker's laryngitis, here's an alternative to sugary "candy" cough drops and alcohol- and additive-rich decongestants:

Ginger Lozenges

Peel and cut a fresh ginger root into paper-thin "lozenges." Suck throughout the day to relieve hoarseness and freshen "sick" breath. To double your pleasure, alternate with cups of hot ginger and mint tea.

Ginger Juice Gargle

Brew a double-strength cup of ginger tea, cool, and gargle as needed.

Benefits healing zones: 2, 3, 4, 7, 10

Also see: Cancer, Common Cold, Herbs, Coronary Heart Disease, Indigestion, Juices

GRAPEFRUIT

Think pink when you think grapefruit. The grapefruit is believed to be either a Barbados hybrid of the pommelo or a native of China. But all grapefruit weren't created equal. The juice of a fresh pink grapefruit has 27 times more beta-carotene than the white variety. But both supply the antioxidants lycopene and vitamin C and are richer in potassium than tangerines or blueberries, with half the calories of bananas. Even better, the fiber they contain in the form of pectin lowers blood cholesterol and reduces arterial plaque as effectively as prescription drugs, says Dr. James Cerda, professor of gastroenterology at the University of Florida and a leading researcher on the citrus-cholesterol connection. As stated earlier, this is significant when you consider that each 1% reduction in cholesterol cuts the risk of heart disease by 2%.

The lycopene in pink grapefruit is important for reproductive function. Women with high levels of this substance typically have a fivefold decrease in risk of cervical dysplasia. According to natural healers, it's also as effective as quinine in treating infection and relieving pain. But to benefit, eat the grapefruit pulp, including, when possible, the membranes that separate the sections and the white interior of the rind. The therapeutic pectin resides in the cell walls, or "juice sacs."

TIP: To quick-peel a whole grapefruit, plunge into boiling water for 60 seconds to loosen peel.

Grapefruit bored? Reach for a pommelo (meaning "big lemon"). The largest member of the citrus family, it has a sweet, sensual flavor (due to its deficiency of a substance called naringen, which gives ordinary grapefruit its tartness). Ranging from the size of a small cantaloupe to that of a basketball, the flesh is fragrant, juicy, translucent to clear (white variety) or pink to rose red (pink variety). (Candied pommelo peel is sometimes served as petit fours in China.) Pommelos are high in vitamin C and potassium. They keep up to one week refrigerated.

Beta-carotene Pommelo Gimlet for One

Combine ½ cup freshly squeezed pommelo juice in the blender with four fresh strawberries. Add two to three crushed ice cubes. Blend until frothy. Sip for a fast breakfast or a snack.

Variation: Substitute ½ cup pink grapefruit juice for pommelo.

Benefits healing zones: 2, 6, 7

Also see: Lemons, Oranges, Juices

GRAPES, RAISINS, AND OTHER DRIED FRUITS

What's power food for an ageless body and a timeless mind? Dried fruits are as good as and sometimes better nutritional bets than fresh because dehydration concentrates nutrients.

America's favorite can't-stop-after-one finger food, grapes (and raisins) were cultivated as far back as 5000 B.C. Today they are the #1 fruit crop grown globally and fall into three categories: Old World, North American, and hybrid.

Old World grapes account for over 95% of the crop grown worldwide and are used as table grapes, raisins, and wine. North Americans (including the Concord and the Niagara) are used for juice and table grapes (but not raisins), while hybrids are a cross between Old World and North American grapes and are used primarily for wine. *Note:* European grapes have five times the vitamin C of American varieties.

To keep your munch-a-bunch passion alive, play the field. Here are 10 picks for your fruit bowl:

Cardinal/Emperor (large, dark red seeded grapes)

Flame (seedless, medium to large red grapes)

Ribier (large, blue-black with seeds)

Tokay/Queen (large, bright red, seeded)

Almeria (large, golden)

Calmeria (longish, light green)

Perlette/Thompson (green, seedless, compact clusters).

Both raisins and grapes supply fiber, potassium, and vitamins A, B, and C (grapes have more than raisins). They are low in fat, sodium, and cholesterol and are one of the four top fruit sources of phosphorus.

CURES FROM THE VINE

In folk healing, grapes and raisins have been used to counter dyspepsia, liver and kidney disorders, tuberculosis, and hemorrhoids. The ancient Persians believed that dried grapes eaten before breakfast improved the memory.

Raisins are blood purifiers and builders, recommended for internal cleansing. Grapes can be eaten, seeds and all, or juiced to benefit from their flavonoid antioxidants that treat venous disorders, including varicose veins and atherosclerosis. Sun-dried grapes (raisins) even rival dried beans as fiber suppliers for healthy heart and bowel function and weight control. Dried fruits like raisins appear to help inactivate the viruses responsible for polio and herpes infections, indicate studies by Canadian researchers. Grapes' tannins (the pucker-up acids also found in tea leaves and wine) help fight tooth decay, and the ellagic acid in grapes is regarded as a factor in lowering the risk of some cancers.

Grapes should be wrapped in biodegradable, nonplastic storage bags (see Mail Order Sources) and kept refrigerated. Rinse under cold water before eating.

RAISINS AND OTHER DRIED FRUITS
To Go

Rotate your stock to stay out of the same-old dried-fruit rut. Stock up on newer varieties such as dried papayas, cherries, blueberries, and other-than Myrna figs.

Keep a variety of dried fruits on hand for backpocket snacks, portable desserts, candy bar substitutes, and quick, single-bite breakfasts.

TIP: Backpocket a toothbrush to counter the sugar residue a dried fruit chew can leave on your teeth.

Dry your own fruits. A dehydrator will pay for itself in less than a year if you want to satisfy a sweet tooth holistically. Or if you want to do it yourself, here's a recipe in the right direction.

Oven-Dried Grapes

> *4 cups seedless white or red grapes (or a mixture), cut in half*
> *¾ teaspoon Super Healing Salt (see p. 276) or salt substitute*
> *Freshly ground pepper to taste (optional)*

Preheat oven to 200 degrees. Spread grapes onto two baking sheets. Bake for 1½ hours. Remove from the oven and season to taste. Bake until grapes shrink to one quarter their original size (but stay juicy). Cool on baking sheets.

Transfer to tight container and refrigerate.

Makes 1 cup.

Benefits healing zones: 1, 5, 7, 8

Also See: Hemorrhoids, Coronary Heart Disease, Basic Dieting Facts and Advice, Cancer

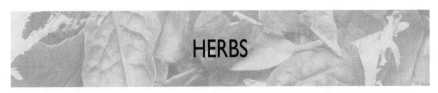

HERBS

A cup of herb tea is the original what-a-relief-it-is hot drink. In their healing manifestations, herb teas are called tisanes or infusers. They were brewed long before coffee and cocoa and, in fact, well before recorded history—and with good reason.

According to studies at the National Institutes of Health in the Netherlands, men who consumed the highest amounts of flavonoids in foods like apples and drinks like tea had half the heart attack rate of tea teetotalers. The flavonoids in tea protect the heart by preventing the formation of plaque (which clogs the arteries), by lowering cholesterol, or by lowering blood pressure.

Enhanced vitamin and mineral absorption is a second good reason to consider an herbal brew when you pause to refresh. See the table of a few of the hidden nutrients in 10 herbs that suit us to a tea.

If your health is in the red for any reason, have a cup of herb tea that ups your EGCD. In Shitzouha, Japan, where unfermented green tea is drunk daily, the cancer rate is lower than in any other region of Japan. Green tea's cancer-inhibiting secret ingredient appears to be Epigallo-

HERBS
Their Hidden Nutrients

Herb	VITAMIN A	B_1/B_2	C	E	Calcium	Iron	Potassium	Magnesium
Alfalfa	•	•	•	•	•	•	•	•
Catnip		•				•	•	•
Cayenne	•	•	•		•	•	•	
Chamomile	•	•			•	•	•	•
Lemon grass	•				•	•	•	•
Parsley	•	•	•			•	•	•
Peppermint	•	•	•		•	•	•	•
Raspberry leaf	•	•	•	•	•	•	•	•
Red clover	•	•	•		•		•	•
Rosehips	•	•	•	•	•	•	•	•

catechin gullate (EGGD), which interacts with the initiator cell to prevent tumors. Studies at Rutgers University and the University of California at Berkeley support these findings and add that the flavonoid antioxidant catechin in green tea also helps lower cholesterol and kills *Streptococcus metans,* the bacteria responsible for cavities. Green tea is also a vitamin C enhancer, improving your body's ability to assimilate ascorbic acid in healing amounts.

TIP: To experience fully the sensuality of green tea, which is customarily sipped straight—without milk or sugar—you must be open to its unique fragrances, color (from near clear to yellow, gold, and transparent green), and nuanced flavors. Use hot, not boiling water to preserve nutrients.

FIVE TO-A-TEA BENEFITS

Above all, a healing herbal tea offers drug-tree relief without caffeine, excess calories, carbonation, tannic acid, or unnecessary synthetic additives. But before you pour, here are a few tips.

TASTERS' TIPS: Before You Pour

1. Choose your tea. Green tea, oolong tea, and black tea all come from the leaves and buds of the evergreen shrub, *Camellia siensis,* but are differently processed. Green teas are the freshest, youngest, and least processed of all sinensis leaves. They are steamed and rolled and dried without fermentation. Oolong and black teas are produced by a fermentation process that converts some of the tannins (which account for tea's astringency) into coloring compounds. Oolong tea, an intermediate between green and black types, is semifermented. A fourth type is twig tea (kukicha tea or bancha tea, made from young branches of the tea plant), which is lower in caffeine than green or black. If you're avoiding caffeine, ask before you buy. To determine whether any herb is your cup of tea, open and sniff.

2. What's your pleasure? Are you drinking herb tea to enhance health or for a specific healing benefit? Check out a tea's therapeutic action before you fill your cup (see "One Minute Healers").

3. Choose your tea format—loose leaves, roots, or bark allow you to experience the full texture and color of the herb, but they aren't as convenient as bags; tinctures are 4 to 10 times stronger and enter

the bloodstream more rapidly, while pressed or tableted herbs, like bags, are ideal for the mover and sipper.

4. Choose your method. A medicinal cup of tea for super healing should be brewed longer than a recreational cup. Here's how. With leaves or flowers (of mint, lemon balm, lavender, chamomile, etc.), make an infusion (pour 1 pint of almost boiling water over 2½ ounces of fresh or 1 ounce dried herbs), let steep for 2-3 minutes; remove bag or tea ball, or strain if loose.

With bark, berries, or roots (willow, valerian, etc.), make a decoction by putting an ounce of dried (or 2 ounces of fresh) herbs into a pot with 1½ pints of cold water. Simmer over low heat for 10 to 20 minutes.

Tips on Healthful Sweeteners and Lighteners

Honey's healthier because it contains caffeic acid esters, a possible anticarcinogen. Or consider unbleached, unrefined white sugar (see Mail Order Sources), red maple sugar or syrup, or a natural fruit/grain sweetener such as dry date sugar or rice syrup.

For half-and-half alternatives, try skimmed condensed milk, low-fat rice or soy milk, or a homemade dairy alternatives (p. 74).

HERBAL HINTS

1. Herbal ice cubes: Fill ice cube trays with tap water; insert herbal sprig or flowers or berries in each cube. Freeze. *Variation:* Fill trays with leftover herb tea or lemonade or fruit juice before inserting herbs.

2. Fill a plant mister with leftover tea (chamomile, yarrow, or lemon mint) and spritz face two times morning and night as a refreshing complexion clarifier.

3. Use green tea (where flavor is compatible) to replace a portion of any fresh juiced vegetable combination or as part of the liquid in baking and cooking. Keep green tea in cubes in freezer to use in mineral water, lemonade, fruit juice coolers, ice tea, or mini cubes to use as healing hardcandy alternatives.

4. Looking for a Pekoe-tea counterfeit without the caffeine? Try red raspberry or combine equal parts alfalfa, mint, and red clover.

5. For hot and cold healing throughout the day, keep one refrigerated pitcher and one hot thermos at the ready.

6. Now that you've made the transition to healthy herbs, look for
   environmentally healthy packaging—organically grown herbs
   and oxygen-not-chlorine-bleached tea bags without strings, tags,
   and staples.*

ONE-MINUTE HEALERS

Try the following healing teas (use dried leaves unless otherwise directed):

Herb	Healing Efect
Alfalfa	For both low and high blood sugar; kidney, bladder disorders
Angelica (also Dong Quai and licorice)	Helps normalize menstruation and hormonal balance
Bilberry tea (use bilberry extract)	Improves circulatory health, vision, and cerebral function
Burdock root (use root or tincture)	Helps acne and related skin disorders
Cayenne (Red pepper)	Speeds weight loss; improves circulation
Chamomile	Provides relief from constipation, insomnia, stress, and heartburn
Cherry bark licorice tea	Provides relief from asthma, viral infection, and menstrual difficulties (licorice)
Dandelion leaf	Reduces edema (caused by water retention); normalizes Brody's sodium balance
Gingko Biloba (rich in vitamin C and bioflavonoids)	Fights viral and respiratory infections; aids mental alertness

---

* See Mail Order Sources.

Herb	Healing Effect
Golden Seal, Garlic, Ginseng tea germanium, calcium, magnesium, and B complex; avoid Chinese ginseng, which is an endangered species)	Rejuvenates all 10 healing zones; helps normalize (rich in all bodily functions; stimulates cerebral function; acts as an antistress agent
Green tea (*Camellia sinensis*) *Note:* Never boil; pour hot water over leaves, steep for five minutes. For maximum healing, drink 3 to 5 cups daily	Aids in cancer prevention; fights hypertension; reduces cholesterol; fights cavities; enhances vitamin C action
Horsetail (silica)	Regenerates nails; aids kidney function; promotes bladder healing
Ma-huang	Relieves fatigue and depression; aids weight loss
Marjoram	Relieves seasickness
Peppermint (also cinnamon)	Relieves nausea, and indigestion; fights respiratory infections
Raspberry leaf	Relieves diarrhea; eases childbirth pain and cramps
Red clover	Relieves arthritis and headaches
Rosemary	Relieves fatigue and depression; improves memory; relieves arthritis
Sage	Soothes sore throat, indigestion, diarrhea, and bronchitis
Spearmint	Relieves mental stress and headaches
Valerian	Fights insomnia; reduces stress
White willow bark or birch	Relieves headaches, migraines, and muscular pain

In addition, try these recipes:

10 Sprigs Tea

Pour hot water over 10 sprigs of parsley and steep for 5 minutes. Strain and flavor with lemon.

Ten sprigs of parsley provide 10% of your RDA for beta-carotene and 15% of your RDA for vitamin C.

For 10-Sprigs Tea Plus, pour hot green tea over parsley. Green tea contains vitamin-C-enhancing polyphenols.

40-Wink Four-Herb Tea

> *½ ounce hops*
>
> *1 ounce valerian*
>
> *3 ounces chamomile*
>
> *1 ounce passion flower*

Mix the 4 ingredients. Use 1 teaspoon per cup hot water. Steep for 20 minutes. Drink ¼ cup each 30 minutes until drowsy.

Sleep pillow

Stuff dried hops, rose, chamomile, and lavender into a linen pillow case to create a sleep pillow.

ONE-MINUTE OLFACTORY HEALERS

What's good when ingested is often just as healing when inhaled. Here are 15 super healing botanical whiffs.
Directions:

- ◆ Use only pure essential aromatherapy oils. Keep them in an airtight bottle and store in a dry, cool cupboard.

- ◆ To use, add three to five drops to bath water or mix with a carrier, such as wheat germ or sesame oil, and massage on temples, neck, chest, and other sensitive spots.

Note: Once you've got your nose in the air, keep it up. The longer you use aromatherapy oils, the stronger your scentual senses will become.

Scent	Healing Benefits
Basil	Stimulates memory; reduces insomnia, depression, and fatigue.
Chamomile	Soothes inflamed skin, headache, insomnia, and toothache. Balances female reproductive system. Calms anger.
Cinnamon bark	Stimulates circulation. Fights flu and infectious diseases.
Clove buds	Heals respiratory system, infectious diseases, toothaches; stimulates memory; reduces nervous fatigue.
Eucalyptus	Balances energy. Heals respiratory system. Expectorant for asthma and bronchitis.
Geranium	Uplifting; relieves nervous tension.
Lemon	Uplifting; balances, counters stress.
Peppermint	Stimulates metabolism and nervous system. Eases nausea, vomiting. Soothes fever. Relieves muscular pain, depression, and stress.
Rose	Aphrodisiac. Regulates feminine reproductive system. Emotionally uplifting.
Rosemary	Rejuvenating, uplifting; relieves stress.
Sandalwood	Elevates mood; reduces depression.
Spearmint	Alleviates digestion, depression, and mental fatigue.
Thyme	Stimulates metabolism. Fights intestinal infections.

Benefits healing zones: All.

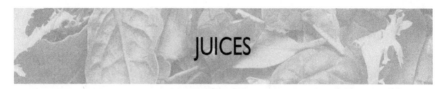

JUICES

You could be on your way to better health and weight loss if you get juiced. According to the late Dr. Bircher-Benner, founder of the famous Swiss Nutrition Clinic that bears his name, fresh juices are the most therapeutic food substances on earth (along with sprouts), offering a synergistic concentration of healing nutrients that nourish every cell of the body, enhance overall health, and prevent a wide spectrum of ills from acne to zinc deficiency. And juicing is no born-yesterday healing notion. The practice of raw juices healing therapy developed in the nineteenth century as a treatment for cancer. Regularly using a variety of plant foods may even reduce or eliminate your need for supplements. This is no surprise, considering the liquid assets of any raw juice cocktail. Unlike solid foods, which may take two to eight hours to digest and assimilate, ½ pound of carrots (one 8-ounce glass of carrot juice)—which provides 48,000 IU of anticancer beta-carotene, vitamin C, bone-building calcium, and antiaging trace minerals such as silicon and sulphur for healthy skin, teeth, and nails—is instantly released into the bloodstream for instant energy and cellular repair. Pump up the healing volume with some juiced green kale and you get an additional 17,500 IU of pro-vitamin A (beta-carotene) and bonus amounts of calcium, vitamin C, and iron.

KEY TO FATIGUE CONTROL/ANTIAGING

Raw juice is alive with organic catalysts called enzymes (destroyed when food is cooked), which increase the rate at which foods are broken down and absorbed (which is why a super healing diet that lives up to its name should consist of at least 50 to 75% of raw meals that heal.) Raw juice is the key to doubling your energy, according to the Hippocratic Health Institute, and slowing—or even reversing—aging and the onset of the degenerative disease process.

There's no faster way than juice fasting to support your immune system through a wide variety of healing processes. Juices exert a free-radical-quenching effect on tissues, membranes, and the bloodstream, clearing your system of environmental toxins.

Fast, Safe Weight Loss

Juice fasting is the fastest, safest way to lose 5 to 10 pounds without sacrificing essential feel-good nutrients, such as the antioxidant vitamin C complex (the highest concentration of C is found in fresh juices), energizing potassium, calcium, and the anticancer, antitoxin antioxidants.

EIGHT TIPS FOR GETTING JUICED

◆ Use organic fruits and vegetables, or carefully wash and/or peel using a vegetable brush and a soap specifically formulated to remove pesticide residue. (*Note:* Tropical fruits are often imported from countries where carcinogenic sprays are still in use; therefore, they should be peeled.)

◆ To avoid possible toxins (natural or added), discard citrus skins, rhubarb greens, and the seeds of apples (which contain trace amounts of cyanide). Avoid juicing fleshy low-water fruits such as avocados and bananas unless your juicer is designed to process them.

◆ A healthy daily down-the-hatch dose is 1 to 4 cups of juice. (More than 1 cup is better when healing is a high priority.) Drink all juices immediately after processing for maximum benefits, or freeze surplus as ice cubes for fast conversion.

◆ Health affirmation #1: Have 1 cup of juice for every three to four glasses of water daily. Health affirmation #2: Juice-fast one day a month to cleanse and rejuvenate all 10 healing zones.

◆ Dilute strong-flavored fruit and vegetable juices (beets, onions, lemons, turnips, collard greens) with spring water or mild juices or teas (3:1 ratio).

◆ Juice twice as many vegetables as fruits. Fruit, in general, is less easily tolerated by the organs of digestion and elimination than vegetables.

◆ Size up your servings according to the following chart:

	Amount	Makes
Fruits		
Apples	I medium	1/4 cup juice
Grapes, seedless	2 cups	I cup juice
Peaches (ripe)	2 whole	I cup nectar
Pineapple	I whole, peeled and speared	2 cups juice
Strawberries	2 cups	I cup nectar
Fresh Herbs		
Parsley leaves	2 cups	1/4 cup juice
Watercress	I pound	1/4 cup juice

◆ Use juice boosters for more nutrition. Seven good ones to use in extract form (1-3 drops per 8 oz. serving): gota kola, ginseng, nettles, fo-ti, passion flower, astragalus, liquid or powdered kelp or dulse. Or add 1 teaspoon of aloe vera gel or liquid or ½ to 1 teaspoon of powdered vitamin C; or juice lentil, alfalfa, or clover sprouts with vegetables, or cereal grass powder (wheat, barley, kamut, etc.).

◆ Recycle the remains of your juicing day: Pulp from fruits and sweet vegetables adds fiber, minerals, flavor, and texture to baked goods and desserts and reduces or eliminates the need for sweetening. Use carrot pulp for moister meatless meatloaves apple pulp for sugarfree cakes and sweet breads. Try making a Health Slaw: Layer carrot and lemon pulp, sprinkle with coconut, toasted seeds, or sprouts and a dash of vinaigrette. Beauty bonus: Beauty and body masks, eye compresses, and assorted natural complexion-corrective creams can be concocted by combining vegetable or fruit pulp with egg yolk (for oily skin) or whipped cream (for dry skin), or Fuller's earth (for all skin types) to make a simple astringent mask.

TIPS FOR JUICE FASTING

1. Get your doctor's approval, especially if you have a serious health condition, before beginning any fast.

2. Fast with juice—not water. Water fasting releases too many toxins and too few of the detoxifying nutrients—such as vitamins C and E and beta-carotene—needed to neutralize them.

3. Fast for one to five days. For longer fasts, consult a medical professional and only do so after getting a go-ahead from your physician or nutritionist.

4. Fortify your liquid meals with protein or milk powder if you suffer from low blood sugar (hypoglycemia) or low weight.

5. Use these six super cleansers as starters and staples: beets (no more than 2 to 3 ounces the first day, increasing gradually to 6 ounces); cabbage; lemon; carrot; celery; and apple with sprouts and wheat germ as boosters. Drink one daily cup of detoxifying herbal tea—dandelion, goldenseal, comfrey, and nettle, for example—increasing to two on the second or third day (this can be healing and empowering). Drink the herbal tea separately or combine with vegetable juices to cleanse the liver and kidneys. Steep ½ teaspoon of each herb in a pint of water, and strain. Add lemon.

6. Consider natural bulking agents. One or two teaspoons of psyllium seed added to each glass of juice once or twice a day is a safe, natural aid to elimination.

7. Do it right. Your day-before-the-fast diet should contain raw fruits and vegetables and vegetable broth, homemade vegetable soups, or steamed vegetables. After the fast; abstain from meat, milk, fish, and grains until the fifth day.

The juice fast below can be followed for one to five consecutive days and modified as suggested. One serving of beet or cabbage juice per day is recommended to cleanse the system.

Here's a 12-recipe, four-day juice fast plan:

Choose any three liquid meals a day (each recipe makes two to three small servings), rotating them for a balanced intake of complementary fruits and vegetables. All juices may be diluted or supplemented with boosters Each 6-ounce meal-in-a-glass cocktail supplies about 100 to 200 calories. The following recipes make three to four servings.

Juicy Fruit Juicer #1

> *2 firm peaches or 4 apricots, diced and pitted*
>
> *½ lime or lemon*
>
> *1 ripe banana, peeled*
>
> *1 tablespoon brewer's (nutritional) yeast*

Juice peaches or apricots and lime or lemon. Combine juices, banana, and yeast in blender or processor, and liquefy until smooth. Dilute as needed with water or mild tea. (2 servings)

A.M. *Energizer*

> *Handful of parsley or cress, including stems*
> *5 cubed carrots, greens removed*
> *1 small apple or pear, seeded, peeled*
> *3 lettuce or spinach leaves*

Bunch up parsley, chop coarsely, push through chopper stems and all with carrots and apple (pear). (2 servings)

Cleansing Cocktail

> *¼-inch slice ginger root, diced*
> *1 small beet, with or without leaves*
> *1 small apple, cubed, seeded*
> *4 carrots, greens removed*

Push ginger, beet, and apple through chopper with carrots. Dilute if desired. (2 servings)

Spring Tonic #1

> *Handful dandelion greens (unsprayed)*
> *3 pineapple rings*
> *3 radishes, red or white, or ¼ cup clover sprouts*

Bunch up greens and push through chopper, alternating with pineapple and radishes and sprouts. (1 serving)

Sweet Red-Pepper Juice Plus

> *8 medium-size red bell peppers, stemmed, seeded, and deribbed*
> *4 tomatoes*

Pass the peppers through a juice extractor. Strain through a fine-mesh sieve. Skim off the foam.

Separately, pass tomatoes through juice extractor. Let stand overnight. Place fine-mesh sieve over a large bowl and let the juice drip through. Stir from time to time. Takes about one hour. Combine with red-pepper juice.

Spring Tonic #2

> *2 parsley sprigs*
> *Small handful wheatgrass or alfalfa sprouts*

4 to 6 carrots, greens removed

2 stalks celery

$^1/_2$ cup broccoli florets or 1/2 beet

Bunch up parsley and wheatgrass, and push through chopper with carrots, celery, apple, and beet.

Ginger Ade

$^1/_4$-inch slice ginger root

4 stalks fresh rhubarb

1 diced pear

Sparkling water

Push ginger through chopper with pear. Pour juice into ice-filled glass. Fill glass to top with sparkling water.

Variation: In place of ginger, use a wedge of prickly pear. (1 serving)

Juicy Fruit Juicer #2

$^1/_2$ pineapple, peeled, diced

$^1/_2$ apple, seeded, diced

$^1/_4$-inch slice ginger root

Push pineapple through chopper with apple and ginger. (3 servings)

Grasshopper Juicer #1

$^1/_2$-inch wedge green cabbage, cubed or shredded

2 small green apples, seeded

1 bunch parsley or coriander (Chinese parsley), stems removed

$^1/_4$ cup lentil sprouts (optional)

Put cabbage, apples, and parsley through chopper. Dilute to desired consistency. (2 servings)

Grasshopper Juicer #2

Handful spinach

4 or 5 carrots, or 2 carrots and 2 parsnips, cubed, greens removed

1 handful alfalfa sprouts

Green tea, 4 oz. (or healing tea of your choice)

Bunch up spinach and push through chopper with carrots. Dilute with tea. (2 servings)

Juicy Fruit Juicer #3

½ cantaloupe, with rind

5 or 6 strawberries

Push cantaloupe and strawberries through chopper.

Variation: For appetite-stimulating body cleansing, substitute raspberries for strawberries. (2 servings)

Watermelon OJ

4-inch slice watermelon, with white of rind

2 peeled oranges (or tangerines or tangelos)

Kiwi slices

Juice watermelon and oranges or tangerines. Garnish with kiwi.

Variation: Substitute cantaloupe for watermelon, kiwis for citrus, and garnish with lemon slices. (1 serving)

TWO JUICER SHOPPER TIPS

♦ Assess your needs before you buy. Electric juicers operate on different mechanical principles—either centrifugal, centrifugal with pulp ejector, masticating, or masticating with hydraulic press. The five features to look for: volume of juice produced; noise level; vibration level; ease of operation; ease of cleaning.

♦ Plan to do some serious juicing? Look into the Vita-mixer™, which even juices bananas and avocados, incorporates rather than discarding the fiber-rich pulp, and makes frozen yogurt and 60-second smoothies. Call 1-800-848-2649 for information.

♦ Juicing without a juicer on the road or haven't got the juicing wherewithal? Look into the three next-best things: freeze dried, ready to reconstitute vegetable combination powders (carrot, broccoli, etc.) (2 tablespoons in water produces an instant energizer). Or stock up on the European bottled 13-fruit multijuices that are 90% juice, 10% pulp, with no preservatives and enriched with vitamins and antioxidants (sold at health food stores) or see sources; or use a food processor to purée produce, and then process through a fine-mesh strainer.

TO YOUR HEALTH
12 SUPER HEALING JUICE COMBINATIONS

Disorder	Super Healing Juices
Asthma	Celery and papaya juice; celery, endive, and carrot juice
Bladder ailments	Celery and pomegranate juice. (Pomegranate juice is the best for the bladder.) Also good: shavegrass herb tea
High blood pressure	Carrot, parsley, and celery juice; lime juice and whey powder; grape juice and carrot; celery/grapefruit juice
Colds and sinus; sore throat	Celery and grapefruit juice; watercress and apple juice; coconut and carrot juice
Constipation; stomach ulcers	Celery with a little sweet cream; spinach and grapefruit juice
Diarrhea	Carrot and blackberry juice
Indigestion	Coconut milk, fig juice, parsley juice, and carrot juice
Insomnia	Lettuce and celery juice
Kidney (bladder) problems	Black currant juice with juniper berry tea; pomegranate juice and goat whey; celery and pomegranate juice

Disorder	Super Healing Juices
Stress	Celery, carrot, and prune juice; lettuce and tomato juice; radish or prune juice
Reducing	Parsley, grape, and pineapple juice
All-purpose tonic	*Celery, parsley, spinach, and carrot juice*

Benefit healing zones: All

Also see: Water, Basic Dieting Facts and Advice, Antioxidants, Carrots, Citrus Fruits, Parsley, Apples, Celery

The following chart indicates the vitamin C, beta-carotene, and calorie content of some common juices available in supermarkets. As you can see, fresh is best.

Juice	Calories	Beta-carotene (mg)	Vitamin C (mg)
Apple, canned/bottled, fortified	115	0	100
Apricot nectar, canned	140	2.0	1*
Carrot, canned	100	38.0	22
Cranberry cocktail	144	0	90
Grape, canned/bottled	155	0	0.2*
Grapefruit, white, fresh	96	0	94
Pink, fresh	96	0.7	94
White, carton	100	0	70
White, frozen	102	0	83
Orange, fresh	110	0.3	124
Carton	110	0.2	82
Frozen	112	0.2	97
Canned	104	0.3	86
Papaya nectar, canned	140	0.2	8
Pineapple, canned	140	0	27
Prune, canned	180	0	11
Tomato, canned	40	0.8	45
Vegetable juice, canned	47	1.8	36

*Vitamin C may be added. If so, it will say on the label.

(RDAs or suggested amounts for beta-carotene 5-6 mg, for vitamin C 60 mg. per day.)

Benefits healing zones: All

Also See: Water, Herbs, Basic Dieting Facts and Advice, Fatigue, Antioxidants

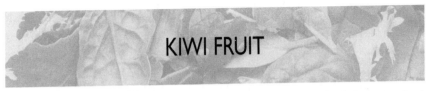

KIWI FRUIT

Over the course of your lifetime, you will spend a total of six years just eating. Why not make all those years of grabbing a bite the best of your life? An occasional kiwi could help.

The kiwi fruit is native to China. According to legend, a New Zealand nun who was a missionary to China is said to have sent seeds back to her convent in New England, and from there cultivation soon spread.

The kiwi sold commercially in the U.S. is *Actinidia chinensis* (*Yantao* in China). Westerners who had discovered it in China called it the Chinese gooseberry, while New Zealanders named it after the kiwi bird. Trained on trellises or arbors like grapes, the fuzzy fruits emerge from white flowers on the female vines. The kiwi's flavor has been described as a cross between a melon, strawberry, and banana.

THE KIWI KEY TO WEIGHT LOSS

One exotic-flavored kiwi has fewer calories than a tangerine, no fat or sodium, and vitamin C—120% of your daily quota. Kiwis also supply four times as much fiber as grapefruit for appetite appeasement and normal bowel functions.

THREE CARDIOVASCULAR FITNESS FACTORS

A kiwi fruit cup for breakfast or dessert provides magnesium, potassium and fiber—three keys to lower cholesterol, normal blood pressure, and stronger arteries. Magnesium, the "forgotten mineral," also helps protect skeletal growth and repair.

KISS A KIWI FOR DENTAL HEALTH

Bleeding gums? Periodontal disease? Loose tooth? Try a little kiwi juice in your morning orange juice and have a kiwi fruit salad instead of cake to boost your protective dose of ascorbic acid. Known as the "hidden toothbrush," vitamin C also helps reduce plaque build-up and keep teeth and gums healthy with less brushing.

Buying, Storing, and Using

Kiwis should be firm and give slightly when pressed. Refrigerated, they keep up to one week.

Enjoy kiwis plain or in fruit salads or juice. Best juice partners: grapes, apples, and oranges.

Kiwi Snow Cone

> *1 cup kiwi juice*
>
> *1 cup orange or white grape juice*
>
> *20 cracked ice cubes (regular or green tea)*

In blender, process half the juice and ice rubes until slushy.

Pour into chilled cups and repeat with remaining mixture. Makes four to five servings.

Variation: Use crushed green tea cubes in place of crushed ice. Or use 1 cup Granny Smith apple juice in place of orange or grape juice.

Benefits healing zones: 2, 3, 5

Also see: Vitamin C, Juices, Basic Dieting Facts and Advice, Coronary Heart Disease

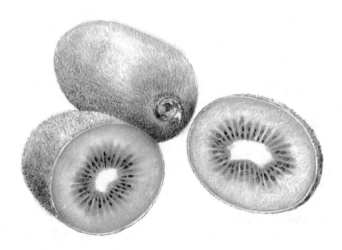

LEAFY GREENS

If you have seen the future, you know it's leafy green.

Lettuce is America's favorite green. It has been cultivated for more than 2,500 years and is one of the earliest known vegetables. Columbus carried lettuce seeds to the Bahamas in 1493. American colonists first received lettuce plantings from Ponce de Leon, and lettuce moved west with the Spanish padres who established missions along the California coast.

Salad days start with iceburg, Boston, and Romaine. But if you're super healing smart, you'll keep going with collard, arugula, amaranth, mesclun (mixed baby lettuce, edible flowers and herbs), and dozens more of the common garden variety greens.

Greens in general are a super healing source of vitamin A-carotene (hidden by the chlorophyll pigment that makes greens green), B-complex vitamins, folate, vitamins A and C, iron, and calcium (ounce for ounce, dandelion greens, collard, and other dark greens have as much or more calcium than cow's milk). On the downside, spinach, sorrel, beet greens and Swiss chard contain oxalates, which interfere with the body's uptake of iron and calcium (to compensate, add a calcium-rich, creamy dressing (see dairy substitutes) and add a vitamin-C-rich fruit or vegetable to enhance iron absorption). (Oxalate-free greens include turnip, kale, and curly endive.)

In general, the darker the leaf, the heftier the vitamin A—up to 50 times more than the more popular pale greens. It's the tip that contains the most A (up to 20 times more) and twice as much iron as the fibrous rib.

But all leafy greens weren't created equal, and a lettuce lover's life isn't complete without including a good cross section of them throughout the nutritional year. Best bets: Romaine for triple the calcium and iron and nine times the vitamin A of iceberg (nutritionally, although iceberg is the only green that can be shredded, sliced, wedged or cored and stuffed whole, or separated into spreadable bread-like slices, it has less A, B, C, E, and essential minerals than any other common lettuce). Mustard, turnip, and collards (cabbage-family greens) are richer in C than citrus, with 500% more calcium than iceberg. Dandelion greens have 40% more vitamin C than tomatoes, six times more iron, and four times the vitamin B_2 of iceberg and 20% more beta-carotene. Amaranth is a good choice, too. Also known as summer spinach or Chinese spinach, amaranth was one of the staple foods of the Aztecs. Cultivated in the Far East and in the tropics, it surpasses broccoli and potatoes in nutritional value, supplies more calcium and vitamin C than spinach, kale, or lettuce, has only 10 calories a bunch; and is richer in protein than other greens. It's a spinach-flavored treat in raw or cooked salads.

Or consider Swiss chard, which looks like spinach but tastes like beet greens and is just the leaf to turn to for hypertension prevention—with almost 500 mg of potassium per ½ cup, plus magnesium and almost as much fiber as dried beans. Or try the spinach-flavored specialty green purslane, a widely grown edible weed that is actually a vitamin supplement in the wild and a potent source of vitamin C, beta-carotene, glucathione (the pesticide-detoxifying antioxidant), vitamin E, and the omega-3 fatty acids (that lower cholesterol).

Nature's other worthiest weeds? Lamb's quarters (usually cooked); groundnut; kudzu; evening primrose; burdock; pigweed; watercress.

PROTECT YOUR INTESTINAL AND REPRODUCTIVE POTENTIAL

Greens are a Grade-A source of the insoluble fibers cellulose and lignin, which increase stool bulk and help relieve constipation and diverticulosis while reducing colon cancer risk by speeding up elimination. Greens also help prevent fatigue and anemia thanks to their folate, which builds red blood cells and contributes to gene building. They also help prevent loblastic anemia, a side-effect of contraceptive use.

MORE LEAFY GREEN CURES

Leafy greens are often the answer to insomnia, which, says the University of Texas Medical Center, can be caused by deficiencies of iron and copper, two top salad-bowl trace minerals. Field greens such as dandelion—which are high in potassium, calcium, iron, vitamin A, B-complex vitamins, vitamins C and E, glycosides, and inulin—stimulate all the glands in the body. Dandelion is useful in treating asthma, diabetes, hypoglycemia, skin diseases, arthritis, and more. Its most time-honored use has been for liver disorders (hepatitis, swelling of the liver, and jaundice) and, because of its diuretic effect, was once called "piss-a-bed." In

Oriental medicine, dandelion is used to treat infections, pneumonia, liver disease, and breast cancer.

Total Tonic

Looking for a tonic leaf to green you clean? Turn to watercress, which the poet William Cowpers called a cheap but wholesome salad from a brook and which Greeks commended as a brain food. With more minerals and vitamins than high-scorer spinach, watercress supplies beta-carotene, vitamins B, C, and E and, so goes the story, was brought to North America because of its vitamin C value for sailors and settlers. Watercress soup was used by the Chinese to treat canker sores, blisters in the mouth, swollen gums, bad teeth, and foul breath. Eaten cold, watercress is thought to relieve hot flashes. Watercress boiled with apple cider vinegar is recommended as a moist dressing for headaches; a watercress infusion is said to soothe eczema and dermatitis; and watercress tea is a time-honored diuretic and expectorant. High in sulphur (the substance that contributes the plant's bite), which cleans the bloodstream and maintains pancreatic health, watercress also provides manganese (which nourishes the pituitary glands), copper, magnesium, sodium, potassium, plenty of bone- and teeth-forming calcium, and iron.

Leaves of Longevity

Salad greens are also antiaging eats. In Shakespeare's time, salads were known as fountains of youth and eaten as spring tonics. The French gastronome Brillat-Savarin, called salad that food that "freshens without enfeebling and fortifies without irritating...and makes us younger" (while novelist Alexander Dumas favored Romaine above all other lettuce).

One reason for the beneficial effects of greens is the B-complex vitamins, which contribute to the health and growth of hair, nails, and skin. A second reason is the combination of beta-carotene and vitamin C, which protect the body's immune system from the viruses and diseases of aging.

Because of its vitamin K and beta-carotene, a lettuce juice cocktail is a good tone-up for the digestive system. And thanks to the calming compound lactucarium it's an aid to sleep.

Crohn's disease? Kidney stones? Ulcers? Lettuce is good therapy since it provides three nutrients for intestinal fortitude and uric acid reduction: vitamin K (70% of the RDA), beta-carotene, and folate.

Buying, Storing, and Using

Iceberg is the best keeper (four to seven days), and spinach is the worst (one to two days). Wrap all fresh greens loosely and store in a vegetable crisper. To prevent spoilage, store greens between 32 and 42 degrees Fahrenheit, and store away from ethylene-producing fruits such as apples, which cause leaf browning.

Calorie cutting? Use leaves (spinach, Romaine) instead of chips for dips and as sliced bread substitutes.

Greens are best served immediately after tossing, at near room temperature, on chilled plates.

The younger the green, the tastier it is. Maturity turns most greens bitter and tough.

The five better-cooked-than-raw leafy greens: dandelion, chickory, burdock, lambs quarters, chard. There are three ways to cook them: (1)steam, drain, and toss in hot oil with herbs and lemon juice; (2) steam and toss to flavor rice and other whole grains; or (3) blanch outer leaves and use in place of cabbage to wrap vegetable, grain, and bean fillings.

One average head of lettuce (about 1¼ pounds) will provide the following quantities:

Shredded	2½ quarts
Rafts*	3 to 4 rafts
Chunks*	21/2 to 3 quarts
Wedges	4 to 6 wedges
Torn pieces	2½ quarts
Cups	5 to 6 cups

Try making Lettuce Cups: Place a head of iceberg lettuce on a work surface. Gently separate leaves and lift from head. Fill with any main-dish salad mixtures, sandwich fillings, or fruit or vegetable combinations.

Six Quick-Fix Salt-Free Dressings

- ♦ Rice vinegar with crushed coriander seed and freshly ground pepper

---

* Cabbage-type lettuce.

◆ Apple cider vinegar with freshly grated nutmeg or cinnamon

◆ Flavored vinegars (such as tarragon, basil, garlic, raspberry, or blueberry) with freshly grated citrus peel

◆ Low-fat yogurt with crushed mustard seed and minced fresh herbs

◆ Buttermilk, Dijon mustard, and toasted poppy seeds

◆ Red wine vinegar with garlic, purée of roasted sweet red pepper, and a pinch of dry mustard

TIPS FOR SALAD LOVERS

TIPS FOR TOSSERS: Edible flowers are best in Bibb or Boston lettuce and dressed with fruity vinaigrette. Endive and arugula are tasty with robust vinaigrette, while anything goes with looseleaf or crisp-headed varieties.

Treat yourself to twice-as-nutritious mesclun (derived from the Latin *miscellarum*) salad once in a while (also known as European or Continental salad): Toss a blend of 8 to 12 baby lettuces, herbs, and edible flowers.

TIP FOR SALAD GARDENERS: Sow tiny pinches of seeds of mixed greens in cell packs of potting soil, and when they come up, plug them directly into the garden on 8- or 10-inch centers. Each clump will quickly become a little salad ready to be cut and served.

Try these salad recipes:

Super Healing Bittersweet Salad

1 bunch dandelion leaves, baby mustard greens, arugula, or watercress

1 head radicchio

2 Belgian endives

2 tablespoons fresh mint leaves

3 tablespoons extra-virgin olive oil

7 tablespoons balsamic vinegar

4 tablespoons shavings of Parmesan cheese

Freshly ground black pepper

Rinse and dry the dandelion, mustard greens, arugula, or watercress. Remove and discard all heavy stems. Pull apart the leaves from the head of radicchio and tear them into bite-size pieces. Add to the salad bowl. Slice the endive horizontally about ½-inch thick and add the slices to the bowl, breaking them up. Add the mint leaves.

Beat oil and vinegar together, pour over salad ingredients, and toss.

Divide salad among four plates. Add cheese. Season with pepper.

Makes four servings.

Variation: Substitute ½ cup amaranth for radicchio.

Super Healing Salad Bars

> *1 batch homemade whole grain biscuit dough*
>
> *or*
>
> *1 batch whole grain biscuit mix, prepared according to package directions*
>
> *2 tablespoons minced fresh herbs (dill, chives, tarragon, parsley, fresh coriander—Chinese parsley), or 2 teaspoons dried*
>
> *1 egg white, beaten*
>
> *3 tablespoons sesame seeds, chia, or flaxseeds*
>
> *½ cup fresh carrot or tomato juice or vegetale juice*

Preheat oven to 350 degrees. On a lightly floured surface, briefly knead minced herbs into biscuit dough. Roll out dough to ¼-inch thickness. With a knife, cut out bars of dough about 5 inches long and 2 inches wide.

Twist each strip loosely to form a twisted bar and place on a lightly greased cookie sheet. Brush each twist with beaten egg white and sprinkle with seeds. Bake 12 to 15 minutes until golden and crisp.

Makes 12 bars.

Serve with any super healing salad.

More Greens Than Grains Tabbouli

Combine cooled, cooked bulgur with finely chopped tomatoes, cucumbers, scallions, fresh parsley, mint, and/or cilantro (the salad should be more greens than grain, but vary proportions to taste); add a generous amount of lemon juice and a little (or no) olive oil, and chill. To serve, scoop salad into lettuce leaves.

Variation: Use kasha or barley instead of bulgur.

Benefits healing zones: All

Also see: Cruciferous Vegetables, Vegetarian, Herbs, Basic Dieting Facts and Advice

LEMONS/LIMES

Lemons are number 7 on America's List of Best Loved Fruits (ahead of peaches and strawberries and just behind melons and grapes). We put the squeeze on one million metric tons of *citrus limonia* a year (just behind Turkey, the world's leading* lemon grower).

Lemons date back to ancient Asia (3,000 years ago). Botanically, the term *citrus* applies to a group of evergreen trees and shrubs belonging to the rue family, distinguished by their glossy leaves and white or pink flowers. The *citrus limonia* is native to Southeast Asia.

THE LEMON
Symbol of Love, Juicy Fruit, Scurvy Cure

Nature's miracle fruit has been treasured throughout history for its unique aroma, color, flavor, and chemical properties, and for good reasons. Lemons, which came to America with Christopher Columbus on his second voyage to the New World, predate roses as symbols of love and fidelity. A chronicler for the English East India Company recorded that "oranges and lemons of which we made good store of water [juice], which is the best remedy against scurvy." (Scurvy, a common sailor's disease in the days of Vasco da Gama, is a severely debilitating and demoralizing vitamin C deficiency disease characterized by swelling of the gums, slow healing, and extreme lethargy.)

When French cooking came of age, so did the cuisine of the lemon. The world-famous chef, Pierre François de la Varennes, author of *Patissier François* and the founding father of Franco-Italian cuisine, pioneered the preparation of sauces made exclusively of vinegar, meat drippings, and lemons, which were an expensive luxury in mid-seventeenth-century France. But America takes the cake for the first lemon desserts. The recipe for the first lemon cheesecake appeared in 1728 in colonial homemaker E. Smith's *Compleat Housewife,* and lemon meringue pie was introduced soon thereafter.

---

* Followed by Italy, Greece and Spain.

MIRACLE BODY CLEANSER AND NORMALIZER

Nutritionally, the lemon constitutes one of nature's seven top sources of potassium (the other six are watercress, mint leaves, sunflower seeds, bananas, oranges, and potatoes), a mineral that promotes clear thinking, aids in normalizing blood pressure, and works with sodium to regulate the body's water balance. Lemons are also nature's top sources of citric acid, a life essential found in the cells of all living creatures. Because both lemons and limes contain 5 to 6% citric acid compared with oranges (1.5%) and grapefruit (1 to 2%) and both are acid fruits (along with cranberries, loganberries, pineapples, and strawberries), they are a top-rated germicide.

Lemons are especially tonic and act as cleansers when toxicity exists in the liver, kidneys, bowels, lungs, or skin.

TREATING FOUR COMMON COMPLAINTS FROM A TEACUP

A lemon tea will help loosen catarrh and ease digestion, and a lemon drink taken with the yolk of a raw egg is an excellent natural laxative. Lemons, like all citric foods, are a natural therapy for treating fever, says the Nutrition and Dietary Consultants Association.

NUTRITIONAL BENEFITS

Lemons also provide modest amounts of nondairy calcium for healthy bones and teeth; magnesium, an aid in forming albumen in the blood; plus enzymes, iron, phosphorus, and copper. Fresh lemon juice has only 4 calories a tablespoon and just a trace of sodium. More importantly, just a single tablespoon of lemon juice one tenth of your daily requirement for vitamin C, according to the National Center for Nutrition and Dietetics. Indeed, the lemon is one of nature's five best sources of ascorbic acid (also found in gooseberries, raspberries, kiwis, strawberries, and other citrus fruits), a nutrient that the Linus Pauling Institute calls "the miracle metabolite" (this accounts for its unique ability to "spoilproof" vegetables and fruits, especially apples, avocados, and bananas, and protect the natural colors of fruits and vegetables from the effects of oxidation). Lemon juice also prevents berries from graying in the jam-making process.

HEALING EFFECTS OF LEMONS

The other ascorbic-acid-bearing portions of the lemon, in addition to the juice, include the albedo—the white, slightly bitter-tasting inner portion of the outer peel—and the flavedo, the exterior peel, which contains the flavor-rich sacs whose riches are released by shredding, slicing, and grating. Both the albedo and the flavedo also supply pectin—the ingredient that makes jelly gel—and bioflavonoids. Lemons are the world's richest source of this antioxidant, which helps regulate body temperature, making the lemon a first-rate thirst quencher. (Even better, try a half-and-half combination of rosemary tea and chilled lemonade on hot, humid days.)

Bioflavonoids, either alone or in conjunction with vitamin C and other nutrients, contribute to the cellular integrity of the capillary and vascular systems. In addition, they appear to have an antiviral and anti-inflammatory action, which makes them a valuable nutritional defense against colds and flu, threats to the immune system, and inflammatory disorders such as arthritis and rheumatic fever. They also speed wound healing.

Mellow Yellow Medicine

The lemon is also a first-rate insect-bite repellent, not just because of its citric and ascorbic acid content but because of the organic citrus compound azadirachtin, a potent natural insect repellent which is secreted by the skin of the lemon. Azadirachtin belongs to a family of "limonoids," which give some citrus fruits their bitter taste.

Beauty Benefits

Cosmetically, the lemon has been valued since biblical times as a bleach and an internal and external astringent. Empresses in the Chinese court and Queen Elizabeth I of England used elixirs of honey, water, and lemon as a daily beauty drink.

LIMES' GIFT OF COOLING

Like the lemon, limes are a native of southeastern Asia and were probably first used by Indians and Arabs during the period of Mohammedan expansion in A.D. 570–900. Limes were part of the island cuisine of Haiti in the 1500s and spread from the West Indies to Florida.

Limes have been grown in California and Florida since the early days of the citrus industry. After the great freeze in Florida of 1894–1895, when the lemon industry was almost totally destroyed, California began growing virtually all the lemons in the United States. Florida's lime industry has since expanded, and now Florida grows most of the limes used in this country. California is second in production, and Mexico is a close third. Florida, California, and Mexico produce the lion's share of limes used globally.

With a Twist of Lime

Limes help relieve arthritic pain, and a drink of lime juice is said to cool the brain and nervous system (limes were traditionally used to treat brain fever). Limes are a therapeutic intervention for hot tempers and negative emotions.

Buying, Storing, and Using Limes

The principal variety of lime grown in the United States is the seedless, large-fruited acid lime called the Florida Persian, which is very acid but full flavored. The Mexican lime has a strong-flavored, very acid juice but is not grown in this country. The single sweet lime is not imported into the United States.

Look for limes that are a bright green and heavy for their size. Fully ripe, yellow limes lack a high acid content. Limes can be used as a lemon substitute. Like lemons, limes are high in vitamin C, a good source of vitamin B, and rich in potassium. Store limes in a cool, dry place.

Limes' natural flavor is enhanced when combined with other juices. Add to melons to bring out their natural flavor. A few drops of fresh lime juice improves the flavor of consommé and jellied soups and subacid fruits like peaches, apples, pears, and plums.

TIP: Both lemons and limes may cause intestinal gas, especially if drunk or chewed in excessively large amounts, and their acid can erode tooth enamel. Both can produce contact dermatitis (the oil in the peel is the culprit) and allergic headaches in sensitized individuals.

Buying, Storing, and Using Lemons

1. Know what you'll get from what you've got: 6 medium lemons = 1 cup juice; 1 medium lemon = 3 tablespoons juice; 1 medium lemon = 3 teaspoons grated peel and ¼ cup pulp. The average lemon or lime yields about 2½ tablespoons of juice (trained) 1 tablespoon of grated peel, and ¼ cup of pulp.

2. Buy lemons ready to use or home-cure your own. Like oranges and grapefruit, lemons are one of the 12 fruits that don't ripen after picking. According to Sunkist Growers of Van Nuys, California, lemons are usually cured a few days by pickers, a waiting period that "tenderizes" them. To home-cure your own store-bought or home-grown "greenies" and double the juice yield, give them a five-day rest in a warm kitchen, plunge into warm water, dry, and give them a gentle massage on the kitchen counter before slicing or juicing.

3. Don't accept second best. A good lemon is firm and heavy for its size. Lemons that are pale or green were picked too soon. Coarse or rough skins indicate a high-on-pulp low-on-juice fruit. Also pass up fruit with punctured or shriveled skin, soft spots, and hardened rinds. And think thin. A thick peel is a tipoff that your lemon was picked past its prime.

4. What you see and what you get: Lemons that look "too good to be true" usually have been waxed and given a chemical dip to lengthen their shelf life. Unless your lemon wears a certified organic sticker, be sure to wash well with soapy warm water before using the peel.

5. Plan ahead. Lemons and limes stay fresh for 7 to 10 days. Chilled uncovered, shelf life is 10 days to two weeks. And don't give every bad lemon the raspberry. A worse-for-wear lemon can be rejuvenated by soaking in water for 10 minutes before juicing.

6. Coddle your citrus. A relaxed-to-the-max lemon or lime yields the most juice. So does a warm one. The best live-longer temperature

for a lemon is 55 to 58 degrees Fahrenheit—10 degrees warmer than the ideal keeping temperature for an orange. Before juicing, gently press and roll the fruit and cut in half, and prick the insides, twisting with the tines of a fork first. Or bake a batch in a low to moderate oven just long enough to heat through. Then roll, press, and juice.

7. Grate before squeezing. A lemon or lime is easiest to grate when it's firm and whole. Grated peel can be stored in a plastic bag for future use, or dry thoroughly and bottle in spice jars. Use the stem end of a lemon when a recipe calls for half; you'll get better juice mileage.

8. Maximize juice yield with your microwave. Prick a lemon (or lime) and microwave on high for 15 seconds. Cool for one to two minutes, roll, and juice. For fast-track drying, grate the peel, place in a glass bowl, microwave on high for 30 to 50 seconds (stirring once), and freeze.

9. Freeze your bounty. Surplus freshly squeezed juice can be frozen in a container or ice cube trays and then stored in plastic bags and used for lemonade or recipes calling for 1 to 6 tablespoons of juice. Extra citrus can also be frozen whole and then thawed in the microwave and juiced as needed (CAUTION: This is an emergency measure only; freezing dries out the inner pulp). Frozen juice keeps for four months.

10. Best way to enjoy lemons in your salad-a-day diet: Peel and then blenderize a whole lemon, seeds and all. Add a spoonful to homemade salad dressings (where appropriate). *Variation:* Substitute a lime or grapefruit for lemon.

11. Best ways to enjoy lemons wherever you go? Keep bowls of fresh lemons (or limes) throughout the house for fragrance and eye appeal.

MORE HINTS AND TIPS

♦ *To reduce a fever.* Lemon and lime juice promotes perspiration and helps block pain. When lemon juice is heated, salicylic acid (a painkiller)—the chemical precursor of aspirin's active ingredient—is produced. A folk remedy for influenza prescribes baking a lemon for 20 minutes. Then slice, squeeze, add a glass of tepid tea (preferably boneset, a source of calcium which enhances acid take-up), and drink every half hour.

♦ *For flu.* The juice of half a lemon in warm water morning, noon, and night helps eliminate toxins and ease aches.

♦ *To prevent or relieve colds/coughs.* Drink lemon juice straight or mixed with honey or fruit juice. Take the equivalent of 2,000 mg daily to nip a cold in the bud.

♦ *Lemon and lime wash and dry.* In hazy, hot, and humid weather, a cut lemon or lime rubbed over face and hands is a clean-up pick-me-up.

♦ *Alligator skin.* Bend an elbow and set it down in a squeezed lemon or lime half twice a day.

♦ *Body toddy.* To use lemon juice as an astringent body pack, mix juice with oatmeal or prepare this decoction: Slice two lemons and two oranges or four lemons, and simmer these in 2 quarts water for 30 minutes. Cool, sieve, and sponge mixture slowly and gently all over your body. To make a body toddy mud, add moistened oatmeal and mix to pasty consistency.

♦ *Nicotine nails.* Rub half a lemon or lime over stained nails, remove lemon pulp, and with remaining rind rub one nail at a time until they come clean.

♦ *Citrus set 'n' go.* Use fresh lemon juice to set your hair. The drying period lasts longer, but so does your set. When you run out of lemons, use bottled lemon juice.

♦ *Lemon hair rinse.* Squeeze juice out of two big lemons, strain, and dilute with 1 cup of warm water. Comb juice through hair. (Avoid getting any on your skin; it can promote burning and mottled skin.) After 15 minutes, rinse hair thoroughly with warm water or chamomile tea.

♦ *The eye-drop alternative.* Use one drop of fresh lemon or lime juice diluted in 1 ounce warm water. Use as an eyewash.

◆ *To reduce corns.* Apply lemon or lime juice directly.

◆ *For smoker's cough.* Pour 1 quart boiling water over 4 tablespoons of whole flaxseed and steep for three hours. Strain, add the juice of two lemons, and sweeten to taste (crystals of rock candy are used in the original remedy). Use a tablespoonful as needed. (Adapted from the *Universal Cookery Book,* published in 1988.)

◆ *To cure hiccups.* Dip a lemon wedge in salt and suck on it, says Dr. Varro E. Taylor, former dean of pharmacological sciences at Purdue University and author of *Hoosier Home Remedies* (Purdue University Press). Or try a long suck on a "citrus Lifesaver®" (a cube of sugar saturated in lemon or lime juice).

◆ *For energy.* Three tablespoons of fresh lemon or lime juice in a half glass of warm water before breakfast daily for one week is a better-than-coffee energizer; it also stimulates and cleanses the gallbladder.

◆ *To relieve a sunburn.* Out of aloe? A slice of lemon or lime on a fresh sunburn will prevent blistering.

◆ *Scratch-and-sniff bug repellent.* Rub undiluted lemon juice on skin to help prevent mosquito and other insect bites and to reduce swelling and itching if bitten.

◆ *Lemon lickety split elixir.* To get rid of a charley horse, apply the following: Chunk two peeled lemons, a lime, two oranges, and one small grapefruit and purée with 1 teaspoon cream of tartar. Refrigerate in a covered jar. Take 2 tablespoons with 2 tablespoons water two times daily, morning and night.

◆ *Nontoxic way to freshen laundry.* Presoak in lemon-juice-scented water (¼ cup to each gallon).

Try these lemon and lime recipes:

Super Healing Citrus Scrub

> *1 cup orange and lemon peel (air dried in an uncovered basket until brittle)*
>
> *1 cup uncooked oatmeal*

1 cup blanched almonds

Blend ingredients to a coarse powder in a blender or food processor. To use, shake a bit of the scrub into your palm and mix the grains to a paste with a few drops of warm water.

Pat on face with circular upward motion. Rinse off, pat dry.

Variation: Substitute lime or tangerine peel for orange or lemon. Use 1 cup cashews in place of almonds. Substitute wheat or rice flakes for oats.

Clear Conscience Cheesecake (crustless)

32-ounce carton sugar-free vanilla-flavored, low-fat yogurt

1 tablespoon lemon juice

2 tablespoons sugar or honey (or to taste)

1 tablespoon cornstarch

1 teaspoon vanilla or lemon extract (for extra-lemony flavor)

2 eggs, lightly beaten

Preheat oven to 325 degrees. Lightly grease an 8-inch pie pan or 7-inch spring-form pan.

Place yogurt in a medium-size bowl. Add sweetener, cornstarch, lemon juice, and vanilla. Stir in the eggs. mixing gently with a fork or wire whisk until well blended.

Pour into prepared pan, and smooth top with a spatula. Bake until center is set (20 to 25 minutes for a pie pan or 45 to 55 minutes for a springform).

Cool on a wire rack and chill.

Makes eight servings, about 99 calories each.

Citrus Sprinkles (for acid indigestion)

Take the peel from a large organic or well-scrubbed* grapefruit, leaving pith behind (the citrus oils and bioflavonoids it contains are stomach soothers). Place on wax paper and dry in a low oven overnight. Grind in a seed mill or

---

* See Mail Order Sources for organic suppliers and toxin removal products.

blender until gritty. Sprinkle ½ teaspoon on tongue. Suck on sprinkles, then chew slowly. Repeat as needed.

Variation: Substitute orange, tangerine, or tangelo peel.

Alka-Settler

Combine ¼ cup lemon juice, to 4 cups sparkling mineral water, and ½ to 1 teaspoon bicarbonate of soda. (Baking soda is an effective and nonallergenic systemic neutralizer—basically an antacid without aspirin, caffeine, or assorted additives.) Sip as needed while fizzy.

Variation: For a high-C version, add one crushed vitamin C tablet or ½ teaspoon vitamin C powder.

You can see from the following chart how nutritious lemons and limes are.

LEMON/LIME NUTRITION IN A NUTSHELL

	1 Lemon (2½ " Diameter)	1 Tablespoon Fresh Lemon/Lime Juice
Calories	22.0 calories	4.0 calories
Protein	1.3 grams	0.1 grams
Fat	trace	0.0 grams
Carbohydrates	11.6 grams	1.3 grams
Calcium	66.0 mg	1.0 mg
Phosphorus	16.0 mg	1.0 mg
Iron	0.8 mg	0.0 mg
Sodium	3.0 mg	0.0 mg
Potassium	157.0 mg	19.0 mg
Vitamin A	32.0 IU	3.0 IU
Thiamin	0.1 mg	trace
Riboflavin	trace	trace
Niacin	0.2 mg	trace
Ascorbic acid	83.2 mg	4.0–7.0 mg

Source: Agriculture Handbook No. 8-9, *Composition of Foods,* United States Department of Agriculture, Human Nutrition Information Service.

Benefits healing zones: 1, 3, 4, 7

Also see: Vitamin C, Antioxidants, Juices, Common Cold, Grapefruit

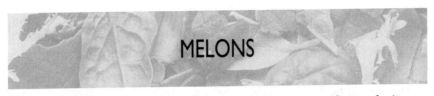

MELONS

High-speed healing may be only a melonade or cantaloupe fruit cup away. Melons—in all their variety, from the everyday cantaloupe to the late summer crenshaw and casaba and Persia- and Africa-indigenous watermelon (members of the gourd family, which also includes squash and cucumber)—are all nutritional ammunition in the fight against a wide variety of health disorders.

According to the Center for Science in the Public Interest, it's not bananas that rate as our top-banana fruits, and little wonder. Half a cantaloupe has twice the antioxidant vitamin C content of cabbage (and more than orange juice; next best vitamin C choice—crenshaw, honeydew) plus folicin, B vitamins, and fiber.

The cantaloupe is named after the castle of Cantalupo in Italy, where this Armenian musk melon was first cultivated for a sixteenth-century pope. Next in line nutritionally are the honeydew (with half a day's RDA of vitamin C) and watermelon* (with goodly amounts of fiber, vitamin C, and beta-carotene and the fewest calories of all).

YOUR MORNING MELON
For Cardiovascular and Anticancer Protection

Research by South American and German medical teams suggests that the substance called odenosene (also found in onions and garlic) in cantaloupe has anticoagulant properties (that is, the ability to inhibit blood platelet clotting and thus reduce risk of stroke and cardiovascular diseases). With zero grams of fat and sodium, melons rank as A-1 diet and heart-protective foods.

Melons are also rich in carotenoids, one of the important food-derived anticancer nutrients. Diets rich in melons (and other orange fruits and vegetables) provide seven times more protection from often fatal cancer than low-carotene diets, according to population studies. One cup of cantaloupe has 3 mg of carotene which is converted by the body to 5,160 IU of vitamin A (more than the RDA).

---

* "When one has tasted watermelon, he knows what angels eat," observed Mark Twain.

To double your nutritional benefits, drizzle your morning melon with honey. According to researchers at the American Health Foundation, the caffeic acids in natural honey have cancer-deterring capabilities.

SUPER HEALING 60-CALORIE FRUIT CUP

Dieting? Don't stop dishing up dessert; just make it melon. High in water (70 to 90%), low calorie (average of 60 per 1 cup, diced), and high in fiber, melon can be puréed into guilt-free smoothies, puddings, and ices. To make Melon Pepsickles, for example, combine 2 cups diced and seeded watermelon, 1 cup fresh or canned papaya, and 1 cup fresh cantaloupe and purée in a blender. Transfer to paper cups. Freeze until slushy. Insert popsickle sticks or tongue depressors. Peel off cups and eat.

MELON MAGIC
Eight Folk Remedies

◆ For heat rash, rub skin with watermelon rind.

◆ To prevent or reduce the discomfort of measles, drink a vitamin A-rich carrot/cantaloupe juice.

◆ To lower blood pressure, have watermelon seed tea a half hour before meals, three times daily.

◆ Melon has been used to treat hepatitis (China), irregular menstrual cycles (Philippines), edema (India), and reproductive disorders (Africa) and to improve kidney function (international).

Buying, Storing, and Using

With the exception of honeydews, melons don't ripen after picking but benefit from two days' holding before refrigeration, so look for vine-ripened fruits. Aroma is a guide to a good melon—except for casabas, which are odorless—this means a fuller, sweeter flavor. Melons should be of uniform shape, and undamaged. A ripe melon should yield to the touch at the stem end and rattle when shaken or sound slightly hollow when thumped. Try these melon uses:

◆ Cube or ball melon and toss with fruit and/or grain salads.

◆ Purée for low-calorie smoothies and cold summer soups.

◆ Use melon "milk" as a nondairy cereal topping.

Best juice partners: grapes, celery, berries, tropical fruits, and ginger.

Watermelon Lemonade

> *2 cups watermelon chunks, seeds removed*
>
> *3 cups pineapple juice*
>
> *Juice of one lemon*

Put everything in a blender and process. Pour over ice. Makes four small servings.

Honeydew Ice

> *8 cups peeled, seeded, and cubed honeydew melon*
>
> *4 tablespoons fresh lime juice*
>
> *2 teaspoon grated lime zest*

Combine ingredients in a blender and purée until smooth. Freeze in an ice cream maker according to manufacturer's instructions. Let "ripen" in the freezer an hour before serving.

Only 60 calories a cup. 10 servings.

Variation: Substitute cantaloupe or Persian for honeydew and use lemon or kiwi juice in place of lime.

Melon and More Fruit Salad

> *1 small cantaloupe*
>
> *1 cup watermelon, diced*
>
> *1 cup blueberries and ¹/₂ cup red raspberries*
>
> *1 cup strawberries, sliced*
>
> *1 cup nonfat plain yogurt*
>
> *¹/₄ cup orange juice*
>
> *2 tablespoons lime juice*
>
> *1 tablespoon honey (optional)*
>
> *Pinch of ground cloves (optional)*
>
> *1 head Bibb lettuce, washed*
>
> *¹/₂ cup nasturtium, pansy, or marigold petals*

Slice melon in half, remove seeds, and scoop out flesh with a melon ball scoop. Combine cantaloupe, watermelon, blueberries, raspberries, and strawberries.

Dressing: Blend yogurt, orange and lime juice, honey, and cloves.

Divide lettuce between four plates. Spoon some of fruit mixture onto each plate and top with dressing. Garnish with fresh flower petals or herb sprigs.

Makes four servings.

Benefits healing zones: 2, 6, 7

Also see: Basic Dieting Facts and Advice, Beta-carotene, Vitamin C

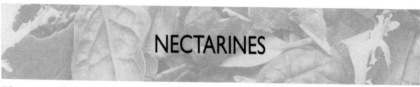

NECTARINES

There are 8 bones in each wrist and if you're like most of us, you keep them busy reaching for off-limits snacks. Reaching for a 67-calorie nectarine makes better nutritional sense.

The nectarine dates back to the beginning of the Christian era. In the sixteenth and seventeenth centuries, the nectarine was called "nucipersica" because of its resemblance to a walnut (the word *nectarine* is derived from the Greek *nekter,* the drink of the gods in Greek and Roman mythology).

The nectarine is actually a smooth-skinned peach, and nectarines can be grown from peach stones, and vice versa. Peach and nectarine trees can produce half peach/half nectarine hybrids. The trees, leaves, and seeds of peaches and nectarines are indistinguishable, but the nectarine is fuzz-free, smaller, firmer, and has a finer aroma and richer flavor. Like peaches, nectarines are available as clingstone or free, and flesh may be red, yellow, or white.

Nectarines may be used in any of the ways peaches are used—fresh as a table fruit, stewed, baked, or made into preserves, jams, and ice cream. They can be canned and dried.

In the eastern United States, nectarines are not grown as successfully as peaches. For this reason, virtually the entire commercial nectarine crop is grown in California. Nectarines are on the market June through September from domestic sources and January through March from abroad.

PROTECTIVE BENEFITS OF THE "PRETENDER PEACH"

Do you suffer from subpar digestion, poor vision, lowered immunity, or kidney stones? Do you need pollution protection? With their generous levels of beta-carotene, vitamin A, potassium, magnesium, and 12% of your RDA for ascorbic acid, nectarines are nutritionally a good bet. Their beta-carotene improves your body's uptake and synthesis of protein, while magnesium aids in energy production.

Dieter's Fruit

Two nectarines or 8 ounces of pure nectarine juice provide fewer than 100 calories for a pure-energy lift.

Buying, Storing, and Using

Look for the three top varieties: Quetta, a large, deep-colored clingstone; John Rivers, a medium-sized, highly crimson freestone; and Gower, a medium-sized, highly colored freestone fruit, which is the earliest on market shelves.

To speed-peel, dip nectarines in warm water for one minute. The peel will slip off easily.

Nectarines are a well-digested and -assimilated subacid fruit and can be used like peaches—dried, stewed, baked, canned, puréed into preserves, or grilled as fruit kebobs or added as nutrient boosters to muffin batters. Best juice partners: lemons, limes, and green grapes.

Try these recipes:

Nectarine Skin Tightener Mask

> *1 fresh ripe nectarine*
>
> *1 egg white*

Whip together in a blender until smooth. Smooth mixture all over the face. Leave for 30 minutes, then rinse off with cool water.

The beta-carotene fruit acids in nectarines help skin maintain elasticity and prevent dry skin.

Ketchup

> *1 tablespoon vegetable oil*
>
> *1 large onion, thinly sliced*

4 ripe nectarines

¹/₄ cup brown sugar, packed

3 tablespoons molasses

2 tablespoons white sugar

¹/₂ teaspoon freshly ground black pepper

¹/₄ teaspoon allspice

¹/₂ cup white vinegar

2 tablespoons fresh lemon juice

In a large pot, heat the oil over medium heat until hot but not smoking. Add onion and sauté for five minutes. Add the nectarines and cook an additional four minutes, stirring. Add remaining ingredients except the lemon juice, and simmer over low heat for one hour, stirring. (If necessary, add a small amount of water to prevent the mixture from burning.)

Remove from heat, add lemon juice, and purée. Ketchup will keep, covered and refrigerated, for several weeks.

Yield: 24 servings, about 35 calories a tablespoon.

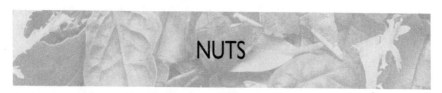

NUTS

A nut is one natural food that's all it's cracked up to be—and then some.

There are 300 nuts grown globally. Most are top sources of thiamine and folate for the health of the nervous system; iron, magnesium, and zinc to fight fatigue and stress and build endocrinal health; antiaging E, the polyunsaturated fat that helps lower cholesterol; calcium and potassium, which normalize blood pressure; lecithin, which feeds the nerves and glands and maintains reproductive zone health; and, above all, protein (eating nuts with such foods as milk, grains, or rice makes nuts a complete protein, containing all essential amino acids).

How does the protein content of nuts stack up? One pound of peanuts has as much protein as 7.4 pints of milk. And 5.8 pints of milk would be needed to match the protein content of 1 pound of black walnuts. Peanuts, with 26.2% protein, have more protein than cheddar cheese, which has 25% protein. Butternuts have 27.9%; almonds, beechnuts, pistachios, and walnuts all have around 20% protein. By comparison, a boiled egg has 11.4% and raisins 2.6% protein.

Nuts are also high in EFAs (essential fatty acids), which the body uses for energy, ocular and dermal health, and heart muscle (up to 60% of the heart's muscle nourishment comes from EFAs). Best sources: pecans, with 70.7% EFAs, and Brazil nuts, butternuts, almonds, and pistachios, with more than 59% EFAs.

ANTICANCER AND OTHER BENEFITS IN A NUTSHELL

Nuts are a top source of the antioxidants called protease inhibitors (eight have been isolated thus far; potatoes are another source), substances which block or slow the growth of cancer by interfering with cancer-causing proteases (protein-splitting enzymes). Inhibitors, say researchers at Louisiana State University Medical Center, help control blood clotting and prevent many types of viruses from being activated— without the side-effects of antiviral drugs.

Nuts are also rich in the anticancer antioxidants selenium and the polyphenols. Take nuts to heart for a headache, too. According to researcher Dr. Ivan Danhof, professor of physiology at the University of Texas Medical School at Dallas, chewing 10 to 12 almonds may put enough painkilling salicylate into your bloodstream to provide relief without the stomach-lining distress of aspirin. (Other salicylate-rich foods are potatoes and apricots.) Nuts also give you something OTC painkillers don't—protein, potassium, and moderate amounts of the unsaturated fats that feed your skin and remedy weak fingernails.

Nuts even provide hangover prevention. West African healers prescribe peanut butter before partying, while a snack of six raw almonds is one American Indian nostrum for the morning after.

WHAT'S GOOD FOR WHAT
A Few Nutritional Facts About Nuts

The world's biggest seed food, the coconut palm, *Kalpa Vriksha* (which in Sanskrit means "tree which gives all that is necessary for living"), is classified biologically as a drupe (single-seeded, fleshy fruit). The coconut palm is a good whole-body cleanser. Solid, preservative-free coconut oil makes a replenishing skin cream and is a vegetarian substitute for lard, used in moderation.

Pistachio nuts, related to mangos and poison ivy, are 20% richer in protein than most nuts and are a good source of calcium, iron, and thiamine. They are used in China to treat diarrhea. In Pakistan, pistachio oil is used for asthma and reproductive disorders. (Pistachios can be used to replace almonds in recipes.)

Almonds are 19% protein, contain nutrients from every basic food group, and provide more calcium than any other common nut (1 ounce = ¼ cup milk). Almonds eaten in 1-ounce doses two to three times daily are reputed to have anticancer properties. (If nothing else, they have a better phosphorus-to-iron ratio than any other nut, which makes them easier to assimilate.) Did you know that there are 70 biblical references to this ancient nut, a symbol of happiness in pre-Biblical times?

Peanuts (which are, botanically speaking, underground legumes, not nuts at all) are higher in protein (26%) than most meats (1 tablespoon of peanut butter has 5 grams protein—more than ham or chicken salad), more iron than cottage cheese, more vitamin D than hamburger, and as much fiber as a slice of whole wheat bread. They top the list of foods that cause the least dramatic rise in blood sugar and insulin. Peanut oil is used in treating arthritis pain (in the form of a once-a-week massage).

Walnuts were favored by King Solomon in biblical times and were considered the "royal" nut of ancient Rome. In addition, walnuts are a good-luck food. Walnuts are the nut of choice for vegetarian nut-loafs and burgers.

Buying, Storing, and Using

Store nuts in the shell to protect from light and heat, which causes rancidity. (Unshelled nuts will keep at room temperature for up to a week.) Whole nuts keep better than pieces. Unroasted, unsalted nuts have a longer storage life than roasted, salted varieties. Refrigerate shelled nuts for up to three months in tightly closed containers, or freeze.

Buy nuts raw and roast them yourself (roasting enhances flavor). Up to 72% of a nut's thiamine is lost in commercial processing, plus 25% of the vitamin B_6. Salted nuts have 82 times more sodium than raw.

To roast, spread nuts on an ungreased, shallow pan. Bake in 350-degree oven for 5 to 12 minutes or until lightly browned. Nuts continue to darken after removing from oven. Cool and then refrigerate.

Nuts can be chopped, ½ cup at a time, in the blender on high speed. Sliver or slice nuts while still warm from blanching with a thin, sharp knife. Do not use a blender or food processor to grind; use a hand-operated Mouli grater (or nut mill).

NUT KNOW-HOW

Don't have a nutcracker? Place walnuts or pecans on end, hold by seam, and strike with a hammer on pointed end. Hard shells (Brazil nuts) are easier to open if you freeze first.

A pecan lover's shell-shucking trick: Pour boiling water over unshelled nuts and soak overnight. Drain. Giving the small end of the nut a tap with hammer does the rest.

To blanch: Nuts with a thin inner skin can be removed by pouring boiling water over the nuts. Drain and slip skins off. Dry on paper towels.

A pound of unshelled nuts equals (about) ½ pound shelled. One pound unshelled will yield the following:

Almonds, unblanched, whole	6⅓ oz.	1¼ cups
blanched, slivered	4½ oz.	1 cup
Brazil nuts, whole	4½ oz.	1½ cups
Cashews, whole	4½ oz.	1 cup
Hazelnuts or Filberts, whole	7⅓ oz.	1½ cups
Macadamias, whole	5⅓ oz.	1¼ cups
Peanuts, whole, roasted	11⅔ oz	2⅓ cups
Pecans, halves	8½ oz.	2¼ cups
Pistachios, unshelled	14 oz.	3⅔ cups
Walnuts, halves	7¼ oz.	2 cups

Nuts add flavor as well as crunch. Many of your favorite foods will taste even better when you add nuts. Here are some suggestions:

- ◆ Serve sour cream with nuts on baked potatoes.
- ◆ Try slivered/sliced nuts in tossed salads.
- ◆ Use ground toasted pumpkin or squash seeds to authenticate your next molé sauce.*

---

* Mexican chocolate sauce

- Sprinkle cupcakes with crushed nuts before baking and you can skip the frosting.
- Blend peanut butter (about 1 tablespoon per serving), into cream soups.

NUT LOVERS' TIPS

Dieter's PB&J: Spread sparing amount of fresh peanut butter on sliced apples. A tablespoon of curry sauce adds a flavor spike.

Snack, but put a cap on it. Here's the per-ounce calorie cost (whole, unroasted).

Almonds	170
Brazil nuts	185
Cashews, roasted	159
Chestnuts	70
Hazelnuts	180
Macadamias	196
Peanuts, roasted	165
Pecans halves	195
Pistachios	170
Pine nuts	146
Walnuts, halves	185

Soak, then snack. Presoaked nuts may not crunch, but a brief bath (8 to 12 hours) activates growth forces, makes complex starches more digestible, and improves nutrient content, says the Seeds for Life Foundation. (After soaking, drain, dry at room temperature, and eat or refrigerate. Best candidates: almonds, cashews.)

Alternate your inventory of nuts, nutbutter, and oils. Try pine nut butter (slightly sweet), crisp roasted macadamias from Hawaii, black walnut oil (see Mail Order Sources) instead of olive on salads.

Switch to full-flavored low fat coconut oil for popcorn (3 table-spoons coconut oil per each ½ cup of kernels). You can skip the butter and salt.

Try this recipe:

Almond Milk

> *2 cups blanched almonds*
> *2 cups water*
> *6 pitted dates*

Put all ingredients in blender and process for two minutes or until smooth. Strain. (To thin, add more water.)

Makes 2½ cups.

Variations: Make "chocolate milk" by adding 1 teaspoon carob or cocoa powder per cup. Use cashews or pine nuts instead of almonds.

TIP: To get the best "brain boost," drink milk before eating.

Benefits healing zones: 2, 3, 5, 9

Also see: Walnuts, Antioxidants, Sprouts, Vegetarian Foods

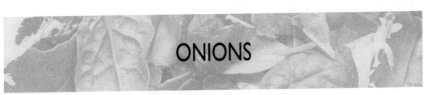

ONIONS

What's true about garlic is just as true in large part of the onion, another aromatic member of the 500-strong allium family (and second cousin to the lily), a family which includes the globe onion, Welsh onion, shallot, scallion, leek, chives, and such oddball *allium cepas* as the wild Southern European leek (potent enough to burn the tongue when eaten raw) and the sweet-as-apples Vidalias of Georgia in the United States.

The onion is a native of central Asia with a 3,000-year history as a people's pharmaceutical to treat everything from the common cold to cancer. Poet Robert Louis Stevenson once dubbed the lowly onion "the rose among roots"—and with good reason.

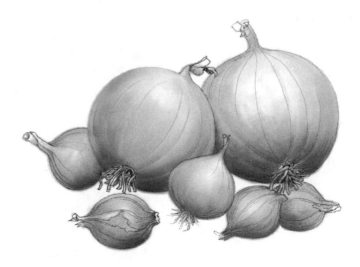

PHARMACEUTICAL OF THE PHARAOHS

Onions (the only vegetable that reduces us to tears) have a long history of healing. The Egyptian medical papyrus Codex Ebero listed over 8,000 onion-alleviated ailments. In ancient Greece, Hippocrates prescribed onion as a diuretic, wound healer, and pneumonia fighter. In the Far East, onions were used for infections, hypertension, and more. In the Old Testament, the onion is one of the half-dozen foods the Hebrew people pined for after leaving the Promised Land. Leeks (oversized scallion lookalikes smell of both onion *and* garlic), have been the Welsh national symbol for centuries.

ONION SOUP RX FOR VASCULAR AND PANCREATIC HEALTH

Like garlic, onion helps prevent thrombosis and reduces hypertension, says the American Heart Association, because of the prostaglandin A2 factor it contains. According to Dr. Victor Gurewich of Tufts University, the juice of one white or yellow onion a day can raise your good HDL cholesterol by 30% over time. Onions are also prescribed to stimulate a weak heart. But remember the benefit is in the bite. Mild red onions lack the HDL-elevating effect of yellow or Bermuda onions.

25+ SECRET INGREDIENTS THAT FIGHT CANCER AND DIABETES

According to population studies by the National Cancer Institute, various chemicals in onions appear to inhibit the growth of cancerous cells, especially in the gastrointestinal system, and fight against leukemia. Onions contain 25 active compounds, the antioxidant flavonoids (including quercetin, which is, says the University of Munich's Dr. Walter Dorsch, a potent carcinogen deactivator) the antioxidants coumarin and ellagic acid, plus the fiber pectin (also found in grains and fruits).

Onions also lower blood sugar as effectively as some prescription diabetic drugs, thanks to their allyl propyl disulphide (APDS) content.

ONION RING ANTIBIOTIC/ANTIASTHMA

The sulphurous compounds and mustard oils in onions help prevent the inflammatory response that leads to asthma attacks and other respiratory disorders. (In traditional Chinese medicines, onions and garlic were used to treat tuberculosis; an old Spanish Basque remedy to still whooping and smoker's or asthmatic coughs calls for peeling and slicing two Spanish onions, covering them with dark honey, storing in a covered container overnight, and straining the next morning. Dilute syrup with water and lemon juice and take at two-hour intervals to heal the throat.

Drinking onion juice before exposure to irritants reduces bronchial asthma attacks by about 50%, according to German researchers, and onion oil used topically can reduce swelling and inflammation.

AN ONION A DAY FOR HYPERTHERMIC RELIEF, HEALTHY HAIR, AND MORE

Onions are just what the holistic beautician ordered for conditioning your hair, improving scalp circulation, and preventing hair loss. Put 2½ cups of lightly packed onion skins into a pan with 1 quart of boiling water. Cover, steep for 50 minutes, and then strain through a sieve. After shampooing, towel dry. Use the onion skin rinse, and then rinse with clear water to condition, soften, and enhance natural highlights.

And there shouldn't be a dry eye in the house if you're after relief for hypothermia. According to experiments at the University of Puerto Rico in San Juan, applying a poultice of grated onion laced with cayenne to the heel of each foot—until warmth returns—is an effective way to relieve shivers and chills.

BELIEVE-IT-OR-NOT REMEDIES

An onion cocktail can soothe the digestion or work as a side-effect-free diuretic (to boost antiedema power, combine with dandelion tea and celery or artichoke juice), aid in healing an enlarged prostate, and help eradicate brown spots of aging (use topically). A sliced raw onion beneath your pillow even enjoys a reputation as an insomnia buster.

And thanks to the substance allicin, onions have wound-healing antibiotic properties and are often used in naturopathic eye, ear, and nose drop preparations.

NUTRITIONAL PROFILE

Nutritionally, onions are natural uppers—providing beta-carotene, vitamin A, potassium, vitamins B_1 and B_2 and vitamin C. Onions contain no fat, little sodium, and only 40 calories per medium-sized onion globe.

Buying, Storing, and Using

The only way to test your onion-lovers' potential is to try them all. Start with the sweeter-eating varieties such as Georgia Vidalias (which are higher in vitamin C, have the sugar content of apples, and produce no afterbreath) or the Hawaiian Mauis or Walla Walla varieties (a.k.a. "French onions" after the *fin de siècle* farmer who developed them), which are said to make delicious alternatives to jelly in a P&J sandwich. And don't overlook shallots—the garlic-shaped, delicate-flavored scallions—or the grass-like, onion-flavored chives, a perennial in grass roots remedies for sinus, cold, and flu complaints.

Globe onions should be clean, dry, and hard with smooth, intact skins (avoid misshapen bulbs and onions that show any sign of sprouting). Green onions should have bright green tops. Only leeks and scallions need refrigeration. Other varieties should be dry, at room temperature.

Two ways to turn your onions into non-tear-jerkers:

♦ Refrigerate an hour or more before using.

♦ Bag them and whack the bag against a wall or other hard surface to free the offensive volatile oils before peeling.

Try these uses:

◆ Make your own onion starters by recycling the cores of dry onion bulbs. Plant the core (with root knob and top shoot intact) in a small clay pot, and water. Each "mother bulb" will send up a handful of onion shoots for salad. Keep cutting and planting for year-round cuttings.

◆ Chewing on raw parsley, dill, or fennel seeds when eating onions will combat onion or garlic afterbreath. (Ancient Greek hedonists substituted rose petals or jasmine buds.)

◆ Shallots retain their flavor and shape better than globe onions and can be used in place of garlic or regular onions in cooking.

◆ Onion eater's vitamin C? Try allium cepa, the homeopathic ascorbic acid.

◆ Grated onion, onion juice, or dried onion flakes or powder can pinch hit for salt in salads and prepared dishes.

◆ Onions' best juice partners: garlic, parsley, and any root vegetable.

Try this recipe:

Onion Burgers

1¹/₃ cups sunflower seeds (or a combination of seeds and peanuts)

2 cups cooked soybeans

2 large globe onions, coarsely grated

3 tablespoons soy sauce

Bran, dry bread crumbs, or cracker crumbs

Preheat oven to 350 degrees. In a processor or blender, grind seeds (or seeds and nuts) to a fine meal. Grind beans to a dry pulp, combine with seeds, and add soy sauce and mix to blend. (If the mixture is too soft, add bran or crumbs.)

Form into oval patties using about ½-cup mixture for each.

Bake in a greased pan for 20 minutes, or broil 3 inches from heat for five to eight minutes per side. Serve on whole wheat buns. Tasty topped with Super Healing Salsa or Super Healing Hummus (see pp. 157 and 256).

Makes five to six servings.

Benefits healing zones: 2, 3, 4, 7

Also see: Garlic, Coronary Heart Disease, Cancer, Common Cold, Halitosis, and Mail Order Sources

ORANGES
(and Tangerines)

Did you know that when you start your day the O.J. way you're actually eating or drinking the juice of a 20-million-year-old berry—one of the five or six most important fruits in the world?*

Oranges, once known as "apples of the sun," are thought to have originated in southeast Asia and did not arrive in Europe until the Middle Ages. Oranges were said to be food of Mohammedans—they were only eaten by those who intended to become members of that faith, and their eating was proscribed for all nonbelievers. The Arabs introduced oranges into Europe in the sixteenth century.

In England, oranges were boiled or stewed (as were most fruits and vegetables before the eighteenth century) as a sauce or side dish and used as an elegant breath freshener by the gentry. A delicacy was boiled turtle steak served with melted butter, cayenne pepper, and orange juice. The aromatic potential of the orange did not go unnoticed; flowers and rind were used in tea, and Elizabethan noblemen had the custom of holding an orange peel to their nose while riding to Westminster Hall, probably because of the stench in the streets. This became a custom, and even today judges in London perform the rite once a year. By the seventeenth century in England, oranges were being cultivated avidly in greenhouses called orangeries and served raw with meat dishes.

America's California orange industry originated with a grove or four hundred trees in San Gabriel Mission, California, in 1804.

HEALING FROM HAIRLINE TO HEARTBEAT

Raw or cooked, juiced or eaten whole, oranges have a long history of healing. In the twelfth century, orange peel was brewed as a tonic tea for the digestion (just as citrus rind, oil and flowers are still used in sedatives and digestive preparations). In seventeenth-century Italy, ferment-

---

* The name *orange* probably derives from the Old French word for gold, *auranja*.

ed orange flowers were prescribed as a heart medicine. Clove-spiked citrus fruits were carried to ward off the Plague; and in Arabia, dried, oil-soaked oranges were used to reverse graying hair.

Today, oranges are beneficial in healing all disorders of the respiratory system (thanks to their abundant electrolyte minerals—potassium, calcium, sodium and magnesium) as well as in preventing and alleviating asthma and viral and staph infections and destroying the bacteria connected with many sexually transmitted diseases (STDs), says the Preventative Medical Research Institute.

CITRUS SOLUTION TO LOWER CHOLESTEROL AND LESS CANCER

The combination of those elements plus fiber (pectin) accounts for the orange's ability to stabilize blood cholesterol. Researchers at the Institute of Agriculture and Food Science at the University of Florida in Gainesville have found that oranges, grapefruits, and tangerines are excellent preventive and curative foods against heart disease and cancer. The vitamin C and bioflavonoids from oranges act directly to prevent

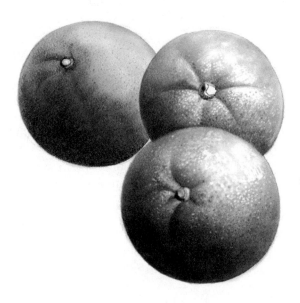

clumping of red blood cells, which can cause heart attacks. The antioxidants coumarin, monoterpene, and selenium in citrus fruits promote better circulation and distribution of oxygen to the tissues and cells of the body—factors that figure in the prevention of cancer.

Oranges (and other citrus fruits) also contain phenolic acids, antioxidants that prevent free radical damage and neutralize carcinogens like nitrosamines that are formed in the stomach when nitrite from food combines with naturally occurring enzymes. They also promote production of gluthanione, an amino acid which is one of the body's most potent detoxifiers.

"PEEL AN ORANGE, SMOKE NO MORE" AND OTHER ORANGE AIDS

The peel of an orange applied spongy side to the skin and bound with a bandage is said to help reduce the swelling of a sprain. Two small oranges and half a grapefruit, blended skin, seeds, and all and diluted with water, is said to cure a charley horse (muscle stiffness). Tea brewed from citrus peel is a natural flatulence antidote.

In many countries, the inner white peel of an orange is kept intact and both fruit and peel are eaten together as a natural laxative. According to the Linus Pauling Institute, eating one orange per day (bioflavonoid-rich pith and all) helps prevent nose bleeds and weakens the urge to smoke.

THE VITAMIN COCKTAIL THAT DOUBLES AS A GARGLE

An orange a day also supplies your vitamin C requirement and eaten with an iron-supplying meal it doubles your absorption of that healthy heart–higher energy mineral. Oranges also supply folate and are a better source of calcium than whole wheat bread, broccoli, or sweet potatoes.

All citrus juices, because of their vitamin C and acidity, make first-rate, alcohol-free germicidal gargles and mouthwashes (dilute with mineral water).

Best O.J. juice partners: Combine tart and sweet citrus juices in a 1:5 ratio (eg., lime/tangerine). Or combine a tart citrus fruit with a sweet noncitrus (eg., kumquat/pear or grapefruit/apple).

Buying, Storing, and Using

◆ Buy your oranges (tangerines and tangelos and kumquats) ripe. Citrus are among the 12 fruits that do not ripen after picking (along with berries, cherries, and plums). But ripe doesn't necessarily mean carrot-orange. Green oranges are routinely gassed, dyed and waxed for cosmetic purposes. A green orange (green indicates the presence of chlorophyll) is probably the best buy in the bin.

◆ Consider organic or low-residue oranges if you plan to use the peel as well as the pulp and the juice. (The dozens of pesticides and fungicides with which oranges are routinely sprayed include two suspected carcinogens, dicarb and parathion.)

◆ Oranges are categorized as sweet or bitter (sour). Sweet oranges for eating and juicing include the Jaffa, Valencia, and Maltese (blood orange); sour oranges (Seville) are used largely in marmalades, and Mediterranean Bergamot is used solely for cosmetic purposes.

◆ The heavier the fruit, the juicier. Thicker-skinned varieties are the easiest to peel and seedless navels the easiest to eat out of hand. According to folk wisdom, the older the tree, the more super healing the-fruit.

◆ Looking for an elite orange to feast on? Try crimson-fleshed, intensely flavored blood oranges from Italy and California, prized for their complex, berry-like taste. The red pigments in the rind and flesh of blood oranges, called anthocyanins, produce a deep-violet to red-streaked flesh and a tangy, thick-textured juice. These are tasty in endive salads and in sorbets, fruit soups, and tarts.

Juicer's Tips

Once opened or squeezed, citrus juice stays fresh for about one week. As orange juice loses its flavor, it loses its vitamin C (to rejuvenate, add the juice of half a fresh lemon to the pitcher or carton).

Beware of juice blends. Priced 15% higher than the pure thing, store-bought blends (such as Five-Alive™) are only 60% reconstituted orange and other citrus juices. The remaining 40% is sugar, corn sweetener, and water. But that's not all you lose. Take a look at the following chart.

ONE CUP OF INSTANT POWDERED ORANGE BREAKFAST DRINK		ONE CUP OF PURE, FRESH ORANGE JUICE	
Ingredient	Function	Nutrient	Function
Sugar	Empty calories	Water (88%)	Maintains body temperature, hydrates bloodstream, maintains function of hormones and all body systems
Citric acid	By chemicalized fermentation process, can damage teeth and bone enamel	Calories (110)	Healthful energy and natural vitality for vigor and strength
Natural flavor	Actually, concocted flavor from real or artificial sources duplicating the natural citrus taste	Protein (2 g)	Builds, maintains, and repairs all body tissues. Supplies energy and helps form antibodies as well as enzymes, and hormones.
Gum arabic (vegetable gum)	Plant gum that may cause allergic or intestinal reaction	Carbohydrates (26 g)	Supplies energy and helps body use fats more effectively. Aids digestion by adding bulk.
Sodium (also known as sodium biphosphate)	Used as an emulsifier and sequestrant that binds and inactivates minerals	Calcium (27 mg)	Builds bones and teeth and helps blood clot. Normalizes heart rhythm.

Source: Natural Food and Farming Association

If you're an ardent orange sucker, keep your toothbrush handy. Orange juice can do more damage to the teeth than cola, says Dr. Mario S. Rodriguez, associate professor of periodontics at the Louisiana State University School of Dentistry in New Orleans. Citric acid has the potential to dissolve dental enamel faster than the phosphoric acid in cola drinks. "Citric acid has a specific affinity for calcium, and teeth are made up primarily of calcium," says the National Institute for Dental Research.

Don't overdo the peels, either; they secrete a vitamin antagonist that neutralizes some of the health effects of vitamin A when eaten in excess.

Note: Oranges and other citrus are off limits on oxalic, acid-free diets and for allergy sufferers sensitive to pollen and salicylate.

MISCELLANEOUS CITRUS FRUITS

These include the tangerine and the tangelo (which provide twice the vitamin A and calcium of oranges) and ugli fruit (an ugly duckling cousin of the pommelo which is used in many island cultures for respiratory ills and for clearing the liver, is the only citrus source of iodine, and provides bioflavonoids and calcium).

Kumquats are the smallest of all citrus fruits and a tart mini-fruit source of trace elements that fight autoimmune disorders, such as Crohn's disease and arthritis. Cultivated in China and Japan for thousands of years, kumquats are usually eaten skin and all (their rinds are sweet while the pulps are tart and juicy).

Named after the city of Tangier in North Africa, the small, loose-skinned tangerine is actually a variety of Mandarin orange. The juicy segments, which separate readily, are dark and have a sweet, delicate flavor. The skin ripens to a deep orange-red and is popular in Chinese folk medicine.

Super Healing Orange Lemonade

> *½ cup fresh lemon juice*
>
> *½ cup fresh orange juice*
>
> *2 to 4 tablespoons natural sugar (optional)*
>
> *1½ cups cold sparkling mineral water*

Juice fruits and mix juices. Add sugar so that taste is sweet-tart. Refrigerate, covered. For each drink, use ½ cup of juice mix in a glass; add ice and ½ cup water.

Makes three servings.

Variation: Use a pommelo or tangelo in place of orange juice, or grapefruit in place of lemon.

TIP: For a pure from-the-pantry skin freshener, dilute ½ cup fresh grapefruit juice with 1 cup water. Mist two to four times daily to stimulate and clear skin.

Benefits healing zones: 1, 3, 4, 7

Also see: Lemons, Common Cold, Vitamin C, Juices, Beta-carotene

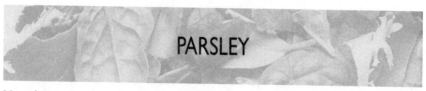

PARSLEY

No plate of super healing protection is complete without a red-hot antioxidant on it, and parsley—by sprig, bunch or teacupful—more than fills the bill.

FROM MAGIC TO MEDICINAL HERB

Parsley, (a relative of rosemary and cilantro) thought to have originated in Southern Europe, was once thought to possess magical properties (along with sage, rosemary, and thyme—the four famous herbs of *Gammer Gurton's Garland*). The ancient Greeks wore garlands of parsley, believing that it would excite the brain and stimulate the appetite. Parsley was a sacred herb of burial among the Romans, placed on graves and served at funeral banquets (which is probably the origin of its use as a garnish). The famous herbalist Culpepper prescribed parsley for stomach disorders, as did Beatrix Potter, who tells us in Peter Rabbit, "First he ate some French beans and then he ate some radishes and then, feeling rather sick, he went to look for parsley." Parsley seed poultices were just what the holistic healer ordered for banishing freckles and curing snakebite in the Middle Ages. Boiled parsley root was even regarded as an antidote for epilepsy before the turn of the century.

Today there are over 30 varieties, some grown only for the stems, others only for the root. It is one of the few herbs used universally. So popular is parsley in the Middle East, it is served as a salad green.

FERTILITY SYMBOLISM

Among gardeners, parsley was originally cultivated as a garden border herb along with rue (thus the expression, "We are at parsley and rue"). And it is still honored as the herb that best symbolizes the arrival of spring and rebirth. (Fertility is often symbolized by a parsley-entwined carrot.) Parsley even enjoyed a reputation in the Middle Ages as a minor aphrodisiac.

A WOMAN'S CUP OF TEA

Parsley's vitamin A (beta-carotene) content makes it a good teacup tonic for the complexion and a good diuretic or anti-PMS aid. As nature's top-rated leafy green source of iron, parsley fights iron-deficiency anemia, one of the five most common health problems among premenopausal women. Parsley also provides plenty of folate, the vitamin that's needed at double the usual dose during pregnancy. A good source of vegetable calcium (the mineral women are most commonly deficient in), parsley also provides chlorophyll, the "youth factor" nutrient that slows aging.

CANCER AND CARDIOVASCULAR PROTECTION

Parsley's antitumor prowess comes from six sources, say Natural Health Clinic researchers at Boston College. Parsley contains beta-carotene (10,000 IU per ½ cup), vitamin C (10 sprigs provide 15% of your vitamin C RDA), plus the four antioxidants coumarins, flavonoids, monoterpene, and polyacetylene, which appear to block the synthesis of cancer-promoting prostaglandins. As a bonus, all six of these elements strengthen the immune and cardiovascular systems.

FOUR MINERALS FOR FOUR ILLS

According to the American Nutritional Medical Association, the potassium, calcium, phosphorous, and iodine in parsley seed, root and leaf help heal kidney and urinary tract infections, raise energy levels, and ease the

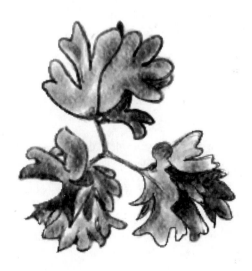

discomfort of rheumatism. Last but not least, parsley is a super munch-a-bunch food with less than 20 calories per cup.

Buying, Storing, and Using

A biennial herb that can reach 3 feet, and will grow in almost any climate, common parsley varieties include the Italian (fern or single leaved), Extra Curled Dwarf, Emerald, Moss Curled or Green Velvet, Italian, Hamburg, and French. Look for fresh, bright green sprigs, (the fresher the variety, the better the flavor) and to encourage daily use, do the following:

- ♦ Keep two parsley bouquets (flat leaved and curly) in a water-filled vase in the refrigerator for impulse nibbling (its a natural breath freshener) and to toss into salads, soups and prepared dishes.

- ♦ Toss 1 cup chopped parsley into any mixed combination of salad greens.

- ♦ Stir handfuls of parsley into yogurt, add lemon juice, and use as a potato topper or dip.

- ♦ Make parsley pesto once a month and use as a sauce for pasta, rice, meatless burgers, and nut loaves.

- ♦ Add one chopped cupful parsley to any salsa, tomato, or primavera sauce.

- ♦ The freeze-dried parsley alternative: For more flavor and nutrition, freeze whole parsley in bunches. When diced parsley is needed, make thin shavings from the frozen bunch to use in cooked dishes, etc. Frozen parsley provides more flavor and nutrition than dried.

Try this recipe:

Parsley Pesto

Blend 1 cup chopped parsley (curly, flat leaved or a combination) with 3 tablespoons virgin olive oil, one clove garlic, 2 tablespoons fresh grated Parmesan cheese and a pinch French tarragon (a good salt substitute). Add 2 tablespoons hot water (or 2 tablespoons parsley tea). (Optional: Add ¼ teaspoon red pepper flakes.) Toss with ½ pound of hot whole grain pasta and serve hot.

Benefits healing zones: 2, 3, 5, 6, 9

Also see: PMS/Menopause, Cancer, Juices, Beta-carotene, Herbs

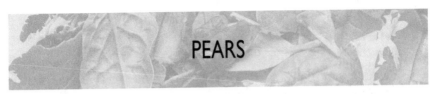

PEARS

What do Shakespeare, Chaucer, and old-fashioned patience have in common? They are all paired with pears. The former two doted on the now dusky pears of yesteryear, and the latter is what you need to raise a fruit bowl crop of edible modern-day Bartletts, Boscs, or Anjous.

Unlike other fruits, pears must be harvested when they are mature but not ripe (they turn gritty and mushy left on the tree). Picked and shipped while hard as potatoes, they must be carefully watched and coddled to develop correctly.

Wild pears, which are native to southeastern Europe and western Asia, were small, hard, and sour. In the eighteenth century, the Belgians introduced the "butter pears" (with soft, sweet flesh) that prevail today.

The first colonists brought pears to America, and some are still grown in New York and neighboring states. But close to 95% of the American crop is grown in northern California, Oregon, and Washington.

Although there are up to 120 varieties of pears grown globally, here's a primer of everyday pears.

♦ *Bartlett.* Bell shaped, with thin green skin that turns yellow when ripe; flesh is fine textured, white, The preeminent pear of summer, it bruises easily and is highly perishable. Derived from an English seedling found growing wild in 1770, acquired by Enoch Bartlett in Massachusetts in 1817, who named it after himself. (The Williams Bon Chretien in Europe and the bumpy Packham are similar.)

♦ *Anjou.* In France known as the Beurré d'Anjou, this is a plump oval pear which remains light green when ripe. Keeps up to seven months in storage, but its hardiness means it can take up to two weeks to ripen. A good one is mildly juicy with spicy cream color. Good for cooking.

♦ *Bosc.* Tawny, cinnamon, or russet with light green or gold and an elegant tapering neck. Lightly perfumed flesh is yellowish white. Keeps its shape well when cooked.

♦ *Comice.* Considered the sweetest and juiciest pear. Originated in France in 1849 as the Doyenné du Comice (meaning "top of the show"). Has light green skin which turns yellow when ripe. Can be eaten with a knife and fork. The delicate flavor is best enjoyed with the grainy skin removed.

♦ *Seckel.* A mini-pear with rich, spicy flavor; olive or russet skin tinged with crimson. Discovered growing wild near Philadelphia in the late eighteenth century.

♦ *Forelle.* In its native Germany called the Trout because of its speckles. Skin is rich red blush against yellow-green. Juicy white flesh and thick, delicious (sometimes tart) skin.

♦ *Winter Nellis.* Roundish, rather small, with a sweet, creamy and spicy flesh. A Belgian immigrant with splotchy gray russet and green skin. Good for eating or baking.

PICK A PEAR, PROTECT YOUR HEART AND ARTERIES

What's true of the apple is, for the most part, true of the pear, which is low in calories, fat, and sodium. Pears do, however, offer more water-soluble fiber than apples (including pectin) and they supply more potassium for normal bowel function and cholesterol lowering. A single 98-calorie Bartlett has as much fiber as a bowl of whole grain cereal. Pears also get a small gold star for folic acid, which is essential for blood formation.

Buying, Storing, and Using

Look for firm, full fruit with no cuts or soft spots. Picked too early, pears never develop good flavor; picked too late, they turn brown and watery at the core. Stored too long, they die and never soften. Handle pears gently; even rock-like pears bruise easily. Or look for fruit which are ready to eat in a day or two (most take three to seven days to arrive at their peak).

When ripe, a pear will yield to gentle pressure at the stem end. Some (notably Bartletts) change color and become fragrant when ripe. Pears ripen from the center out, so when they are soft all over they will be mushy. Pears pass quickly from firm to overripe (a state the English call "sleepy").

To hurry ripening, place pears in a paper bag at room temperature with a ripe banana (a ripening agent), or insert a nail in the bottom of the fruit to stimulate the production of ethylene.

Ripe pears can be refrigerated for two to three days but should be brought to room temperature for eating.

Pears taste best paired with nuts (almonds, pecans, chestnuts) and blue cheeses. Or toss with bitter greens (dandelion, arugula, chicory). Pears are also delicious poached in alcohol-free pink wine. For maximum fiber and vitamin C, eat raw, skin and all (but scrupulously prewashed). Pears eaten with iron-rich foods such as nuts, seeds, or grains increase your intake of vitamin C (the two nutrients potentiate one another). To get twice as many nutrients (with the exception of vitamin C, which is lost in dehydration), snack on dried pears as a snack substitute.

Best juicing pears: Bosc and Comice (use firm, not soft, type). Best juice partners: Plums, lemon, cranberry, raspberries.

Pear-bored? Grab an Asian apple-pear. The taste is buttery, the texture is crisp as a potato, and it's twice as juicy as American types. Or try a Forelle Seckel, famous for its streaking and delicate flavor, or the gift-giver's favorite, the Riviera Comice—smooth enough to eat with a spoon and worth the twice-the-price tag.

Look for pear cider (Perry) and lemon pear butter and pear plum marmalade at specialty food stores.

Try this recipe:

Pear Salsa

3 medium firm pears, peeled and seeded

Juice of one lime

2 tablespoons red onion, minced

3 tablespoons cilantro, chopped

¼ teaspoon salt

Dash of cayenne pepper

Combine all ingredients in food processor or blender. Process until pureed but slightly lumpy. Serve warm or cold over grain patties, soyburgers, and nut loaves.

Benefits healing zones: 1, 2, 7, 8

Also see: Coronary Heart Disease, Juices, Digestion, Antioxidants

PEPPER

What's red and green and bred all over? Common garden peppers. All eight of the common capsicum* varieties that come from the same two species (and the same single genus), *Capsicum frutesceus,* or *C. annum,* are hot stuff as botanical helpers and healers: cayenne (red pepper); red chile (source of chili powder); paprika, jalapeños, and serranos (the extra hot Thai peppers), habañeros (home to the scotch bonnets, second hottest); and red and green bell peppers (the mildest). The pepper family has 150 to 200 members in all (the Hungarian variety from which paprika is processed is generally unavailable, but authentic powdered paprika is a superior source of vitamin C and beta-carotene). Other types include the white, purple, chocolate brown, and the ornamental types (which though rarely eaten are also edible).

PEPPERY PAIN FOR HEALING

Ironically, the chemical substance capsaicin that gives peppers their bite,** or pain-producing potential, is what makes them effective painkillers: This healing substance, which has been the subject of more than 600 clinical studies over a quarter of a century, reduces sensitivity to pain caused by heat, chemicals, injuries, and more by selectively depressing the production and release of a chemical called "substance P" in the nerves that transmits pain. (The effect, says capsicum researcher Charles N. Ellis, M.D., professor and associate chair of the department of dermatology at the University of Michigan Medical School, is specific to the nerves located near the skin's surface and inside the mouth.) This discovery has led to the development of a topically applied capsaicin cream treatment for shingles (herpes zoster), neuropathy (which afflicts 50% of all diabetics), and the itch of psoriasis. Healing has been reported in 66% of all study participants. (Cayenne is officially listed for use as

---

* Capsaicin comes from the Greek word kapto, meaning "I bite."

** Peppers also belong to the solanaceae or nightshade family, along with tomatoes, potatoes, and eggplant.

a non-narcotic local stimulant for the stomach, intestines, and digestion by the U.S. Dispensary.)

Capsaicin puts not just skin-deep pain in its place but osteoarthritic and rheumatoid arthritic inflammation as well, report Scandinavian and Swedish researchers—by increasing DNA synthesis and triggering production of pain-depressing collagenase and prostaglandin. In one U.S. study at the University of Rochester pepper extracts applied externally four times a day reduced pain by one third to one half and produced relief in 80% of the subjects within 14 days.

Capsaicin-based creams have been successful where other drug-based therapies have failed—in PMPS (postmasectomy pain syndrome), for example, and in treating athletic injuries. A rural American folk remedy for animal bites calls for the repeated application of fried, wilted patches of red pepper.

EMPOWERMENT PEPPER FOR CARDIOVASCULAR HEALTH

An occasional pickled pepper may be one way to improve the ratio of your HDL to LDL cholesterol, reports the Linus Pauling Heart Foundation—by improving the efficiency of the liver enzyme responsible for fat metabolism and by stimulating the circulation.

HOT PEPPER PRESCRIPTION FOR SIX COMMON ILLS

Peppering your diet with peppers can provide relief from a cold or sinusitis because capsaicin exerts an expectorant effect, increasing lung secretion and facilitating elimination of mucus. Try a half-and-half cocktail of green pepper/carrot juice.

Cayenne and other hot peppers are also used by herbalists as anti-asthma aids, to heal acne, and as a somatic aid (when insomnia is pain triggered). Peppers reportedly even have aphrodisiac properties, says the American Herb Guild.

TAKING PEPPERS TO HEART
For Your Heart and for Hurry-Up Weight Loss

Capsaicin's ability to stimulate the circulation also accounts for its usefulness as an anti-hypertensive aid, and this blood-pressure-regulating benefit may account for the low incidence of thrombosis in chile-pepper-producing and -consuming populations such as Mexico and

Thailand. Peppers also help prevent copper deficiency, which is often a factor in atherosclerosis. Cayenne and turmeric—both curry-blend herbs—appear to have vascular healing properties.

Peppers may be an A-1 ration for reducers and a healthy alternative to dangerous appetite suppressants. In clinical studies at the University of Arizona Medical School, the addition of hot chile peppers to a meal increased the metabolism at a rate stimulating a sweat sufficient to burn off a 700-calorie meal. Cayenne peppers, as a bonus, also increase the liver enzymes responsible for fat metabolism, reducing the rate of weight gain.

THE MSG/ARTIFICIAL PRESERVATIVE ALTERNATIVE

The capsaicin in capsicums, says the Natural Foods and Farming Association, even helps slow down and prevent the oxidation of vegetable oil, which can lead to potentially carcinogenic toxicity. When oil is heated with pepper, this oxidation process is slowed. (To antioxidate your own cooking oil, slip a sliced pepper in each bottle after opening.) Cooking with a dash of pepper has a second bonus—it enhances the flavor of other foods, but without the risk of chemical additives like MSG.

WHY PUT PEPPERS ON THE MENU

Nutritionally, peppers have as much calcium-boosting vitamin C (including the bioflavonoid complex, which is concentrated in the membrane and seeds) as oranges and grapefruit—½ cup satisfies 50% of your minimum daily requirement for the prevention of acidosis and respiratory disorders. Peppers also contain growth-promoting, anticancer beta-carotene vitamin A (fully ripened red bell peppers have 10 times more vitamin A than green peppers, and red and yellow peppers provide more vitamin C than green types) and four essential minerals—phosphorus, iron, sodium, and magnesium (the latter is one of the three minerals in which American diets are most deficient). Peppers are also sources of vitamin B_6, folate (the B vitamin most women's diets are shortest on), and silicon, the trace mineral for healthy nails and hair, skin, and teeth. Peppers are also a source of the antioxidant pigment lycopene, which helps decrease the risk of birth defects and prompts a five fold decrease in the women's cancer called cervical dysplasia in nonpregnant women, according to the American Nutritional Consultants Association.

Buying, Storing, and Using

◆ The smaller and redder a pepper, the hotter it's likely to be and the more beta-carotene it's likely to supply.

◆ Bell peppers, the best choice for stuffing and general use, are sweeter and fruitier than other types and may be green (the mildest) or red (the Spanish called these "pimientas"), yellow gold, orange, purple, or even black. The next best all-purpose varieties are the larger Anaheim and Poblano chile peppers.

◆ Look for the firm, shiny, and unblemished peppers. And if you're a big-time pickled pepper eater, buy from local farm stands, buy certified "low-residue produce," or buy organic peppers from a co-op. Peppers are among the many crops routinely treated with wax compounds to prolong shelf life. These coatings are laced with unremovable, hazardous pesticides and fungicides, says Americans for Safe Food.

◆ Lightly wrap in a cloth and refrigerate peppers and use within one week. Or slice and dry a few pounds (peppers keep indefinitely) for future use.

◆ Always wear gloves or wash hands, knives, and cutting board thoroughly with soapy water when handling hotter varieties. To tame the firehouse effect before cooking or juicing, remove the membranes and seeds (bearing in mind that you are also losing some big healing benefits). To douse a fiery aftertaste, reach for milk or yogurt, not beer or water.

◆ To maximize vitamin C benefits, eat pepper with an iron-source food (i.e., grain or bean-stuffed green peppers or stir-fried grains and pepper).

◆ A bit of red or green pepper (seeds and all) is a perfect way to add healing nutrients and a salt-free spice to any fresh vegetable juice cocktail.

◆ Try a tablespoon or two of diced habañeros and jalapeños (use these hot chile peppers sparingly) in tropical fruit cocktails or juices with mango, passion fruit, or pineapple juice. Or juice red and green peppers and dilute with juiced tomatoes or carrots for a bonus dividend of beta-carotene. (To tame the fiery flavor of juiced chile peppers in advance, add crushed ice.)

◆ Use cayenne pepper or red paprika (or the green paprika in the following recipe) as a mineral-boosting salt substitute.

Try the following recipes:

Vitamin P (Green) Paprika

(This recipe utilizes the vitamin P parts of the bell pepper that are usually discarded. They are the richest in the entire vitamin C complex.)

Remove only the stem from two or three large, unblemished, unwaxed, ripe bell peppers.

Slice thinly, retaining seeds. Spread on a wax-paper-lined cookie sheet. Dry in a very low oven (with door propped slightly open), dry using your food dryer following manufacturer's instructions, or dry on racks in a well-ventilated attic.

When completely dried, process in blender or food processor (seeds and slices both) to a paprika powder. Store in spice jars and keep in a dry cupboard.

Capsicum Citrus Coleslaw

> *1 cup chopped (red or green) bell pepper (or ¹/₂ cup each)*
>
> *6 tangerines, peeled and diced, membrane removed*

Toss with 1 cup grated cabbage, ¹/₃ cup grapefruit juice, and ¹/₂ cup sprouted alfalfa or sunflower seeds.

Let flavors meld in refrigerator for half an hour. Season with cayenne or paprika. Serve on a bed of grated red cabbage with yogurt or Super Healing Mayo (p. 360).

Variation: Substitute kiwi fruit for tangerines and one diced mild chile pepper for the bell.

Green Salad with Red Pepper Dressing

Salad:

> *1 large head romaine lettuce, washed and torn*
>
> *1 cucumber, sliced*
>
> *1 red bell pepper, seeded and sliced*
>
> *1 tomato, cored and chopped*

Dressing:

> *2 ounces tofu*
>
> *³/₄ cup roasted and peeled red bell pepper*

1 tablespoon apple juice concentrate

½ cup chopped, peeled tomatoes

2 tablespoons vinegar

¼ teaspoon salt-free Dijon-style mustard

2 teaspoons minced garlic

¼ teaspoon black pepper

Place salad ingredients in bowl. Blend dressing until smooth. Pour over salad. (The dressing also makes a good marinade for cooked bean salad.)

Roasted Red Pepper Purée Plus

3 medium-sized carrots, peeled and cut into 1-inch rounds

2 roasted red peppers, coarsely chopped

4 teaspoons low-fat yogurt

¼ teaspoon ground mace

Super Healing Salt (p. 276) to taste

Place the carrots in a medium-sized saucepan and cover with water. Bring to a boil over a medium-high heat. Reduce heat and simmer until tender, about 10 minutes. Drain well.

Place the carrots in a food processor with the roasted red peppers. Process until smooth, stopping to scrape down the sides of the bowl. Add the yogurt and mace. Thin with milk or broth. Season to taste.

Makes two servings.

Variation: Substitute 2 teaspoons walnut oil for yogurt.

Serve for a light winter supper, use to thicken pan juices for sauces, use as a condiment, or thin with milk for a velvety soup.

TIPS: Can't get your capsicum fill? Grow your own with ideas from *The Pepper Garden* by Dave Dewitt and Paul W. Bosland (available from Ten Speed Press, P.O. Box 7123, Berkeley, CA 94707, 800-841-2665.

Looking for out-of-the-ordinary peppers from seeds or seedlings? Write to Horticultural Enterprises, Box 810082, Dallas, TX 75381 for a catalog. Or write to Peter Pepper Seeds, c/o H. W. Alfrey, P.O. Box 415, Knoxville, TN 37901.

Benefits healing zones: 2, 4, 6, 7

Also see: **Vitamin C, Aspirin Alternatives, Herbs/One-Minute Healers, Common Cold**

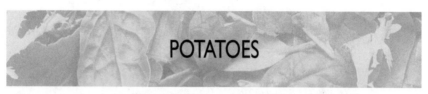

POTATOES

Will a potato a day keep the doctor away? It couldn't hurt if you're out to beat obesity, premature aging, arthritis, and even cancer.

We eat enough spuds annually, according to the USDA (over 300 tons), to cover a four-lane superhighway circling the earth six times.

Potatoes (all several hundred of the varieties grown worldwide*) are members of the *solanaceae* (nightshade) family, along with egg-plants and tomatoes, and are natives of Bolivia and Peru, where they have been cultivated for over 7,000 years. Ever since Spanish explorers took potatoes home from South America in the sixteenth century (in South America the Quechua Indians of Peru have more words for potatoes than Eskimos have for snow), potatoes have occupied an important position in European cuisines. Potatoes grow in more countries today than any food crop except corn and top America's vegetable hit parade (lettuce is second on the list).

SPUD NUTRITION

Potatoes are rich in potassium, vitamin C (they are the second top source after oranges), energizing complex carbohydrates, and fiber for blood sugar and blood pressure control (a baked spud, skin and all, has as much fiber as a ⅓-cup serving of oat bran). They also contain vitamins B_1, B_2, and B_3 and small amounts of protein and iron.

FIRST CHOICE FOR DIETERS, DIABETICS, AND HYPERTENSION CONTROL

Potatoes are tubers to take to heart if you have hypertension, a blood sugar disorder, or take potassium-depleting diuretics. Potatoes supply potassium (twice as much potassium as a banana, as much as a ½ cup of bran) and fiber, which all three conditions require.

---

* See Mail Order Sources for choices.

Potatoes make a good filling substitute for fatty foods in your diet. (Remember, once your total fat level drops below 25% of your daily calories, cholesterol deposition is likely to stop, say researchers.)

Potatoes are also a good source of both blood-building iron and immunity-enhancing vitamins—a vitamin/mineral duo that potentiate each other—plus vitamins B_1, B_2, and B_3, and calcium. Watching calories? An Idaho potato has no more calories than an apple.

ANTICANCER/ANTIVIRAL

Potatoes' protease-inhibiting compounds neutralize viruses and carcinogens even more effectively than those in soybeans and are considered the best source of this phytochemical. Potato skins are also rich in the chlorogenic polyphenol, which helps prevent the cell mutation that can lead to cancer.

POTATO PEELER PHARMACEUTICAL

Shredded raw potato compresses, as well as raw potato juice, are reputed to relieve the pain of arthritis and rheumatism as well as ordinary sprains and bruises and first-degree burns (leave compress in place 15 minutes or longer). A grated red potato compress applied to eyes is said to remove dark circles and, mixed with whipped cream, retard wrinkling.

Potato peel dressings (poultices of boiled potato peelings) are said to promote wound healing, prevent infection, and reduce pain and bacterial contamination.

MASHED POTATO BEAUTIFIER

Mashed potatoes (unbuttered) are the basis of an old-fashioned formula for keeping hands soft and white. Boil potatoes until soft and mash with a bit of milk or yogurt until thick and creamy. Add a few drops of glycerine. Massage hands daily with the mixture. The formula keeps three days refrigerated.

SWEET POTATOES

According to the Cancer Information Service, one serving per day of fruits or vegetables rich in beta-carotene can substantially reduce your risk of heart attack and stroke—by 20 to 40%. A good way to get that health insurance is to help yourself to a sweet potato (24,880 IU of beta-carotene each serving). They're also low in calories (130 per medium), are fat free, and provide half your day's RDA for vitamin C.

Curiously enough, sweet potatoes are not related to the white potato at all but are a member of the Mexican and South American *convolvulaceae* family.

Sweet potatoes are also a good source of vitamin A (essential for normal nerve function) and potassium (keeps the blood pressure down).

Sweet potatoes are tasty baked with pineapple or apple rings, or mashed. Or use sweet potatoes in place of white potatoes in potato salad. (Even better, look for the antiobesity, anticancer, antiaging Mexican yam, the sweet potato's close cousin.)

Buying, Storing, and Using

◆ Avoid potatoes that are wilted, leathery, green, discolored, or show signs of sprouting.

◆ To conserve water soluble nutrients, bake or microwave or steam; don't boil or fry.

◆ Store potatoes in nylon hose or mesh bag in a cool spot.

◆ Add any of the following to mashed potatoes: mashed cooked carrot or broccoli; chopped parsley, spinach, scallions; pressed, diced garlic; shredded cheese.

◆ Experiment. At least a half dozen of the hundreds of varieties grown are available (for example, the purple potato, a Peruvian variety grown in California and the Southwest which resembles a slightly moister Russet with a thinner skin and slightly higher levels of B-complex vitamins and potassium (see Mail Order sources). TIP: Letting baked purples rest 10 minutes before serving allows their silvery purple hue to deepen.

Try these potato recipes:

Healing Hotcakes

> *4 medium sweet or white or purple potatoes, peeled and sliced paper thin*
> *1 tablespoon maple syrup or honey*
> *Cracked black pepper*

Coat two large baking sheets with no-stick spray. Take one potato's worth of slices and overlap to create a circle about 6 inches in diameter on one of the sheets. Add more slices to make a smaller circle on top of the first. Continue until all slices are used. Brush the top with the maple syrup or honey. Sprinkle with pepper.

Repeat to make a total of four stacks.

Bake at 400 degrees for 20 to 25 minutes or until golden brown. Carefully slide a spatula underneath each cake to remove it from the sheet. A breakfast pancake alternative or a supper side dish.

Serves four.

Variation: Substitute yams for sweet or white or purple potatoes.

Uses: As a pancake substitute; as a side dish or snack. Supplies vitamin C, beta-carotene, fiber, and vitamin E.

Super Healing Mousseline

> *6 medium-sized sweet potatoes or yams*
> *2 ripe bananas*
> *Juice of 2 oranges, 2 lemons, and 2 limes*
> *1 teaspoon ground ginger*
> *2 tablespoons natural sugar*
> *4 tablespoons butter*
> *Pepper*

Peel the potatoes, put in pan, and cover with cold water. Bring to a boil and cook gently for 30 minutes, until tender. Drain and place in 350°F oven for five minutes to dry. Mash with the bananas using a potato masher, electric mixer, or food processor.

In a large saucepan, combine fruit juices, ginger, and sugar. Pour syrup into the potato mix, add butter and pepper to taste. Whip again. Spoon into individual soufflé cups.

Makes six to eight servings.

Benefits healing zones: 2, 6

Also see: Basic Dieting Facts and Advice, Fatigue, Beta-carotene, Coronary Heart Disease

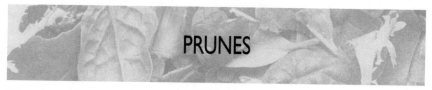

PRUNES

Want to go from tired to tiger? Take a prune to breakfast. Prunes (a.k.a. dried plums) provide the only juice high in iron (30% of an adult male's daily quota). The ancient art of drying plums originated in the Middle East; the Gauls mastered the art before the Roman occupation. The French prune (i.e., the pitless Brignolles) is still considered the best of breed.

NATURE'S NEARLY PERFECT FOOD

High-sugar (30% glucose, 15% fructose, and 2% sucrose) energizers, prunes overall supply 80% of your RDA for seven essential nutrients, including magnesium (more than raisins, apples, and apricots) and potassium (the second best fruit source after raisins). Prunes are near zero in fat. A 3.5-ounce serving provides nearly 4% of your daily quota of vitamin A and 100% of your RDA of immunity-boosting beta-carotene. Prunes are also a top source of B-complex vitamins for fighting fatigue.

NATURE'S HEART-HEALTHY SNACK

Ounce for ounce, prunes provide one third as much iron as an equal serving of liver and are a top-rated source (third best after figs and raisins) of the trace mineral iron, needed to convert the body's store of iron into hemoglobin.

A glass of prune juice in the morning supplies as much potassium as bananas or oranges for both normalizing the heart's rhythms and blood pressure, which is why prunes are frequently prescribed as a hypertensive sweet

Of our eleven favorite fruits, prunes rank second in soluble fiber content (ounce for ounce they have more fiber than dried beans). A handful of prunes a day is a convenient, drug-free way to help lower LDL cholesterol, suggest researchers at the University of California at Davis.

CONSTIPATION CONTROL AND BEYOND
Three Healing Benefits

Prunes are also a source of potent fruit acids that help prevent and control constipation better than any other common food. They are also a source of other ingredients that lower the concentration of fecal bile acids in the body (especially the lithocholic acid associated with increased colon cancer risk). Prunes also supply the trace mineral boron for healthy bones and osteoporosis prevention.

IDEAL DIETERS' AND DIABETICS' SNACK

Prunes' low sodium, low fat, and balanced sugars make them the ideal snack or dessert for weight watchers and insulin-sensitive diabetics.

Prunes are also a perfect fat substitute in baking because they contain a substantial amount of pectin, which traps air in baked goods the way fat traps sugar. Compared to other fruits, prunes contain an unusually high amount of the sugar sorbitol, which helps retain moisture in fat-free foods. Prunes are also a rich source of malic acid, which acts as a flavor enhancer in recipes.

Buying, Storing, and Using

♦ Look for sulfite-free sun-dried* prunes in boxes or bags tightly sealed to prevent oxidation, moisture loss, and insect infestation. Prune size and the presence or absence of pits have no effect on quality or flavor.

♦ Stored in tightly closed containers, prunes remain edible for up to six months. Freeze to double life expectancy.

♦ Eat raw more often than cooked. Soaking and heat processing leaches out nutrients (ounce for ounce, stewed prunes have only one third the vitamins A, B and C, iron and fiber of raw).

♦ Prunes may be sliced or diced and tossed with steamed grains, slit and stuffed with nut or bean butters, juiced as a supplement to morning beverages, or puréed into a bread spread or fat/sugar substitute in baking.

Try the following recipe:

Beta-carotene Prune Butter

Dice 1 cup prunes, combine with ¼ cup apple or grape juice, and purée in blender or food processor until smooth.

Use as a jam/jelly spread or as a fat/sugar substitute in baking.

Variation: Use figs in place of prunes and ¼ cup prune juice instead of apple/grape juice.

Benefits healing zones: 2, 3, 6, 7

Also see: Cancer, Coronary Heart Disease, Fatigue, Diabetes, Juices, Low Blood Pressure

---

* Repeated consumption of sulphur dioxide has been associated with kidney malfunction, destruction of B complex vitamins, and allergic reactions. Sulphur dioxide is often used to conceal defects in the fruit. Similarly, potassium sorbate, another preservative, may cause allergic flare-ups in the form of skin irritations. See Mail Order Sources.

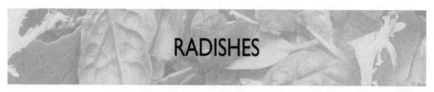

RADISHES

Haven't had a healthy bite in a week? Reach for a *Raphanus sativus*. Radishes are near-zero-in-calories members of the cabbage-mustard family (which also includes such unlikely kin as cauliflower, kale, and turnip). Introduced into Middle Asia from China in prehistoric times, they constituted a dietary staple before the appearance of the Egyptian pyramids.

In the sixteenth century, radishes were eaten with bread or served as a sauce for meat in England. Legend has it that Columbus introduced radishes to the Americas. Radishes appeared in Mexico and Haiti by the mid-1500s and were among the first vegetables grown in colonial gardens. A garden catalog mentions 10 varieties by 1806.

Radishes come in a spectrum of colors and sizes, including the oblong or long, cylindrical or tapered, white, pink, red, purple, and black. The Oriental Daikon can be found growing up to 7 feet in length and 5 pounds in weight. There are other Eastern types grown for cooking and Near Eastern varieties cultivated for greens alone. There is even an oriental variety grown exclusively for the oil from its seeds.

RED AND WHITE CURES

Nutritionally, radishes are a good source of vitamin C, potassium, phosphorus, sulfur and magnesium. Medicinally, a radish juice cocktail daily will stimulate the appetite and do double duty as a safe side-effect free diuretic, even help expel gallstones and flush out the bladder and kidney (try equal parts of radish, green pepper and cucumber; and for double the cleansing benefits, combine with beet juice, suggest natural healers).

RESPIRATORY HEALING AND MORE

Grated, sliced, or juiced, radishes are excellent for loosening catarrhal congestion, especially in the sinuses. Try a teaspoon of pure radish juice at 30-minute intervals to lick laryngitis, suggests the American Association of Naturopathic Physicians.

Black and blue? Grated radish applied as a poultice will stop internal bleeding in a bruise.

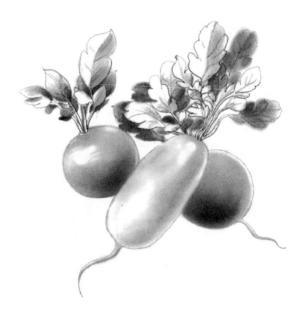

Need an antistress rich-in-nerve-nourishing-B-complex cocktail? Combine equal parts of radish juice and prune juice and a pinch or two of rice polish.

Buying, Storing, and Using

- ◆ Look for roots that are well-formed, smooth, and firm with sturdy greens intact. With greens attached, radishes will keep up to one week in the crisper. To crisp, refrigerate in a bowl of ice water.
- ◆ Radishes are best utilized raw, greens and all, diced or shredded in salads. juiced or pickled. They may also be sprouted. In this form, radishes supply 50 times more vitamin A than an orange and twice the vitamin C of a lemon.
- ◆ Braise young greens briefly and serve with butter as a spinach substitute.
- ◆ Chill and serve French-style with sweet butter and salt, or slice paper-thin, dress with vinaigrette, and eat as a relish, German-style.

Try this recipe:

Pink Radishes

> *3 tablespoons unsalted butter*
>
> *⅓ cup minced scallions*
>
> *3 cups thinly sliced radishes, red or white (or a combination)*
>
> *⅓ cup water or alcohol-free white wine*
>
> *Freshly ground black or white pepper to taste*

Heat butter in saucepan. Add onion and cook, stirring for three minutes. Add radishes and water or wine. Simmer for three to four minutes, shaking pan to prevent sticking. Season with pepper after draining (when radishes will have turned a pale pink). Serve on a bed of raw radish (or watercress) greens. 6-8 servings.

A 3½-ounce serving of raw radishes supplies about 20 calories.

Benefits healing zones: 4, 7

Also see: Cystitis, Juices, Common Cold, Stress, Kidney Stones

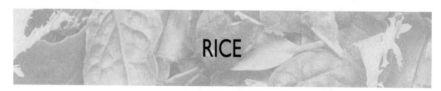

RICE

Rice is more than nice; it is, as the Sanskrit word for this ubiquitous grain puts it, "a sustainer of the human race." Indeed, there are more than 40,000 varieties worldwide, and for two thirds of the world's peoples rice is a life-supportive staple.

THE NEARLY PERFECT FOOD

In its natural state (unprocessed white or brown rice, long and short grain), rice is a premier source of growth nutrients—including B-complex vitamins, iron, and calcium—and comparable in vitamins, minerals, and caloric content to whole wheat, but with a higher quality of proteins. Combined with beans or a soy food or dairy product, rice provides complete protein (comparable to meat, fish, or poultry) and less fat and sodium.

Thanks to its fiber and a compound called gamma-oryzanol, untreated rice bran helps lower serum cholesterol and promotes growth. Like all whole grains, rice is a source of bone- and heart-strengthening calcium. Combine with nuts and seeds for an anti-osteoporosis snack.

SLIMMING DOWN WITH MIRACLE STARCH

A regimen of unsalted rice and whole fruits, a tradition in natural healing since the 1940s, has a fill-you-up-not-out effect, thanks to rice's fatigue-fighting B-complex vitamins and fluid-regulating potassium. It also provides significant amounts of vitamin E for normal heart function. The low sodium content of rice makes it an ideal choice for weight watchers with kidney and blood pressure disorders.

Anticancer Seed

Like all seed foods, rice contains high levels of protease inhibitors (that help prevent or retard the growth of tumors), while rice bran lowers the risk of bowel cancer. Indeed, populations that eat the most rice (along with beans) consistently show the lowest rates of colon, breast, and prostate cancer.

RICE, NOT DRUGS, FOR CONTROL OF DIARRHEA AND INDIGESTION

For 3,000 years, boiled rice preparations have been used by natural healers to treat infant diarrhea by rehydrating the body and increasing stool volume (use 1 teaspoon of salt to 1 liter of water and ¼ cup rice). Rice is also prescribed in Oriental medicine for digestive disorders.

Buying, Storing, and Using

Choose the right rice. Long grain white is fluffier. Short grain white and brown types are chewier and stickier. Pass up "instant" rices, which are deficient in fiber, protein, vitamins, and minerals. In the process of polishing, up to 80% of vitamin B_1, 65% of B_3 (niacin), and 50% of B_6 is lost, along with essential oils. Preferable but not perfect is converted or parboiled rice, which has been steam treated prior to milling. Or treat yourself to the specialty grain (besides Basmati) rices such as Delta Rose, Wehani, wild pecan, and American Texmati, which are 10 times richer in the healing substance 2-acetyle-1-pyrroline (also in nuts and corn), the secret ingredient which produces the "popped corn" aroma and flavor-making compound.

Note: Wild rice—a native North American grain and not a rice at all—is higher in protein, zinc, and magnesium and lower in fat but comparable calorically to brown rice and cooked the same way.

COOKING TIMETABLE

	Water	Time	Yield
Wild Rice			
I cup	3 cups	I hr.	4 cups
White/Brown Rice			
I cup	2 cups	45 min.	3 cups

Nine Success Tips

♦ Use a heavy pot with a tight-fitting lid and stir to assure top-to-bottom doneness.

♦ Cooked rice keeps up to a week refrigerated and reheats in minutes in a microwave.

♦ For a perfect potful every time? Buy a rice cooker (useful in cooking all your whole grain meals). Second best method for the time-pressed—a crock pot or pressure cooker. But pass up the microwave except for reheats (sprinkle 1 teaspoon water over 1 cup of cooked grain, cover, process on high for 2 minutes).

♦ Try woodsy-flavored wild rice in soups, stuffings, salads, or dried fruits.

♦ Leftover rice? Make Potlikker Brittle: Pat warm or cold cooked grain onto wax paper to 1/4-inch thickness. Chill until thoroughly dried to snap off into bite-size snacks.

♦ Rice plus? Sprout it, don't steam it. Sprouting increases water soluble vitamin B complex and fat soluble vitamin E.

♦ For a tastier, more nutritious popcorn alternative, put whole brown rice through your steam popper.

♦ Eating out? Opt for steamed—not fried—rice and save 150 calories and 13 grams of fat per 1-cup serving.

♦ Short and sweet: Stickier short grain rice is better in casseroles or as a sweet side dish such as rice pudding.

Try this recipe:

Steamed Brown Rice Bread

1 cup brown rice flour or rice polish

1 cup white flour

1 cup graham or whole wheat flour

1½ teaspoons baking soda

1 tablespoon vinegar

1 cup nonfat milk

1 cup lowfat sour cream or yogurt

½ cup honey or to taste

1 cup raisins (optional)

Mix together rice flour or polish, white and graham or whole wheat flours, and baking soda.

Combine vinegar, milk, and sour cream or yogurt. Add honey, raisins. Combine two mixtures; stir well.

Fill well-oiled 1-pound coffee cans two thirds full. Cover tightly with foil and steam in a large, lidded pot with a steamer rack for three hours. When bread has cooled (but is still warm), loosen with a table knife and knock from can.

Makes 8 to 10 servings.

Benefits healing zones: 3, 5, 6, 7

Also see: **Bran, Fatigue, Basic Dieting Facts and Advice, Indigestion, Low Blood Pressure, Kidney Stone**

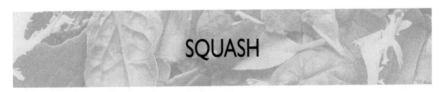

SQUASH

What can you eat a half cup of each day that could lower your risk of lung cancer by 50%—or, even better, a half cup of plus seeds that could protect you from colon, bowel and bladder cancer, kidney disorder, and constipation? The answer is squash, and every form of it—from summer zucchinis to fall pumpkins and multicolored turban and winter pumpkins—is a super healer.

Squash belongs to the gourd or melon family native to Central America of pre-Columbian times and it falls into two major categories:

summer (including white, yellow, bush scallop, crookedneck or straight neck zucchini) and winter squash (including pumpkin, butternut, acorn and Hubbard, and spaghetti).

SQUASH
A Six-Kinds-of-Cancer Fighting Protection

Winter squashes top the list of the 45 vegetables which the Tokyo National Cancer Institute cites as factors in populations where cancer rates are low. In fact, deep-orange squashes are a defense against six forms of cancer (esophageal, stomach, lung, bladder, laryngeal, and prostate), and, with carrots, are the top three foods for prevention and control of lung cancer even among heavy smokers. (Smokers who ate 2½ servings of squash a day were the group with the greatest reduced risk of lung cancer, according to a National Cancer Institute study of nicotine-dependent New Jersey males.)

A high intake of squash and other deep-orange vegetables provides protection from second-hand smoke. Dark yellow vegetables like winter squash are a good source of cancer-fighting nutrients such as vitamin C and beta-carotenes, which block the destructive activity of free radical scavengers, as well as iron for healthy blood, plenty of fiber, complex carbohydrates (the preferred source of calories for diabetics and dieters), potassium and magnesium for a healthy heart, and reproductive health nutrients folate and vitamin B_6.

Summer squashes aren't far behind. One of the lowest calorie counts in the vegetable kingdom (14 per serving) and a respectable fiber content makes zucchini a great staple for weight watchers. In addition to potassium and magnesium used to convert vitamin D into its active form, zucchini provides vitamin C (to improve iron absorption) and folate to improve resistance and prevent reproductive dysfunction.

PUMPKIN SEED POWER

Both pumpkin and squash seeds are nothing to sneeze at. Both are a rich source of protease trypsin inhibitors, which prevent the activation of viruses in the intestinal tract, as well as zinc and essential fatty acids, which protect the prostate gland and reproductive organs.

HAVE A SQUASH, THE HAVE-A-HEART VEGETABLE

Putting a little hot buttered pumpkin* or summer squash on your plate can contribute to peak cardiovascular health. Virtually free of fat and heart-risky sodium, squash supplies beneficial amounts of potassium and magnesium (the twin minerals that help prevent strokes) plus plenty of cholesterol-lowering insoluble fiber (as much as spinach, twice as much as tomatoes) along with vitamin C, the vitamin antioxidant that helps prevent plaque build-up in arteries.

AROUND-THE-WORLD HEALING

Pumpkin seed tea is a Cherokee Indian folk medicine for edema, gout, and kidney stones. In India and parts of Europe, squash pulp is used as a compress to relieve headaches, earaches, neuralgia, and burns. In Ethiopia, pumpkin and squash seeds are used as purgatives and laxatives. Among the Zuni Indians of Arizona, pumpkin seeds and squash flowers are used to heal wounds and scars.

Best juice partners: parsley, celery, and carrot.

Buying, Storing, and Using

For winter varieties, look for firm, brightly colored, unwaxed, unblemished squashes and pumpkins. With the stem on, winter squashes will keep up to two months in a cool, dry place. TIP: Best pie type—blue Hubbard, butternut, and New England pie.

For summer squashes, buy firm, small (tastier) zucchinis and patty pans and refrigerate. Eat raw (unpeeled, seeds and all), steam, or stir-fry briefly. Or add to casseroles, soups, cooked grains, and pasta dishes. Or stuff and bake.

Allergic to grain? Don't pass up pasta. Get it from spaghetti squash. These football-shaped vegetables contain golden strands that resemble angel hair pasta and can be plucked out after the squash is halved and steamed or microwaved.

Make quick gazpacho: Toss two sliced zucchini in the food processor with one tomato, half an onion, one clove of garlic, 1 tablespoon of

---

* For a change of pace, try a mini (single-serving-sized) pumpkin, a sweet-flavored squash/pumpkin hybrid that has 50 calories and plenty of beta-carotene.

lemon juice, and 1 cup of tomato juice. Blend until chunky soup consistency.

Make zucchini bars: Split a zucchini lengthwise, scoop out the center. Sauté an onion and celery with zucchini pulp. Mix in cooked rice and fill hollow zucchini halves. Bake in the oven at 350 degrees for 30 minutes. Top with low-fat grated cheese; bake five minutes more.

Grow your own green or yellow zucchini. Snip the unopened blossoms with a 1-inch stem, dip in egg batter, and quick-cook in hot oil for low-calorie, no-fat fake fried oysters. (Ditto for cucumber blossoms.)

If you're big on pumpkins,* send for the how-to-grow-world-class-giant-pumpkin catalogs from Annedawn Publishing, Box 247-G, Norton, MA 02766 ($14.95 plus $3 shipping and handling).

Six Ways to Use and Cook a Winter Squash

♦ Grate and add to salads, stir-fried vegetable dishes, or cole slaw.

♦ Slice and dice and steam over a pot of boiling water until tender. Sprinkle with cinnamon or nutmeg for extra flavor. When nearly cooked, add chopped greens, and season with lemon.

♦ Slice, dice, and sauté in oil, with or without spices, to bring out the flavor. Toss with other vegetables and water for a bright sauce or soup.

♦ Bake small whole pumpkins for one to two hours until fork easily pierces skin. Open and scoop out the flesh and mash. Or slice in half, scoop out the seeds, oil the cavity, and fill with a cooked grain (herbed buckwheat, millet, or rice). Place in open pan with ½ inch water, cover and bake at 400 degrees until tender. To bake squash quickly, peel and cube, add seasoning, and bake in a covered dish for 30 minutes.

♦ Add 1½ cups of squash cubes to millet, rice, buckwheat, or barley, and simmer together. Squash adds color appeal to side dishes or breakfast cereals.

---

* The world's record for largest pumpkin—827 pounds—is held by a Washington State pumpkin breeder.

◆ Steam, boil or bake squash until soft, then mash, or purée and season—use ginger juice, cinnamon, orange peel, a few cranberries, or tahini—for a mousse-smooth side dish. Or fill a pie shell.

Try the following recipes:

Beta-carotene Purée

1 medium-size butternut squash, peeled and cut into ¹/₂-inch cubes

1¹/₂ teaspoons grated fresh ginger

1 teaspoon grated orange rind

Freshly ground pepper to taste.

Place squash in a medium-size saucepan and cover with cold water. Place over medium-high heat and bring to a boil. Reduce heat, simmer until tender (about 10 minutes). Drain.

Place squash in a food processor with ginger and rind. Process until smooth. Add pepper and serve immediately.

Makes four servings.

Pumpkin-Rice Pudding

2 cups cooked pumpkin or winter squash

1 cup milk or water

3 to 5 tablespoons honey (or to taste)

1 tablespoon tahini or nut butter

1¹/₂ teaspoons pumpkin pie spice

1 or 2 eggs or ¹/₂ cup tofu

2 cups cooked brown rice

¹/₂ cup raisins or currants

Blend pumpkin or squash, milk or water, honey, tahini, pumpkin pie spice, and egg(s) or tofu until smooth. Combine with rice and raisins or currants.

Pour into a greased casserole. Place in a pan of hot water and bake at 350 degrees for one hour or until the knife comes out clean. Serve warm or chilled, with or without yogurt topping.

Makes a good dessert or hearty breakfast. (Six servings)

Benefits healing zones: 2, 3, 6, 9

Also see: Cancer, Beta-carotene, Basic Dieting Facts and Advice

SOYBEANS

If you want to amount to more than a hill of beans, keep soybeans on your menus. In the form of cooked, fresh, or dried whole beans, tofu, tempeh, miso, sprouts, soy, milk or flour, soyas provide more protection from cancer, heart disease, osteoporosis, stress, diabetes, and bowel disorders than any other member of the 5,000-strong pulse-legume family. The soybean is the queen bean in terms of quality and versatility.

PROTEIN FOR WEIGHT AND MOOD CONTROL

Soybeans are 40 to 50% protein (twice as much as ordinary dried beans). In fact, adding a single tablespoon of soy powder to 4 tablespoons of cornmeal doubles the protein of the baked goods made from it. What's more, that protein is rich in mood-boosting antidepressant amino acids and is comparable to meat, eggs, and dairy. Soybeans are the only reliable food source of the natural appetite suppressants and antidepressant amino acid D-phenylalanine, and they are the only phenylalanine food that's low in fat. Soybeans are only 17% fat (100% of it unsaturated). Another antidepressant factor in soybeans is lecithin, which is essential for the health of the nervous system.

MILK A BEAN FOR A BETTER-THAN-DAIRY SOURCE OF MINERALS AND ANTIOXIDANT VITAMINS

Soybean milk* is richer in potassium (an antiaging mineral that increases energy) than cow's milk and has 15 times more iron, 50% less fat, no cholesterol, and calcium with no growth hormones and one tenth the hazardous agricultural residues found in dairy milk. Tofu (along with yogurt) is one of the two best sources of calcium recommended by the Osteoporosis Foundation for meeting adult calcium needs (1,000 mg daily) to prevent osteoporosis, the brittle-bone disorder that affects 25 million Americans (one 4-ounce serving of tofu provides twice the calcium of 1 cup of plain yogurt).

---

* An important part of the Chinese breakfast, according to traditional Oriental medicine, soy milk contributes to *chi*, the universal life energy which is also considered a measure of one's health.

Soybeans provide the antioxidant vitamins A and E and, when sprouted, compare favorably with citrus fruits as a source of antioxidant vitamin C. In addition, soybeans are a source of zinc (a mineral that women are commonly deficient in), which is necessary for the protein synthesis that makes healing possible. (Half a cup of miso or natto soy paste supplies two thirds of your RDA of zinc.)

USING YOUR BEAN TO PROTECT YOUR HEART AND LIVER

In ongoing studies conducted at European health clinics, an eight-week regimen of soy foods in place of animal protein foods produced typical cholesterol reductions of 23 to 25%—similar to those produced by most cholesterol-lowering drugs (results are especially dramatic in cases of Type A hyper-proteinemea, in which there is a higher than average risk of death from heart attack).

Soybeans supply linolenic acid, one of the omega-3 oils, a natural substance that helps lower cholesterol and prevent the risk of coronary disease by as much as 25%. Soybeans are also the richest known source of lecithin, which protects the liver by promoting digestion of fats, prevents fat build-up on artery walls, and helps lower the concentration of cholesterol and other fats in the bloodstream. An unknown factor in lecithin improves the utilization of vitamins E and A. Lecithin also supplies energizing B vitamins, especially inositol and choline, vital to the functioning of the liver. Lecithin is available naturally in soybeans and is sold as a granular or liquid supplement.

Studies indicate that eating soy foods of any type six times a week can reduce high cholesterol by 20% or more and helps age-proof the arteries. Even switching to a semivegetarian diet can reduce your atherosclerosis risk by 50%, says a Duke University/Harvard University study funded by the National Institutes of Health. A soybean-intensive diet even appears to counteract the effects of a high-fat diet.

THE SOYBURGER DEFENSE AGAINST CANCER

A soy-intensive diet is one of the best dietary ways to cancer-proof your body, suggest Japanese studies in which miso (soy paste) soup* once a day reduced the incidence of stomach cancer by 30%.

---

* Drawback: Miso is excessively high in sodium; low-sodium natto is a better soy-base choice.

Breast cancer is also responsive to the antitumor phytochemical isoflavones and 2-phytyosterols in soybeans (including genistein, found *only* in soy). The natural estrogen-like substances* that soybeans contain appear to help normalize elevated female hormone levels (which have been linked to reproductive system cancers), say Italian scientists at the Center for the Study of Hyperlipidemias of the University of Milan.

TWO TYPES OF SOY FIBER FOR FIVE BENEFITS

Soy fiber, say researchers for the American Dietetic Association, provides both the cholesterol-lowering value of soluble fiber plus the bowel and colon protective benefits of insoluble fiber (which also helps prevent or dissolve gallstones and relieves constipation).

Soy protein is the top-rated vegetable food for maintaining normal blood sugar energy levels on the glycemic index compiled by Dr. James Anderson.

Antiviral Action

As if that weren't enough, soybeans are the plant kingdom's primary source of protease inhibitors (also found in nuts, beans, and all seed foods, including grains), a substance that helps control blood clotting and inactivates viruses that trigger gastrointestinal disorders, influenza, pox virus, and retroviruses associated with leukemia, according to researchers at Johns Hopkins University School of Medicine.

Using Your Bean

Soybeans can be roasted like peanuts or chestnuts; baked like kidney beans; steamed or deep fried like dumplings; sprouted like alfalfa; stir-fried like mung beans; cultured into yogurt, cream cheese, or tofu; fermented into counterfeit Camembert cheese or tempeh; sauced to taste like mock veal-, chicken-, or tuna-burgers; and aged into soy sauce, teriyaki, or the miracle high-protein soup, sauce, and gravy base called miso and natto. Other uses include soy spaghetti; soy milk and soybean ice cream for the lactose intolerant; and ground and roasted soybeans, which pinch hit for decaf when perked.

---

*Also found in some 2,000 other plant foods.

Buying, Storing, and Using Soy Products

Tofu: (Also called soybean curd): Tofu is made from curds from ground, cooked soybeans drained and pressed into custard-like cakes. Firm and soft indicate density; silken indicates a very smooth texture. Some types are calcium fortified. Tofu is highly perishable. Refrigerate in water up to four days after opening. Aseptically packaged tofu may be stored at room temperature until opened. Tofu may be sliced, diced, mashed, eaten raw, steamed, baked, or stir-fried. Substitute for ground meat, cottage cheese, or eggs (use 4 ounces puréed soft tofu for each egg in baking).

Tempeh: Tempeh is made from cooked fermented soybeans and is the richest known nonanimal source of vitamin B_{12}; it is also highly digestible. It is available in a variety of flavors; it can be used in dairy case items such as chili, Sloppy Joes, and burgers. Refrigerate up to 10 days or freeze for up to two months. Tempeh is a tasty meat alternative and good in stir-fries, stews, chili, sauces, salads, or as a vegetable stuffing.

Miso and Natto: This is a soy paste rich in B-complex vitamins and iron. The lighter the color, the lighter the flavor. (*Note:* Do not boil, or the digestive enzymes it contains are destroyed.) It is best refrigerated and keeps indefinitely. Use this cheese-flavored condiment to start soups or sauces, as a color or flavor enhancer, as a broth, or tea or coffee substitute.

Soy Milk: This is a noncurdled liquid from cooked, ground soybeans. It is a good high-protein, low-fat alternative to cow's milk and is available as 1% milk and in powdered and flavored forms.

Refrigerate soy milk, as for cow's milk. Aseptically sealed cartons may be stored at room temperature until opened. Substitute equal amounts of soy milk for dairy milk in cooking and baking.

Soy Cheese: Soy cheese is similar to tofu, but more liquid is removed and a solidifier is added. Keep refrigerated. Flavors include cheddar, mozzarella, and spiced jack.

Soy Sauce: Soy sauce is made from soybeans that are salted and fermented with wheat. It is lighter tasting than tamari. Look for low-salt versions.

Store at room temperature for up to six months. Use soy sauce for an Oriental seasoning and dipping sauce. Soy sauce becomes saltier during long storage.

Textured Vegetable Protein (TVP): TVP has a ground meat quality. Simply stir into a dish and cook for 15 minutes. For each cup TVP added, allow 1½ cups extra liquid. Store TVP in an airtight container for up to two months. Use TVP as a protein source in sauces, stews, soups, and casseroles.

By Bean Alone

If you decide to have a bowl of soybeans or a plate of tofu rather than chopped steak, here are a few of the dietary essentials you stand to gain or lose:

	TOFU 4 oz. (½ firm cake)	SOYBEANS 4 oz. (⅝ cup cooked)	HAMBURGER ⅓ lb. raw (4 oz. cooked)
Calories	150	146	298
Carbohydrates (grams)	3	11.8	0
Usable protein (grams)	10	7.6	19.4
Fat (grams)	8	6.2	19.3
Fiber (grams)	0.2	1.7	0
Vitamin A (IU)	0	31	0
Iron (mg)	3.2	3	3.3
Calcium (mg)	53.4	81	8
Sodium (mg)	6.7	25	53.3
Phosphorus (mg)	189	199	249.3

Source: USDA Handbook., 1994, U.S. Dept. of Agriculture

Try these recipes:

Sweet and Sour Soybeans

> 2 tablespoons low-salt soy sauce
>
> 1 tablespoon vinegar
>
> 1 tablespoon cooking wine
>
> 2 teaspoons natural sugar
>
> 1½ tablespoons cornstarch or arrowroot
>
> 5 tablespoons water
>
> 1 cup soybeans, rinsed and soaked for 4 hours or overnight
>
> 1 onion, chopped

2 slices ginger, finely minced

oil for cooking

Mix soy sauce, vinegar, cooking wine, sugar, starch, and water in a cup; set aside.

In a medium pot, combine beans and 5 cups of water and cook until soft (3 hours if stovetop boiling, 15 minutes if pressure cooking). Drain, then place them in cold water to cool. Drain again.

In an oiled skillet, stir-fry the onion and ginger until fragrant. Add beans, stir fry 30 seconds, and add the soy sauce mixture, stirring until the sauce thickens.

Garnish with sliced citrus or fresh grape clusters.

3 servings.

Soy-Citrus Sherbet

1¹/₂ cups 1% light soy milk

1¹/₂ cups fresh orange juice (about 5 oranges) with pulp

1 tablespoon grated orange zest

¹/₄ cup unsweetened orange juice concentrate

Combine all ingredients in a large bowl and chill at least one hour. Freeze mixture in an ice cream maker according to manufacturer's instructions. Let "ripen" one hour in the freezer before serving.

Only 63 calories per ¹/₂ cup serving and 9% total fat from calories.

Benefits healing zones: 2, 3, 5, 6, 7, 8

Also see: Coronary Heart Disease, Cancer, Vegetarian Foods, Osteoporosis

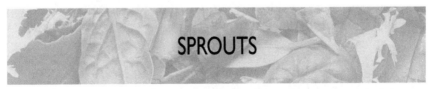

SPROUTS

Tout a sprout! Since they are usually eaten fresh (raw) with all their high-fiber goodness intact, germinated seeds—which have been with us since 2939 B.C.—are a first-rate source of minerals and vitamins A, B, C, D, even G and K. If you don't like vitamin K source foods such as beef liver, sprouts are the answer (vitamin K is the anti-blood-clotting factor nutrient). Sprouts are good fiber foods, good diet foods, and good energy foods. And they cost only 3 cents a cup to grow (1 pound produces 10 cups of food).

800% MORE ANTIOXIDANT VITAMIN C

The vitamin C in sprouted peas increases by as much as 800% in four days over that found in dry peas. In lentils and mung beans, it triples; the B-complex vitamins increase in sprouted wheat from 20% to over 600%, and vitamin E in sprouted wheat increases to 300% in four days. Unsprouted wheat kernels supply only 28 grams of folic acid (the nutrient that protects reproductive functions) but, when sprouted, supply 106 grams.

Studies indicate that ½ cup of soybean sprouts contains as much vitamin C as six glasses of orange juice. Sprouts eaten raw are a storehouse of enzymes, which occur by the billions in the body and perform over 700 separate activities. (Over 100,000 enzyme particles can be found in a single drop of blood.) Once a seed or legume is soaked for four to eight hours—the first step in sprouting—its enzyme factory comes to life. In addition, sprouting facilitates the digestion of hard-to-eat foods. The fats and oils in seeds are converted by the enzyme lipase into carbohydrates when sprouted, making them twice as digestible as the seeds themselves. These are the same factors that break down the fats and oils in body cells. These so-called lipotropic elements are prodigiously prevalent in sprouts.

Sprouting also causes hydrolyzation of protein, the breaking down of protein into its component amino acids—a boon if you are short on hydrochloric acid (common after age 40) and/or have trouble handling protein.

Beans (such as lentils, mung, and soy beans) and grains (such as wheat and rye) contain so-called trypsin inhibitors and phytates, which, if *not* denatured by cooking or sprouting, can interfere with protein digestion in the gut (which is promoted by the enzyme trypsin) and/or with the uptake of minerals.*

---

* Phytic acid, for example, renders zinc biologically unavailable and can produce zinc deficiency syndromes, including stunted growth, retarded development, and anorexia. (This same mineral unavailability occurs when large amounts of rhubarb, berries, or spinach are eaten.)

Nothing's a bigger help in the right weight-watching direction than sprout salads, breads, and stir-fries. Sprouts are rich in lecithin to speed up fat breakdown and reduce cholesterol and are low in calories. One fully packed cup of our most commonly eaten sprouted seed—alfalfa—adds less than 50 calories to your diet.

More important, sprouts are nature's top source of that miracle trace mineral and antioxidant, chlorophyll, which is chemically related to human hemoglobin.

Sprouts are rich in cardiovascular and digestive health-boosting fiber. Bread made from sprouted whole grain, for example, contains 300% more fiber than white bread and 24% more than most whole wheat products.

NATURE'S LOW-CALORIE UPPER

Sprouts even supply aspartic acid, which stimulates natural hormones in the body, says biochemist Dr. Roger Williams. (Aspartic acid is also found in almonds and in pits of apricots and lemons.)

Despite their modest calorie count, sprouts are a high-energy food. The natural sugar they contain is in the monosaccaride form, which enters the bloodstream immediately after rapidly breaking down. Because sprouts are high in enzymes, they are easy to digest.

Buying, Storing, and Using

You can buy sprouts singly or premixed, ready to eat or ready to grow. Any untreated seed, grain, legume, or vegetable can be sprouted (except sunflower seeds, which must be shelled first). Best big and small choices: alfalfa, clover, lentil, mung. One pound of seed yields between six and eight pounds of sprouts.

From Seed to Sprouts

1. Use a large, wide-mouth container, such as a 1-quart Mason jar, plus a square of cheesecloth, gauze, netting, or nylon to cover the jar opening. Put ¼ to ½ cup of dry seeds into jar. (A good beginner's mixture is 3 teaspoons alfalfa plus 5 teaspoons of lentils. A few mung beans or whole wheat may be added.)

2. Fill jar half full with lukewarm water. After six to eight hours, agitate jar, fasten netting in place with a rubber band, and pour off soaking water. Place jar on its side in a warm, dark spot in the

kitchen. Rinse and drain seeds twice a day with tepid water without removing netting. After two days, place container in indirect sunlight to increase chlorophyll content. If you are sprouting a seed that grows leaves (see the following chart), place in indirect sunlight. Sink strainers, colanders, collapsible steamers, and large spice jars with perforated snap-on caps make suitable sprouters, too. So do backpackers' perforated plastic sacks. To hasten sprouts' growth, leave a sterling silver fork or spoon in the jar. Silver contains a growth-promoting substance, sprouting veterans say.

3. Most seeds sprout in three to five days. When the "tails" are about twice as long as the seed itself, they are ready to eat. For maximum nutrition, eat the sprouts raw, eat all of the sprout, and eat it soon. (Sprouts are highly perishable and keep only a few days refrigerated.)

Do's and Don'ts

◆ Do not sprout the seeds of tomatoes, potatoes, or lima beans, which contain a substance that yields hydrocyanic acid when eaten.

◆ Don't freeze sprouts; their nutritional value lies in their freshness. Instead, cover any surplus with cold water and refrigerate for no more than two days.

◆ Don't use anything but chemically untreated (organic), certified edible seeds. Commercial bean seeds for planting are sometimes treated with fungicides that render them inedible.

◆ Don't use water containing fluorine, chlorine, or similar chemicals, which may sterilize the seed's embryo and prevent germination.

◆ When mixing seeds for combo sprouting, the most important consideration is time. Seeds which take approximately the same time to harvest make the best companions.

◆ Know which seeds "green" (sprout leaves, i.e., alfalfa). (Leaf sprouters combine well with seeds, grains, and legumes which don't.) Seeds which can be grown to the green-leaved stage by the common jar or bag method include alfalfa, clover, radish, mustard, fenugreek, cabbage, Chinese cabbage, clover, and turnip.

◆ Don't sprout alfalfa with pumpkin, almond, sunflower, sesame, grains, large beans, or mucilaginous seeds such as flax, chia, and cress. But just about any other partnership gets a grower's green light.

Now that you know how to raise sprouts, how're you going to eat them? Sprouts are best enjoyed out of hand, like peanuts, and provide the most nourishment raw—in salads, slaws, juices, soups, salad dressings, even cold cereal. The best places to put sprouts when you do cook them are breads, casseroles, omelets, pancakes, stir-fries, Sloppy Joes, meatloaves, or even tossed with hot grains and noodles. Here's a sampler to get you started.

SPROUTING CHART

Seed	Method of Sprouting	Amount of Seed for Qt. Jar	Soaking Time (Hrs)	Sprouting Time (Days)	Length at Harvest (Inches)
Alfalfa	Jar/tray	2 T	5–8	4–6	1½–2 G
Buckwheat (unhulled)	soil	—	12–18	8–12	5–7
Clover	Jar/tray	2½ T	6–8	4–6	1½–2 G
Fenugreek	Jar	½ C	8–10	3–5	½–2
Lentil	Jar	¾ C	8–12	2–3	½–¼
Lettuce	Jar	3 T	6–8	4–5	1–1½ G
Mung bean	Jar	⅓ C	12–16	3–5	1–3
Oats	Jar/towel	1½ C	1–2	3	LS
Pea	Jar	2 C	10–15	3	½–¼
Popcorn	Jar	1½ C	12–16	2–3	½
Pumpkin	Jar	1½ C	8–10	2–3	½
Radish	Jar	3 T	6–10	4–5	½ G
Rice	Jar	1½ C	10–12	3–4	LS
Rye	Jar/soil	1 C	10–12	2–3	LS
Sesame	Jar	2 C	8–10	3	LS
Soybean	Jar	¾ C	12–16	3–4	½–2
Sunflower	Jar	1 C	6–12	2–5	½–1½
Wheat (hulled)	Jar/soil	1 C	10–12	2–3	LS

KEY:

G = greened (the sprouts can be put near a window where their leaves will develop chlorophyll and turn green);

LS = length of seed;

C = cup;

T = tablespoon.

Try these recipes:

Mung Foo Yong

>*4 eggs, beaten*
>
>*1 cup mung bean sprouts, coarsely chopped*
>
>*6 sliced scallions (including tops)*
>
>*½ cup celery, shredded*
>
>*Oil, 1 tablespoon*

Heat oil in a heavy pan. Combine ingredients except oil, and sauté on both sides as you would pancakes—one tablespoon at a time. Serve hot with light soy sauce or hot mustard.

Makes two to four servings.

Dessert Stir-Fries
(stir-fried sprouts and fruit)

>*Nut or vegetable oil, 1-2 tablespoons*
>
>*2 cups sprouted wheat, rye, triticale, or rice berries*
>
>*1 large apple, cored, peeled, and shredded*
>
>*Sunflower seeds*
>
>*Pinch allspice*

Preheat wok or skillet. Heat a small amount of oil.

Add sprouted grain, stir-fry for three to four minutes. Add fruit, stir-fry until soft. Stir in seeds and spice. Serve for dessert, breakfast, or snack.

Makes four to five servings.

Grow up to 30 different kinds of seeds simultaneously with a triple-decker grower, sold at most health food stores. Or try a sprouting "tube" that automatically removes hulls. See Mail Order Sources for a selection of organic seeds dealers.

Benefits healing zones: 3, 6

Also see: Basic Dieting Facts and Advice, Vegetarian Foods, Nuts, Seeds

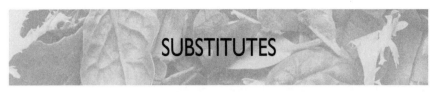

SUBSTITUTES

Is there life after chocolate cessation? Is there a next best thing to regular coffee, white sugar, real creamery butter, or old-fashioned and other foods that contain full-sodium salt and contribute to anxiety, obesity, insomnia, asthma, allergies, depressed immunity, and a whole lot more, but taste, smell, look, or feel too good to give up?

There is, and what's more, the whole-food solution 9 times out of 10 isn't half bad. (Unless otherwise noted, most of the below are "taste swaps" and often a whole lot less caloric.)

101 SUBSTITUTES FOR THE THINGS YOU DON'T, WON'T, OR SHOULDN'T EAT OR DRINK

INSTEAD OF	TRY
Dairy	
Butter	Avocado purée, tahini
Whole milk	Lowfat wheat, rice or soy milk
Cheese, cubed	Cauliflower florets (raw)
Chocolates I	Freeze ripe black cherries in a single layer. Store in plastic bag. Eat while slightly icy.
Chocolates II	Prunes, simmered in sweet alcohol-free wine
Cocoa/Hot chocolate	Prunes puréed in skim milk or carob made with lowfat non dairy milk
Mayonnaise	Plain low-fat yogurt puréed with bit of Dijon mustard; or tofu mayo
Vanilla custard	Puréed cherimoya (tropical fruit)
Fruits	
Cooking Apple	Quince (a hard green relation, for cooking)

(continued on next page)

INSTEAD OF	TRY
Fruits *(cont'd)*	
Apricot	Prickly pear (a tropical dessert fruit)
Cranberry juice*	Pomegranate juice*
Grapefruit	Pommelo or shaddock (oversized citrus fruits)
Lemon, lemon juice	Lemon grass
Lemon rind	Lemon balm, lemon thyme, or lemon verbena (all herbs), (herbs), or tamarind peel
McIntosh apple	Atemoya (Colombian fruit)
Melon juice	Juiced kiwi
Peach custard	Fresh puréed mango
Pineapple/guava	Feijoa (Latin American fruit)
Plums, grapes, apples fruit cup	Diced Carambola (tropical fruit)
Raspberries	Boysenberries
Vegetables & Herbs	
Artichokes	Cardoons (vegetable) or
Bean fajitas (high calorie)	Soy tempeh fajitas (low calorie)
Celery hearts	Cardoon or celeriac (celery root)
Coriander (spice)	Lemon peel and cinnamon
Corn (fresh)	Dumpling squash (raw, diced)
Creamed spinach	Creamed nettles
Cucumber flavor	Borage leaves
Garlic and pine nuts	Shitake mushrooms
Lima beans	Green soybeans
Morels (mushrooms)	Dandelion blossoms (flour and fry in oil)
Potato chips I	Paper-thin slices of raw turnip or jicama (root vegetable)
Potato chips II	Paper-thin slices of raw parsnip or turnip
Potatoes (cold, for salad)	Jerusalem artichoke (peeled, diced)
Sage	Chia seeds
Sage leaves	Chia seeds
Spinach, creamed	Nettles, creamed (wild herb green)

* or vice versa

INSTEAD OF	TRY

Vegetables & Herbs *(cont'd)*

Spinach (raw) — Amaranth leaves (raw)
Chard or beet greens

Miscellaneous

INSTEAD OF	TRY
Anchovies or peanut butter	Miso
Black pepper	Winter savory
Butterless sauce	White wine reduced and whipped with yogurt
Butter and sugar (in baking)	Beta-carotene Prune Butter
Caviar (roe—fish egg)	Caviar provençale (pounded black olives seasoned with pepper and lemon juice)
Chestnuts	Star of Bethlehem bulbs (raw)
Chinese noodles	Whole wheat spaghetti, half cooked, sautéed in oil
Egg salad	Soft tofu, crumbled, seasoned, and combined with soy mayo and grated celery, herbs
Coffee	Sunflower seeds or okra seeds toasted, ground, and perked
Corn meal	Millet (high calcium) or Quinoa (complete protein)
Grape nuts cereal	Alfalfa sprouts, oven dried and crumbled
Nutmeg	Dried tansy leaves
Peanuts in shell or peas in the pod	Soy beans in pods
Pepper	Papaya seeds, dried and ground
Popped corn	Popped wheat or rice (use steam popper) to "puff" all whole grains.**
Salt	Ascorbic acid or calcium ascorbate powder
Sandwich bread	Zucchini or eggplant slices, sliced lengthwise and broiled
Shrimp seasoning	Powdered/crushed sea vegetables (dulse, hiziki, arame)
Toasted wheat germ	Toasted okara (soybean pulp)
Wine, red (cooking)	Cranberry juice and lemon
Wine, white	White grapefruit plus dash white vinegar

* See recipe under Prunes.

** Did you know that mature Fava beans will "pop" when oven dried?

Try this recipe:

No-Tomato Tomato Sauce

½ onion, chopped

2 cloves garlic, minced

1 tablespoon oil

3 medium-size beets, cooked

1½ cups cooked carrots

3 tablespoons apple cider vinegar

½ teaspoon oregano

1 teaspoon kelp or low-sodium salt

¼ cup Tamari soy sauce

Sauté onion and garlic in a large skillet in a little oil until soft. Add the beets and the carrots to the blender. Blend until smooth. Add to onions and garlic in skillet. Heat, then add remaining ingredients. Season to taste. Simmer 30 minutes.

Yield: About 5 cups. Can be used in any recipe calling for tomato sauce. Tasty on pizza.

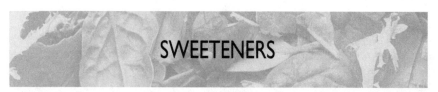

SWEETENERS

Sugar is a honey of a medicine. According to Richard Knutson, M.D., of the Delta Medical Center of Greenville, Mississippi, granulated sugar speeds healing and, as a hydrophilic agent (it absorbs moisture), reduces the swelling that accompanies injury.

Sugar may even be an aspirin alternative. Studies show that something in sucrose causes chemical changes that trigger a salicylate-like lowering of the body's sensitivity to pain.

Sugar gives hair an instant slick (mix with water and comb through), and it's a flavor enhancer. Adding ¼ teaspoon of sugar to recipes stimulates the palate so taste buds get a sharper perception of the spectrum of flavors in a food.

Sugar promotes sleep by boosting serotonin levels in the brain (which is why a sugary glass of Kool-Aid™ is a better nod-off beverage than milk), and a teaspoon of sugar (or honey) keeps cut flowers fresher longer.

A teaspoon of granulated sugar helps interrupt the hiccup cycle (try a pinch on the back of the throat). A sugary soft drink such as ginger ale acts as an active ingredient for an upset stomach and helps to restore digestion to normal.

Ordinary table sugar is also a first-rate first aid for roof-of-the-mouth burn caused by scalding hot coffee, salsa, or pizza.

Sugar's a complexion dew-gooder. Sugar cane's glycolic acid helps keep skin smooth by maintaining the acid/alkaline ratio. (Make a facial scrub by mixing grains with soapy lather. Apply, rinse off.)

Natural sugar-in-the-cane (sold in produce departments) supplies as much calcium per 4-ounces as one glass of whole milk. Peel the "sugar baton" and chew the pulp or use it to sweeten homemade baked goods.

But the bad news? If you're overdoing sugar, you may not only be undoing your dental health, you may be getting a lot less copper than you need to keep your heart healthy (one way to compensate—munch more copper-rich pumpkin seeds and cashews).

Here are a few more sour facts about our favorite recreational sweet.

Sugar is fattening.* Adding 2 tablespoons of sugar to your meals each morning can result in a weight gain of 2 pounds a month or 24 pounds a year. (One quarter cup of sugar is equal to a slice of apple pie, a Danish, or two glazed donuts.)

Sugar causes a rapid rise in the body's glucose levels and an excessive secretion of insulin, followed by an abnormal drop in blood sugar levels and fatigue that's worse than the one that caused you to reach for that sugar-rich sweet or presweetened cereal in the first place.

Sugar slows down the transport of nutrients within the teeth and throughout the body, increases stomach acids, dulls the taste, and burns up large amounts of the B vitamins necessary for energy and proper digestion.

---

* And inescapable. It accounts for 3.4% of a parsnip, 5.94% of a carrot (glucose, fructose, and sucrose), and 6.45% of a beet. Even extracted fruit juices contain as much sugar as chocolate (but juice the whole fruit and you get the bonus of more minerals and fiber to slow down sugar absorption). Vegetables low in sugar include broccoli (1.82%), celery (1.23%), and escarole (0.58%).

Sugar substitutes such as fructose, say USDA researchers, may account for most of the harmful biological effects of sucrose, including impaired insulin response and chromium and copper depletion. Substitutes such as saccharin, a suspected carcinogen, and aspartame (NutraSweet™), which adversely affects brain chemistry, are often worse.

If you must sprinkle with something, switch to maple sugar, date sugar, or minimally processed unbleached cane sugar (see Mail Order Sources). Or try rice syrup, maple syrup, or a "grain sugar" like amazake or barley syrup. Make your own fruit- and grain-based sweeteners (see the following recipes). Or trade your sugar bowl for a honey bear. Honey is the world's oldest sweetener (bees predate humans by 55 to 60 million years), and its main sugars (fructose and glucose), by contrast with table sugar, are absorbed directly into the bloodstream, providing quick energy.

Honey is an easily digested source of carbohydrates and is more palatable than sucrose. The enzymes in natural honey enhance the digestive process, while glucose (dextrose) and dextromaltose, which are found in honey, are superior to other sugars and supply vitamins like B complex and minerals like calcium in small quantities. (Sugar is 100% nutrient free.)

Moreover, honey is a honey of a medicine, useful in preventing infections because its low pH creates an unfavorable environment for bacterial growth. A tablespoon of pure honey is even said to alleviate a hangover and provide hay fever relief. According to Greenwich, Connecticut, environmental ecologist Dr. Anthony Redmond, people with hay fever who eat honey produced in the area where they live are taking in the substance to which they are allergic and develop helpful antibodies to it.

Buying, Storing, and Using

Honey usually is classified and sold as liquid, comb, solid, chunk, and cut comb. Liquid has been extracted from the comb and is free of crystals. Cut comb and comb honey are in their natural wax comb. Liquid honey that has been granulated into solid form is usually sold as creamed, churned, or candied honey. Liquid and cut comb honey packed together is called chunk honey.

Honey is also classified by color and source. Depending on floral source, honey is white or amber. Lighter white honeys are milder in flavor, while darker amber honeys have a more pronounced taste. If a honey is made from one predominant nectar source, it is referred to by that plant name (e.g., orange or clover honey). Darker honeys are generally more nutrient dense than light or clear honeys. Look for the words *unprocessed, unheated,* or *unrefined* on the label.

To retain flavor and color, store honey in a dark, cool place. Freezing helps honey retain flavor but may hasten granulation. To reliquify honey that has granulated, place container in warm water or 200-degree oven until crystals melt.

Like to solar-decant your own honey from the comb? Fill a cheesecloth bag with fresh honeycomb and suspend the sack over a large pan in a sunny window in a warm, unventilated room. Comb will self-separate in a day.

Try these recipes:

Unsugar (Counterfeit Table Sugar)

Sift together ¼ cup each of whey or milk powder (whey powder is the sweeter of the two) and arrowroot starch, and combine with ⅓ cup fine unsweetened coconut meal. You may substitute powdered fructose for ¼ cup of the coconut, if desired.

Enriched variation: Replace coconut meal with ¼ cup finely ground white sesame seeds (sesame meal contains four times more magnesium and 10 times more calcium than sunflower seeds and is an important source of a more easily assimilated form of lecithin than that available from soybeans).

Half-and-Half Honey (calorie reduced)

Blend ⅓ cup water with 1 cup honey for maple-syrup consistency. Or blend ⅕ cup water with 1 cup honey for cane-syrup consistency.

Homemade Honeycombs

Pop 4 cups of corn. Preheat oven to 325 degrees. Combine ⅓ cup natural honey, ¼ cup unsalted butter (or canola oil), and ¼ teaspoon vanilla extract. Heat gently for 10 minutes. Pour over corn and mix well until coated.

Spread on lubricated cookie sheet, and bake at 325 degrees for 15 to 20 minutes. Stir occasionally (or until dry and crispy).

Sprinkle with wheat germ or bran (optional). Cool, and spoon into container or storage bags. Serve with milk or cream or use as a snack.

Benefits healing zones: 4, 6, 7

Also see: Ten Basic Super Healing Recipes, Basic Dieting Facts and Advice; Substitutes

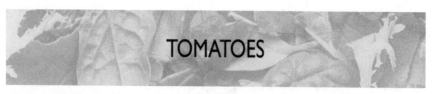

TOMATOES

The tomato is no lemon. If you're typical, you put away better than 70 pounds' worth of this fruit-vegetable, which, like avocados, is really a fruit but is eaten as a vegetable and, along with grapes and eggplants, is in fact botanically classified as a berry.

Known as the "gold" or "love" apple (and considered poisonous), the tomato was discovered in the tropics by Spanish Conquistadors, introduced to Italy in 1522, but not grown in America until the mid-eighteenth century. Like many other fruits and vegetables, tomatoes were ornamental plants and a pharmaceutical food (used in the treatment of diarrhea) before they were included in the culinary scheme of things.

Ordinary freshly juiced tomatoes are still used to rejuvenate the liver, report Japanese researchers at Tokyo University, which may explain our favorite "I-should-have-had-a-V8" vegetable's popularity as an on-the-wagon crutch for teetotalers (combine freshly juiced tomatoes with freshly juiced lemon; drink on the rocks).

TOSSING A TOMATO AT TUMORS

Tomatoes are among the National Cancer Institute's "second line of defense" foods (right behind carrots and broccoli) and one of the three richest known sources of the antioxidant lycopene, a potent anticancer carotenoid (also found in red peppers and pink grapefruit). This, as well as the antioxidants vitamin A and beta- and alphacarotene, may account for the lower stomach cancer rates among tomato-loving Hawaiians, reduced lung cancer incidence in BLT-happy Norwegians and reduced risk of prostate cancer among tomato-eating American males and seniors (who in one study had half the death from cancer of the non-tomato eaters). Lycopene-rich vegetables like tomatoes are also known to provide protection from cancers of the cervix, bladder, and pancreas.

Tomatoes also supply the vitamin antioxidant C and antioxidants P-coumaric, 2-phenol, and chlorogenic acid, which help block the amount of carcinogens formed in the body by nitrosamines, say researchers at Cornell University.

FIGHTING THE-BLAHS WITH A BEEFSTEAK

Because of its vitamins A and C and liver-stimulating mineral salts, a daily tomato cocktail is a beneficial way to fight or prevent energy-deficit disorders including chronic fatigue syndrome, hypoglycemia, anorexia, and mononucleosis. (Season with cayenne pepper or a bit of fresh chile pepper plus fresh lemon or lime juice for extra punch.) A cup of tomato soup or regular gazpacho is good nutritional intervention, say natural healers, for kidney disease.

BLT, HOLD THE B

Tomatoes are ideal diet foods, with an average of 30 calories per tomato, plus the B-complex vitamins, iron, and potassium, which are often missing in weight-loss regimens. Have a BLT, but skip the bacon.

Purely Cosmetic

◆ Try the juice of a fresh tomato (applied as a compress) to bleach freckles.

◆ Use tomato juice to rid your hair of chemical residues (saturate hair, cover with shower cap for 10 minutes, rinse, and shampoo).

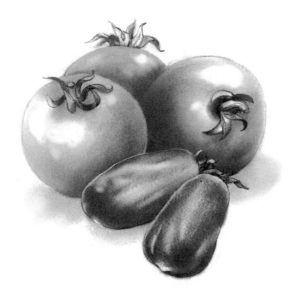

Putting Tomatoes on the Menu for Maternity

Because of their iron, vitamin C, and folate content, tomatoes should be included in the diet of every pregnant woman. As a bonus, they supply fiber to relieve the constipation and hemorrhoids common to pregnancy.

TWO WARNINGS: Tomatoes are a common source of food allergens. Common symptoms: hives, headaches, itching. As members of the nightshade family and salicylate bearers, they are contraindicated for the arthritic and the aspirin sensitive.

Buying, Storing, and Using

- ◆ For optimum taste and nutrition, shop seasonal markets and U-pick or organic farms, or grow your own. (TIP: Red tomatoes have four times the beta-carotene of immature or green tomatoes.)
- ◆ Best taste buys: Pik-red, yellow, cherry, star pak, and roma plum.
- ◆ Buy fewer but better sun-ripened tomatoes. Sun is what develops the flavor compounds inside the seed sacs. (Most supermarket varieties are thick-walled, low-in-gel varieties ripened with ethylene oxide to prolong shelf life.)
- ◆ Buy tomatoes ripe for best taste and most nutrition.
- ◆ Grow your own? Like to have 'em all winter long? Pull up the entire plant before the first frost, and hang upside down in a dark place. Green tomatoes ripen slowly.
- ◆ Use large, ripe tomatoes for juicing, plums for sauce and condiments, and cherry varieties for salads, snacks.
- ◆ Tomatoes can be crushed, puréed, dried into leather, or made into relish, catsup, or marmalade.
- ◆ To boost your uptake of tomato's iron, eat with other iron-rich foods (whole grains, dried beans).
- ◆ To neutralize the acidity of tomato sauces, stir in ½ teaspoon instant coffee dissolved in ½ cup sauce for every 2 cups.
- ◆ To fast-peel, plunge tomatoes into boiling water for 6 to 10 seconds, rinse with cold water.
- ◆ Toss your tomatoes with grains and beans to up your intake of the nonheme iron they contain.
- ◆ Ready for a change of pace tomato? Try the tomatillo, a lemony flavored antique from Aztec times, rich in vitamin A, with only 25

calories a 3.5-ounce serving and a long (up to three weeks) storage life once refrigerated (in a paper-lined dish). To prepare: Remove husks, wash and chop for salads, sauces, gazpachos, or garnishes.

Try these recipes:

Super Healing Salad (onion free)

2 shallots, peeled and finely minced

1/4 cup vinegar

3/4 cup olive oil

3 tomatoes, peeled, seeded, and finely chopped

1 serrano chile, seeded and chopped

1/2 cup chopped fresh basil

2 tablespoons chopped fresh thyme (or 1 tablespoon dried)

2 tablespoons chopped fresh marjoram (or 1 tablespoon dried)

Freshly ground pepper to taste

Whisk shallots with vinegar.

Add oil slowly, continuing to whisk. Stir in remaining ingredients. Blend and serve.

Makes about 2 cups.

Oven-Dried Tomatoes

28 medium-size plum tomatoes (about 4 pounds), core end cut off, halved lengthwise

2 1/2 teaspoons extra-virgin olive oil

1 teaspoon salt substitute

Freshly ground pepper to taste

Preheat the oven to 200 degrees. Lightly coat skin side of each tomato half with olive oil. Place skin side down on large baking sheet. Sprinkle with salt and pepper to taste.

Bake tomatoes until they shrink to about one quarter original size, about 4 to 6 hours (they should stay soft and juicy). Let tomatoes cool on baking sheet. Place in a container, refrigerate.

Makes two cups.

Benefits healing zones: 1, 3, 7

Also see: Cancer, Antioxidants, Prostate, Dieting

VEGETARIAN FOODS

Vegetarianism was good enough for Epicurus, George Bernard Shaw, Leo Tolstoy, the Trappist monks, and Seventh Day Adventists, and it's good enough for the 12 million Americans who are part of the three quarters of the global population who are vegetarians.

A healthier cholesterol reading is one reason. Studies indicate that nothing produces a sharper rise in LDL levels than four weeks on a meat-inclusive regime. In fact, average cholesterol levels typically increase 19% and blood pressure rises 3%, says Dr. Frank M. Sacks of Harvard Medical School's Channing Laboratory. Studies suggest an adverse effect of consumption of beef on cholesterol levels and blood pressure, he concludes. Nevertheless, the average American eats his or her weight in red meat each year, averaging 77 grams a year, or close to 6 tons of animal protein over the course of a lifetime.*

BROWNIE POINTS FOR RED MEAT

In all fairness, meat has its good points. It is a good source of iron and niacin and provides the kind of complete amino-acid-balanced protein that seems readymade for human needs. But it's totally free of fiber and doesn't have anything you can't get from land- and sea-grown plants, which also have a wider array of trace nutrients, more dietary fiber, less saturated fat and sodium, and fewer pesticides and hormone residues. Studies suggest further that a high-fiber diet (preferably meat free) helps prevent every major killer disease, from coronary heart disease to cancer, to AIDS. One 10-year study of 871 fit men revealed that death rates from cancer and from all other causes combined were three times lower for those who ate fiber-rich, plant-based diets than for men who followed low-fiber, meat-rich regimens. A diet containing at least 37 grams of fiber daily—an amount easy to come by on a standard vegetarian diet (cereal grains, beans, fruits, and vegetables)—appears to pro-

---

* Only less than 1% of all Americans seldom or never eat meat, says a recently published study by the National Center for Health Statistics, and 95% of us have yet to sample a meat substitute.

long life by preventing a spectrum of cancers, especially those of the colon, stomach, and prostate.

Need more no-meat-for-me motivation? Consider the fact that environmental pollutants are most concentrated at the top of the food chain in animals that are eaten and in the humans who eat them. According to the Earthsave Foundation, meat eating is a drain on natural resources.*

Another bonus of the vegetarian option is freedom from obesity, which Dr. Scott Grundy, chairman of the American Heart Association's Nutrition Committee and director of the Center for Human Nutrition at the University of Texas Health Science Center at Dallas (*New England Journal of Medicine,* June 10, 1992), says is *the* major causative factor in hypertension, more important even than excess salt.

According to Dr. Antonio M. Gotto, Jr., president-elect of the American Heart Association and professor of medicine at Baylor College of Medicine, data from a combined study by the United States and the former U.S.S.R., show that the more HDL (high-density lipoprotein) you have, the likelier it is your weight is near normal and the lower your risk of coronary artery disease. But the greater your body weight, the lower your good cholesterol and the greater your risk of coronary artery disease.

Because meat is fiber free but high in sodium and saturated fat, even a 6-ounce daily serving could, in the long run, have a negative impact on your general health in spite of other positive habits. For example, research by the Vegetarian Resource Group indicates that if you've exercised vigorously most of your life, by the time you've reached your senior years you'll be 10 times less likely to develop heart disease than your less active friends. But you lose that edge if you've spent a lifetime eating meat.

The good news? Even becoming a halfway- or semivegetarian lets you reclaim some of that edge. In fact, in one study, substituting soy protein for animal protein lowered cholesterol levels even more than a prudent low-fat, low-cholesterol diet that included conservative servings of lean meat.

---

* Over one third of all raw materials consumed—including fossil fuels—are devoted to the production of livestock. Half of the earth's land mass is grazed by livestock, and 64% of U.S. cropland produces livestock feed. Livestock also requires more than half of all water consumed for all purposes in the United States.

Other research indicates that, more importantly, when soy protein concentrate was added to hamburger before cooking, mutagenic activity (changes that predispose cells to cancer) was reduced. Beef-plus-soy burgers, in other words, are good health insurance.

VEGETARIAN BENEFITS

But can all your nutritional needs be met with land- and sea-grown plants and herbs, including vitamin B_{12}? According to conventional wisdom, the only reliable source of vitamin B_{12} is meat. But in fact B_{12}, which prevents anemia and fatigue and promotes red blood formation is found in eggs and dairy products and in fermented soy foods such as tempeh and meat analogs such as fermented rice food called mochi. Sea vegetable proteins, including spirulina and blue-green algae, are also reliable sources, as are herbs such as comfrey.

Here are two simple rules of thumb:

◆ Learn the complementary protein mixtures (i.e., combine two plant protein foods that have opposite amino acid strengths and weaknesses so that they balance one another, creating a complete protein). For example, beans and wheat are twice as beneficial if eaten at the same meal than alone. Combine sunflower seeds and peanuts, and their amino acids combine to produce a high-quality, complete protein (sparing you the necessity of carrying perishable meat and dairy foods on your hiking, camping, or biking outings).

◆ Complement grains with dried beans and wheat germ; or enjoy dried beans with grains, nuts and seeds, and wheat germ; or match nuts and seeds with dried beans and wheat germ. And remember, even though vegetable proteins, unlike meat proteins, are incomplete (low in one or more of the nine essential amino acids), you get the protein you need even if the foods served at any one meal don't contain enough of all nine. The body makes up the shortage by simply dipping into its reserve. Calories and variety are the keys.

If you're not a no-eggs-or-milk vegetarian, to maximize your nutrient uptake from grains, dried beans, and nuts and seeds, add eggs or dairy products (milk, cheese, yogurt, kefir). For example, try granola and kefir and scrambled eggs with sunflower seeds. And use the complete-protein grains, amaranth and quinoa, wherever possible in food combining. Use the following chart as a guide.

VEGETABLE PROTEINS
The Top 20

Food	Protein	Fat	Calories
Black beans, I cup cooked	15	1	227
Bread, 2 slices whole-grain	6	2	140
Brown rice, I cup cooked	5	1	232
Corn, I cup cooked	6	2	178
Corn bread, 2-inch square	3	4	130
Corn tortilla	2	1	67
Cottage cheese, I cup of 1%	28	2	164
Egg, I large	6	2	79
Egg white, I large	3	0	16
Garbanzo beans, I cup cooked	12	3	285
Kidney beans, I cup cooked	15	1	225
Lentils, I cup cooked	18	1	231
Milk, I cup of 1%	11	2	120
Pasta, I cup cooked	7	2	200
Potato, baked with skin	5	1	220
Refried beans, I cup cooked	16	3	270
Split peas, I cup cooked	16	1	231
Tempeh, 1/2 cup	16	6	165
Yogurt, I cup of nonfat	13	0	127
Tofu,* 1/2 cup	20	11	183

* Also available in lowfat and 1% fat versions, as is soy and rice milk.

Note: To figure serving sizes, consider a 3-ounce serving of meat to contain roughly 21 grams of protein. To replace this with a vegetarian source of protein, plan on a generous cup of cooked beans and 1 cup of cooked grain. One cup of cooked lentils served over cornbread, for instance (or refried beans plus 1 cup of cooked rice), is an acceptable substitute for a 3-ounce serving of cooked poultry.

Try these recipes:

Soy Quarter-Pounder

> *2 cups cooked soybeans*
> *2 beaten eggs or 1/2 cup tofu*
> *1/3 cup wheat germ, oat, corn, or rice bran*
> *1/2 cup chopped celery*
> *1 cup grated carrot*

1 tablespoon Worcestershire sauce or light tamari soy sauce

1 tablespoon minced garlic

³/₄ cup grated onion or minced scallion

1 tablespoon cumin or curry powder

Preheat oven to 400 degrees. Coarsely grind soybeans in a blender, food processor, or food mill. Combine with remaining ingredients. With wet hands, shape mixture into generous patties or croquettes.

Bake on a lightly oiled baking sheet for 20 minutes, turning once, or broil for five minutes on each side.

Makes four servings.

Variations: Substitute kidney, pinto, or black beans for soy. Use bread crumbs in place of bran or germ. Replace ½ cup egg with 2 tablespoons nut butter. Roll patties in extra bran for added crispness.

Chili Seitan

½ cup peeled and finely diced onion

½ cup finely diced celery or celery root and ½ cup finely diced green or red bell pepper

2 tablespoons minced garlic

1 tablespoon olive or sesame oil

½ tablespoon chili powder (cayenne)

½ tablespoon ground cumin

1 tablespoon tomato paste or reconstituted dried tomato

2 cups fresh tomatoes (seeded and chopped)

Dash honey or pinch sugar

1 cup (or 15-oz. can) cooked red kidney beans or pinto beans

1 cup drained and chopped seitan (a high-protein meat substitute made from wheat). Look for the new five-minute quick mixes at health food stores.

In a soup pot, sauté onion, celery, bell pepper, and garlic in oil with seasonings over medium heat for 10 minutes, stirring occasionally to prevent burning.

Dissolve tomato paste or dried tomato in chopped tomatoes and add to sautéed vegetables. Add honey or sugar, stir well.

Stir in cooked beans and chopped seitan. Simmer 10 minutes longer. Serve on buns or over steamed grain or pasta.

Makes four generous servings.

Questions about vegetarianism? Write to the Vegetarian Resource Group, P.O. Box 1463, Baltimore, MD 21203; or call (301) 366-VEGE.

Also see: **Coronary Heart Disease, Soybeans, Beans, Whole Grains**

VITAMIN B COMPLEX

The B-complex vitamins are one simple way to stay well, and then some. The getting is good if you get your B from nature's A-1 source, whole foods. All nutrients work most effectively in you-can't-have-one-without-the-other coalitions within the body. The test of whether this physiological teamwork is on target is the health of every one of your 10 target healing zones.

NOT ONE
BUT 12 VITAMINS IN ONE

Vitamin B is an example. It is not one vitamin but a complex of 12 nutrients—from B_1 (thiamine) to B_{15} (pangamic acid) and B_{17} (lactrile). The latter two are sometimes considered interloper members of the spectrum.

The Nuts, Eggs and Whole Grain Super Healing for Schizophrenia, Alcoholism, and Senility

B_3 is a four-star part of the complex also called niacin, niacinamide, or nicotinic acid, it has been used successfully (along with vitamins C and B_6) to treat schizophrenia, alcoholism, senility, learning disabilities, and more. It even makes a good side-effect-free aspirin. Eaten in "protective" amounts, it can also lower your cholesterol and triglycerides and protect you from cancer of the esophagus, gout and kidney disorders. And it isn't hard to do. The RDA is 15 to 20 mg, and a protective dose of 30 mg is the amount in a serving of whole grain cereal with nuts. Have one different type B_3 food every other day and you will have eaten your way through the five commonest sources (eggs, nuts, whole grains, brewer's yeast, and wheat germ) in a week.

The Exerciser's B Vitamin

Vitamin B_2 is a requisite if you run, jump, swim, or exercise in any way, since physical exercise increases your need for riboflavin. B_2 found in the same source foods as B_3 above. Vitamin B_2 is also essential to activate the antioxidant enzyme glutathione.

POWER FOODS FOR PREGNANCY

Vitamin B_6 foods belong on every mother-to-be's menu. For example, 25 mg of B_6 three times a day relieves morning sickness, while 4 mg of folic acid (folate) reduces the risk of newborn spinal and brain defects. Both are found in leafy greens, citrus juices, and whole grains. Folic acid fortification of bread and grain products has been governmentally mandated.

Folic acid is one of the common nutrient deficiencies in the American diet, and a B_6 deficiency can be caused by a lack of magnesium (both nutrients occur in whole grains and leafy greens). Likewise, folate works in concert with B_{12} to regulate cellular division and DNA synthesis and B_{12} is the nutritional factor that prevents pernicious anemia, a deficiency that can lead to impaired nerve function.

Or consider B_1 (thiamine) which promotes carbohydrate utilization for energy, normalizes nerve function and helps prevent fatigue, depression, irritability, and memory loss. You need at least 50 mg daily but 100 mg or more during stress and illness.

REASONS TO KEEP B-VITAMIN FOODS ON THE MENU

The B vitamin individually and as a team are responsible for metabolizing carbohydrates, fat, and proteins; maintaining muscle tone; regulating appetite; building blood; stabilizing circulation; promoting growth; regulating iron absorption; building stress tolerance; forming antibodies; and regulating brain function. Vitamin B, along with protein, assures the proper growth of your nails. Shorting yourself on a regular basis on any of the B-vitamin source foods, from wheat germ and yogurt to nuts and leafy greens, can cause one or more of the following symptoms of deficiency: acne, anemia, appetite loss, bad breath, high cholesterol, poor circulation, constipation, depression, nervousness, insomnia, fatigue, and memory impairment.

What You Eat and What You Get

What you eat may not be what you get because B complex is water soluble (temporarily stored) and thus easily depleted. Alcohol, antacids, aspirin, caffeine and diuretics destroy B_1, B_6, and folic acid, for example, while oral contraceptives interfere with the bioavailability of B_1, B_6, B_{12}, and vitamin C, as does excessive protein consumption.

Try this recipe:

B Complex Nut and Wheat Loaf

> *1 cup chopped walnuts*
>
> *1 cup dried whole wheat crumbs, or 1 cup wheat germ*
>
> *1 cup minced celery*
>
> *$^1/_2$ cup chopped green pepper*
>
> *$^1/_2$ cup chopped onion*
>
> *2 tablespoons vegetable oil*
>
> *1 beaten egg*
>
> *1 cup tomato juice*

Mix all ingredients together, combine well, spoon into oiled loaf pan and bake for one hour at 375 degrees.

Benefits healing zones: All

Also see: **Whole Grains, Nuts, Dairy Substitutes, Soybeans, Leafy Greens**

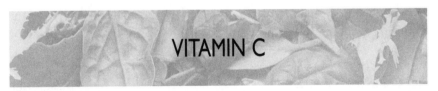

VITAMIN C

What do Brussels sprouts, kiwi fruit, and red clover tea have in common? They are all other-than-OJ sources of vitamin C.

More than a high-impact cold- and flu-fighter, vitamin C (or ascorbic acid)—found in citrus fruits, kiwis, berries, sprouted beans, herb tea, and Brussels sprouts—is a premium, non-toxic antiviral agent vitally important for the manufacture of interferon. It is also an antioxidant which blocks the initiation and promotion of cancer, especially of the oral cavities, pancreas, lungs, breast, and cervix, and prevents the formation of cancer-causing substances such as nitrites and nitrates (found in processed meats and many processed foods). It (vitamin C) prevents free radical damage produced by your metabolism or by the environment (X-rays, ultraviolet light, electromagnetic radiation, etc.), says researcher Bruce N. Ames, Ph.D., of the University of California at Berkeley.

REDUCING CORONARY RISK, CATARACTS, AND ALLERGENS

Vitamin C is also an A-1 cardiovascular nutrient, preventing the plaque that precipitates hardening of the arteries, preventing abnormal blood clotting, and lowering blood pressure. It raises and enhances production of HDL (the good cholesterol). (Blood fat levels are typically two to three times lower when the bloodstream is well fortified with C, says the American Holistic Medical Association.) Ascorbic acid also regenerates vitamin E in the body, reduces blood histamine levels and MSG sensitivity for the allergy prone, and delays development of cataracts.

HOW FRUIT COCKTAIL PROTECTS SPERM COUNT AND IMPROVES BRAIN FUNCTION

If that doesn't motivate you to second helpings of your breakfast fruit cocktail, according to the Linus Pauling Institute of Palo Alto, California, healing doses of C (10 times the RDA of 60 mg) can protect male sperm from genetic damage that can cause inherited diseases or cancer in children.

"C" IS FOR CLEAR THINKING!

Vitamin C plays a major role in brain function. The brain is one of the two organs in the body containing the most vitamin C. Higher blood levels of vitamin C are related to higher IQ scores. According to Michael Lesser, author of *Nutrition and Vitamin Therapy,* large doses of potassium ascorbate (another form of vitamin C) noticeably increase brain activity. Vitamin C also induces production of serotonin, a brain chemical that induces both sleep and positive emotions, and it works with vitamin B_6 to convert the amino acid phenylalanine into norepinephrine, a mood-boosting chemical.

More vitamin-C-rich parsley, papayas, bell peppers, or kiwis* in your meals could also mean more glutathione, a potent amino acid

---

* Calorie for calorie, says the United Fruit Association, this fuzzy-brown-on-the-outside-green-on-the-inside mini fruit is nature's most concentrated source of vitamin C, with twice as much as oranges and four times what you get in a grapefruit half (plus twice the vitamin E of avocados and significant amounts of folic acid, B_6, calcium, and iron).

antioxidant that protects against a range of degenerative diseases. According to the USDA Human Nutrition Research Center at Tufts University, a C-rich diet promotes healthy teeth and gums, prevents periodontal disease, and increases energy and endurance.

A LITTLE OR A LOT?

Why do you need more than the official RDA of 60 mg? Because vitamin C is a multiple-purpose healer essential for the formation of collagen, the substance that binds together the cells of connective tissue, produces new cells and tissues, and prevents viruses from penetrating cell membranes. (Viruses can reproduce only within the cell.) As a major component of scar tissue, vitamin C is especially important in the healing process. Second, it's the body's foremost now-you-have-it-now-you-don't nutrient. It's depleted by water and air (asparagus and oranges lose 50% of their vitamin C in 24 hours at room temperature, for example), alcohol, fluorides, and oral contraceptives, and a single aspirin can triple its excretion rate, as can habitual smoking. (Smokers need at least an additional 100 mg a day, the amount in one large orange or 1½ cups of strawberries.)

At healing doses, (a gram or more a day) says the Pauling Institute, C is a life extender, reducing deaths from cancer and heart disease by 25 to 42% and extending life by six years.

Getting more C pays dividends because every vitamin-C-rich food also supplies bioflavonoids* (best sources—citrus fruit peel and pulp, blackberries, papaya, and buckwheat), which help strengthen capillaries, normalize blood pressure, prevent stroke, and potentiate the value of vitamin C by protecting it from oxidation.

C Without Citrus: 29 Sources

Oranges may be our favorite high-C fruit, but if you're out of them, you aren't out of vitamin C. Did you know, for example, that mangoes have twice as much C as citrus? Or that you get a bonus dose from your foods *without* supplements when you drink green tea (*camelia sinesis*), which, say researchers at Rutgers University, helps the body retain

---

* A group of 800 antioxidants discovered in 1936 by Dr. Albert Szent-Györgyi, the discoverer of vitamin C.

ascorbic acid and enhances vitamin C's antioxidant properties? Or that there is a homeopathic, vitamin C substitute called Aconite derived from the herb monkshood?

Take a look at the following chart. (*Note:* There are seasonal variations in the C content of foods, so opt for in-season, fresh produce, which is the richest source.)

Food	Portion	Milligrams of Vitamin C
Papaya	1 medium	188
Apricots	3	11
Black currants	½ cup	100
Blueberries	1 cup	53
Strawberries	1 cup	85
Cabbage		
Cantaloupe	half	75
Kiwi	1 medium	75
Red pepper	½ cup	64
Banana	1 small	14
Broccoli	¾ cup	61
Mango	1 medium	60
Guava	1 (3 oz.)	
Amaranth, uncooked	4.5 oz.	65
Basil, ground	4.5 oz.	61
Dandelion, uncooked	4.5 oz.	35
Garlic, uncooked	4.5 oz.	15
Mint, uncooked	4.5 oz.	35
Onion, green, uncooked	4.5 oz.	32
Paprika	4.5 oz.	71
Watercress, uncooked	4.5 oz.	79
Acerola cherries	3.5 oz.	1000
Peppers, green	1 medium	125
Grapefruit juice, fresh	2 cup	108
Honeydew melon	½ medium	90
Brussels sprouts	¾ cup	87
Parsley	½ cup	70

TIP: To get everything that's coming to you nutritionally, juice the whole fruit. According to the *USDA Handbook of Foods,* total juicer-type machines utilizing the impact method of extraction give you more nutrition for your time and money—346 mg vitamin C from a pound of lemons rather than 90; 319 mg vitamin C from a pound of oranges rather than 109.

Try this recipe:

High C Tea

> *2 teaspoons any high-C herb (ascorbic acid range in the following herbs per each 100 grams: 35 mg sage and mint; 122 mg parsley; 70 mg cress, rosemary, and basil; 567 mg dried coriander leaf) or green or gunpowder tea, which provides as much C as a glass of orange juice*
>
> *1 small slice lemon or 1 lime or kiwi*

Heat 1½ cups of water. Pour over 1 heaping teaspoon dried herbs. Steep for 7 to 10 minutes. Add citrus or kiwi slices; stir in sweetener if desired. Makes 2 cups.

Benefits healing zones: All

Also see: Lemons, Oranges, Cancer, Herbs, Antioxidants, Common Cold

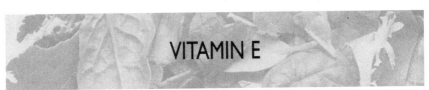

VITAMIN E

Would you make wheat germ, sunflower seeds, oatmeal, and soy oil the sweet spot of your diet if you knew they prevented angina, blood clotting, diabetes, and more? Get out your knife, fork, and baking tins. Vitamin E source foods do all that and more.

HELPING YOUR HEART BY HELPING YOURSELF TO E

Most of us get a scant 25 IU a day of this safe, nontoxic-at-any-dose nutrient*—but at protective levels (100 IU), you can cut the risk of coronary

---

* Vitamin E is fat soluble but, unlike vitamin A, it is not toxic at high levels.

disease by 40%, suggest recent studies of men and women supplement-ed at this level for two to eight years. Since the official RDA is only 15 mg, you can get good results by just tripling this intake using food alone.

While other antioxidant vitamins, such as A and C, are important in preventing heart disease, vitamin E is the one that works hardest for your heart by thinning the blood to prevent abnormal blood clotting and increasing beneficial HDL cholesterol. By improving intermittent clau-dication and angina, E has also been shown to reduce leg pain and increase exercise tolerance.

Vitamin E is particularly important to the circulatory system. When undersupplied, the danger of blood clot formation and heart attacks, strokes, and phlebitis (inflammation of blood vessels) is increased. After heart attacks, vitamin E opens up new channels of blood supply (collateral circulation).

SMOKERS' AND SECOND-HAND SMOKE VICTIMS' PROTECTION

E is the vitamin guardian of lungs, trapping and neutralizing free radicals more effectively than other antioxidants. In conjunction with A, C, and the mineral selenium, it offers special protection for smokers and second-hand smoke victims, conclude studies conducted over the last 20 years.

VITAMIN E TO FIGHT AGING

According to researchers at Harvard Medical School and Brigham and Women's Hospital in Boston, vitamin E boosts the immune response even in the elderly and prevents the pain of osteoarthritis as effectively as anti-inflammatory drugs. Vitamin E at levels 10-fold that of the government's daily quota impacts sexual potency, reproductive health, and the aging process. Vitamin E also contributes to prostaglandin metabolism to pre-vent PMS and circulatory irregularities responsible for night cramps.

Vitamin E also helps prevent complications that worsen sickle cell anemia, Parkinson's disease, cataracts, and Alzheimer's disease. In addi-tion, vitamin E is one of the three top antioxidant defenses against free radical damage and other factors that take their cellular toll, including air pollution, ultraviolet light, and radiation.

Vitamin E is an important exerciser's aid since working out increases the respiration rate, thereby exposing the body to more oxida-tive stress from pollutants, chemicals, and cigarette smoke. Vitamin E also helps prevent injury and, when injury does occur, hastens the for-mation of scar tissue.

EATING YOUR E

While a regulation-sized spinach salad with a vegetable- or nut-oil-based dressing will provide your bare minimum need for vitamin E, a little wheat germ sprinkled on oatmeal for breakfast and some asparagus almondine for lunch would be even better. Nuts and seeds are a superior vitamin E snack.

Note: Increasing the amount of unsaturated vegetable oil in your diet also increases your vitamin E (see the following charts).

15 GOOD DIETARY SOURCES OF VITAMIN E

Food	Portion	% RDA
Wheat germ, toasted	1 tablespoon	29
French vinaigrette dressing	2 tablespoons	22
Blue cheese or Roquefort dressing, regular	2 tablespoons	18
French dressing, regular	2 tablespoons	16
Thousand Island dressing, regular	2 tablespoons	12
Stick margarine	2 tablespoons	9
Soft margarine	2 tablespoons	7

Note: Other good sources: eggs, asparagus, oatmeal, and blackberries.

OILS FOR E
The Seven Top Sources

Oil	E in mg per 100 g
Wheat germ	190.0
Soybean	87.0
Maize (corn)	66.0
Safflower	49.0
Sunflower	27.0
Peanut	22.0
Olive	4.6

Benefits healing zones: All

Also see: Nuts, Coronary Heart Disease, Diabetes, Walnuts, Whole Grains

VITAMIN K

What do green tea, kale, yogurt, and egg yolks have in common? They're all sources of vitamin K, a fat soluble vitamin that helps prevent internal bleeding and hemorrhages, promotes blood clotting, and reduces menstrual flow. Vitamin K also helps prevent osteoporosis by promoting calcium retention and the healing of fractures.

Although the body's K requirement is small (65 to 80 µg daily) and healthy intestinal bacteria manufacture most of that need, a deficiency can be serious, resulting in celiac disease, sprue, or colitis. Prolonged antibiotic or blood thinner therapy, excessive use of mineral oil, and a diet low in calories or high in frozen foods can put you at risk, as can prolonged exposure to radiation or air pollution.

Diarrhea caused by inadequate intestinal bacteria is a deficiency tipoff, as is easy bruising and bleeding.

Good sources of vitamin K include alfalfa, broccoli, spinach, turnip greens, asparagus, and olive oil.

Try this recipe:

Vitamin K Vinaigrette

> *1 cup juiced raw kale*
>
> *2 tablespoons low-fat yogurt**
>
> *4 teaspoons finely chopped scallions*
>
> *2 teaspoons finely chopped fresh basil*
>
> *1 medium clove, peeled and minced*
>
> *Freshly ground pepper*

Whisk kale juice and yogurt together. Add scallions, basil, garlic, and pepper.

Makes 1 cup.

---

*Yogurt promotes the growth of lactobacillus bacteria, which promote vitamin K production.

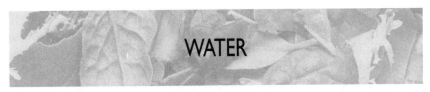

WATER

Healthy water* is integral to health and healing—second, in fact, only to oxygen. Water accounts for 70% of total body weight. And here's what H_2O has to offer.

◆ Every biological process, including control of body temperature, blood pressure, and respiration, depends on water.

◆ Water helps carry away the body's waste products, lubricates joints, and is an antidote for fatigue, which is often only a symptom of H_2O deficit in disguise.

◆ Every body cell needs water to carry out its functions; more than 2 quarts daily are essential to replace what's lost through normal metabolic processes. And while you might survive (if not thrive) for 30 to 45 days without food, without water you'd die in 10 days—or after a 10% water loss, whichever came first.

◆ Water supplies oxygen and nutrients to cells and removes cellular waste through the blood and lymphatic systems. The kidneys eliminate a pint of fluid a day to prevent toxin build-up.

◆ Water also acts as the body's air conditioner by expelling internal heat through perspiration.

◆ Every joint in the body uses water as a lubricant.

◆ Water is a healer. Amounts in excess of six to eight glasses a day are needed to facilitate a rebound faster from colds and other respiratory impairments or the flu. (TIP: Cloudy urine is a sign of a water deficit.)

WHAT'S ON TAP

You don't always get what you need or what you think you're getting out of the tap—or, for that matter, out of the bottle. Here's why.

---

* Free of extraneous chemicals, toxins, etc.

◆ Drinking water in the United States is regulated by the Environmental Protection Agency (EPA), which sets maximum contaminant levels for 30 common contaminants, including organic and inorganic chemicals, metals, bacteria, and radioactive particles.

◆ In areas not regulated by the EPA, where the Safe Drinking Water Act of 1974 doesn't apply, anything could be on tap and probably is. More than 70,000 known contaminants have been found in our water supply.

◆ In addition, the EPA estimates that 42 million Americans drink water dangerously high in lead.

◆ Even clean water can go bad after leaving the treatment plant. Lead pipes in older homes, for example, can leach hazardous amounts of highly toxic lead into tap water. Warning signs that indicate impure water include murkiness and foaming.

So what's your best bet—to shape up your tap water or switch to bottled H_2O? Here are a few more thumbs-up/thumbs-down facts and a few final solutions.

BOTTLED WATER

A recent New York State Department of Health survey of 100 different varieties of bottled waters found that, in general, the bottled waters contained many of the same chemicals as tap water, and at similar levels. Is bottled water really better? (We drink twice as much bottled water today in the United States as we did five years ago.) According to the Bottled Water Association, one out of six U.S. households gives tap water the cold shoulder. But with over 600 domestic and 100 imported brands of bottled and bulk water to choose from, you need a scoreboard to make a healthy choice. According to Food and Drug Administration (FDA) regulations, which took effect in late 1993, all bottled water must meet the same safety standards as the EPA has set for municipal water (for lead contamination the new bottled water standard is even tougher)—or state standards if the source is municipal—and must disclose the levels of any nutrients that are present in significant amounts (e.g., in sodium, calcium, or iron). Unfortunately there are no nationally agreed-on labeling standards. But here's what should be inside the bottle or jug:

- *Bulk drinking water:* Water from an approved source, such as tap water or springs, that's filtered and purified with ozone. Minerals are removed and may or may not be readded.

- *Sparkling (or carbonated) water:* Bottled water that contains natural carbon dioxide from the source or added carbon dioxide.

- *Natural water:* Bottled spring, mineral, or well water from an underground source, not tap water. Natural water has no added dissolved solids and may be filtered.

- *Spring water:* Underground water that naturally flows to the earth's surface under its own pressure. "Natural spring water" means unprocessed in any way.

- *Mineral water:* According to the International Bottled Water Association, mineral waters are usually sparkling and must contain at least 500 parts per million of total dissolved solids. Not all states are enforcing this, as there is no federal guideline.

- *Artesian water:* Well water that naturally surfaces through a constructed hole.

- *Distilled or purified water:* Water that's purified through distillation, ion exchange, reverse osmosis, or another comparable process. Distilled water is vaporized and condensed, leaving behind dissolved minerals. Deionized water is passed through resins that remove most of the minerals.

- *Seltzers and club soda* ("processed" water): Filtered and artificially carbonated tap water regulated by the FDA but not recognized by the International Bottled Water Association. Club soda usually has added sodium, and seltzers may have added sweeteners. Both seltzer and soda are filtered, artificially carbonated tap water unless otherwise indicated.

Getting the Best of the Bottled

1. Call the bottler's 800 number (or long-distance number) and get a list of the contaminants it tests for.

2. Ask about chlorine and fluoride. Most companies don't use chlorine because it can combine with organic materials during the purification process to form carcinogens, says Arnold Pike, D.C., director of the Academy of Nutritional Sciences (usually an aftertaste-free oxygen called ozone is used).

3. Check the source. Water from highly industrialized areas is a bad bet.

4. Consider the option of catalyst-altered water. Developed by chemist John H. Willard, it supplies high concentrations of iron, copper, zinc, calcium, and numerous trace minerals in a unique colloidal suspension which gives it antioxidant properties.

5. Join the Water of the Month Club. Selections from around the world include a French love water with aphrodisiac powers and an Italian antiaging water called Deliziosa. For information, call 1-800-345-5959.

6. Pass up water in polycarbonate resin jugs. Polycarbonate is readily absorbed into the water itself.

FILTER SYSTEMS
The Bottled Water Alternative

Since bottled water can cost 700 to 3,000 times what you get for free, a cost-efficient home water filter is a one-time investment (of about $1,000) that pays for itself. But before you buy,

1. Ask for water system test results from your local EPA Division of Water Quality, or have your water tested. If you have questions, contact the EPA's Safe Drinking Water Hotline at 1-800-426-4791. All filters don't filter out all contaminants, so take the next step:

2. Educate yourself about your four options:

   ♦ Water distillers are the most effective home filtration devices. Water is boiled and vapor condensed, leaving behind most contaminants. The drawback? So many minerals are removed that the water may taste flat. And distillation won't remove chemicals with a lower boiling point than water (but a carbon filter will remove these contaminants).

   ♦ Reverse osmosis devices force water through a semipermeable membrane that traps heavy metals, sediment, bacteria, and radioactive particles. However, they can't rival carbon filters at removing pesticide residues and trihalomethanes. RODs are the most expensive filters, and so are the replacements.

   ♦ Ionizers are commonly used to remove minerals from hard water, and ozone generators are usually used for treating larger amounts of water.

◆ Activated carbon filters are the commonest of the filter systems. Water passes through a granulated or solid carbon block, which traps contaminants in the carbon's pores. Carbon filters are good at removing odors, sediment, chlorine, pesticides, and organic chemicals but not heavy metals (such as lead), radioactive minerals, and bacteria. They also require frequent block replacement.

Three Tips for Filter Users

◆ Write to the Consumers Union, 101 Truman Ave., Yonkers, NY 10703-1057, and request the latest filter performance ratings.

◆ Get a copy of the latest listing of certified water filter models from the National Sanitation Foundation, P.O. Box 1468, Ann Arbor, MI 48106.

◆ Be sure any device you invest in has been quality certified by the Water Quality Association.

FIVE WAYS TO PROTECT YOURSELF FROM TOXIC TAP WATER

1. The highest lead levels occur in the first tap water of the morning. Take a shower before flushing out the faucet used for drinking water; then fill a glass container and place it in the refrigerator for drinking and cooking throughout the day to eliminate the need for reflushing the plumbing when water is needed.

2. Use cold, not hot, water for cooking. Water is higher in lead when heated.

3. Don't boil water longer than five minutes. Boiling concentrates all contaminants, including lead.

4. Eat foods high in iron and rich in calcium to block the body's uptake of lead.

5. Contact the American Council of Independent Laboratories, 1629 K St. N.W., Suite 400, Washington, DC 20006, phone 202-887-5872; or call the EPA's Safe Drinking Water Hotline (800-426-4791) for the name of a lab that will test your water for lead and other contaminants.

WHOLE GRAINS

You can't live by grain alone, but you can survive and thrive if you get whole grains into your daily, weekly, and monthly menus.

Most grains are seed members of the world's most important and prolific crop (there are over 8,000 different species worldwide). Civilization itself took root as a result of the cultivation of cereal grains (named for Ceres, Greek goddess of agriculture), which improved nutrition, increased population growth, and made possible the development of commerce.

Whole grains* are a holistic source of complex carbohydrates, dietary fiber, essential growth minerals, fat-free protein, and B vitamins plus the antioxidants vitamin E and octacosan (concentrated in the germ and the bran). Whole grains protect against the development of chronic degenerative diseases (including cancer, heart disease, diabetes, and varicose veins) and diseases of the colon (including colon cancer, inflammatory bowel disease, hemorrhoids, and diverticulitis).

BAKING FOR BETTER BLOOD PRESSURE

Whole grain bread cereals and casseroles are one reason that vegetarians have significantly lower blood pressure than meat eaters. Eating 20 to 30 grams of raw grain germ a day (oat, wheat, corn, rice) promotes an average cholesterol reduction of almost 8%, says the USDA's Cereal and Crops Research Laboratory and University of Wisconsin chemist Asaf Qureshi. The agent of change appears to be potassium, which also regulates fluid balance in the body and normalizes muscle tone. (Best bran of the bunch: barley, which also supplies two additional cholesterol blockers.) Healthy heart factor #2 is *magnesium,* which provides three-way protection of blood pressure, veins, and arteries. Four top grain sources are rice bran, amaranth, quinoa, and wheat germ.

---

* Why bother with whole grain flour and cereals or whole unpolished brown rice? Because they supply the wheat and bran, which have been removed from refined white flour—a process that leads to losses of 70 to 97% of the B vitamin complex, zinc, chromium, magnesium, potassium, and fiber plus a 25% reduction in the protein that grains are so rich in.

PUTTING THE BRAKE ON CANCER, CONSTIPATION, AND COLON DISORDERS

Whole grain fiber is the top dietary source of fiber—which binds to certain carcinogens and environmental toxins and heavy metals such as lead, resulting in an increased excretion of these toxins from the colon. Fiber also improves regularity by reducing constipation, which is a factor in diseases such as irritable bowel syndrome, Crohn's disease, and diverticulosis.

Just 20 grams of concentrated fiber per day does the job, although the recommended daily amount is 30 to 40 grams, half soluble and half insoluble.

All fibers aren't alike: Insoluble fiber is found in such foods as wheat bran, fruits, and vegetables, while soluble fiber is found in oat bran, rice bran, apples, and dried beans and is associated with reducing blood cholesterol. Both oat and rice bran promote the excretion of bile acids and lower the risk of colon cancer (along with lowering cholesterol).

End the Quest for Rest

Grain-generous menus may save you from sleepless nights since copper and iron—two major minerals grains supply—are often deficient in the sleep deprived, says Washington, D.C. nutritional biochemist Jeffrey Bland (try cream of rice or a steamed mug of rice milk as a nitecap).

GRAINS
Leaner Girth and Good Spirit Insurance

Something sagging spiritually or physically? Whole grains could be your pick-me-up since their high fiber content makes them high-satiety appetite-suppressant foods (popped corn and rice cakes are also the ultimate low-cal filler-up foods, say dieticians) and their high B-complex content makes them natural mood elevators and energizers.

Protein for Vegetarians

Grains such as barley,* amaranth, and triticale are high in lysene, an essential building block of protein missing in most grains, while nutri-

---

*In Victorian times, barley water was a nostrum for an upset stomach and acid indigestion. Or to reverse acid indigestion, chew a handful of rolled oats slowly and then swallow without water.

tion-intense strains such as quinoa and spelt supply all eight essential amino acids and can be used as meat and dairy substitutes. Quinoa's protein content, says the USDA, is a match for whole dried milk. Here's a brief grain alphabet—

Amaranth: Grown for thousands of years by the Aztecs, Africans, Greeks, and Asian Indians and extolled for its life-giving, life-extending properties, this millet-sized seed can be prepared like rice and eaten as cereal or a side dish or ground into cornmeal and used as flour. Amaranth is rich in lysene, the amino acid absent from most grains, and rich in calcium and iron. The leaves are also edible.

Barley: Barley is another ancient grain dating back to the Stone Age and used as an antacid by the Victorians. It is a good source of plant protein, B vitamins and both soluble and insoluble fiber. (Soluble fiber lowers cholesterol, and insoluble promotes bowel regularity.) Avoid pearled barley, a heavily processed version of this grain from which the bran is removed, and look for whole hulled barley ("pot barley") (only the outer husk is removed), which is higher in fiber and all nutrients, or Scotch barley (husk and bran are removed and the grain is coarsely ground). Use in place of rice.

Buckwheat: Actually the fruit of the fagopyrum grass, buckwheat is related to rhubarb. Buckwheat which is called kasha when roasted) is a traditional Eastern European cereal grain with a nutlike flavor, a superior source of fiber, which provides vitamins E and B and protein (try cream of buckwheat to beat the breakfast blahs). It is a good alternative grain for the wheat sensitive.

Bulgur: Bulgar is wheat that has been steamed and dried before grinding. It is a traditional Middle Eastern grain used in pilafs and tabouli and is high in fiber, potassium, and B vitamins.

Couscous: Made from granular semolina wheat, couscous is a good source of fiber, B vitamins (especially folate), and iron. Buy the authentic couscous at a health food store and prepare it properly: It should be steamed in a special couscousiere (a special pot with a built-in colander) or steamed in a heavy pot lined with cheesecloth to prevent seepage. Serve warm as a side dish (add nuts, seeds, or dried fruit) or cold as a pasta salad with tossed vegetables.

Kamut: (Triticum polonicum): An ancient and close relative of the wheatberry, kamut is easier to digest and better tolerated than wheat by the wheat allergic. It is sold as cereal, flour and as a supplemental nutrition booster.

Oatmeal (including oat bran): Oatmeal is high in cholesterol-lowering fiber and B-complex vitamins and low in fat. Look for the old-fashioned long-cooking variety for maximum nutrition.

Quinoa (pronounced keen-wa): Quinoa is actually the fruit of an herb and native to the Andes. It provides all eight essential amino acids plus potassium, iron, and zinc. It is a good, mild-flavored companion to beans and stronger flavored vegetables in casseroles and loaves. It is the least allergenic of all the grains.

Triticale: Triticale is a highly nutritious complete protein hybrid of wheat and rye. It is sold in the form of whole berries, flour, or flakes.

Millet: Millet is a major component of the diet for India, Africa, China, and Russia. Ninety-four percent of the entire world's millet production occurs in Asia. Protein content can vary between 5 and 20%, with an average of 10 to 12%, making millet generally superior to wheat, corn, and rice.

Rye: Rye originated in central Asia. Today Russia is the leading producer of rye (followed by Poland, Germany, and Turkey). Rye contains twice the fiber of wheat germ (6 g) and supplies folate and iron for proper immune function and healthy blood. It is a good source of magnesium for normal blood pressure. To compensate for its denseness in baking, rye should be coupled with lighter (i.e. unbleached white) flours for baking.

Corn: Corn is a good source of complex carbohydrates, essential fatty acids, and vitamin E. It has less protein (of a lower quality) than other grains. Polenta is cooked dried cornmeal (look for whole, un-degerminated versions); white grits are the less nutritious result of grinding degerminated corn kernels.

EIGHT GOOD WAYS TO GO BY THE GRAIN

1. Be a grain brain. You can knead any ground grain into bread, dough fold it into cheese sauces, and use it to fortify waffle and muffin batters. A good grain to begin with: barley, the best choles-

terol lowerer in the category. Or have a whole-grain breakfast in bed: Once a week, fill a wide-mouthed, 1-quart thermos with barley water (to preheat). Bring 1 cup grain and 2 cups water to a boil and put in thermos. Add cereal. Cap. Place on P.M. nightstand to enjoy the next A.M.

2. Take your whole grains straight up. Drinking wheatgrass juice purifies the body, energizes and detoxifies, and even freshens-the breath and clarifies the complexion, says the Hippocratic Health Institute. Just 1 ounce has more nutritional value than 2 pounds of vegetables. Juiced grass (slightly sweet and a good supplement to other fresh juices) is exceptionally rich in vitamins A, C, E, K, and B complex; minerals such as calcium, iron, potassium, magnesium, selenium, sodium, sulfur, zinc, and other trace elements; amino acids; enzymes; and fresh chlorophyll. (Sold fresh in sprouts section, frozen and in powdered supplement form.)

3. Tired of toast? Milk a grain. Check your health food stores for nondairy rice milk in regular, low-fat, and half-and-half nut blend formats.

4. Enjoy the amaranth advantage. According to grain researcher William Brune, Ph.D., at the University of Minnesota, lab animals fed amaranth flour had a twofold increase in good HDL cholesterol, probably due to the high-protein grain's vitamin E-like compound squalene.

5. Pop it, don't boil it. Most whole grains can be popped like corn for snacks or a dry cereal. All you need is a steam popper and dry whole grains. Best candidates: Wheat, rice, triticale, oats.

6. Be a cereal do-it-yourselfer. Did you know that a typical cold cereal can be 40 to 50% fat and 80% sugar? For the same price as a box of readymade cereal, you can buy 8 pounds of whole grain to make 80 bowls of 10 times as super healing hot cereal.

7. Be a "cream of" eater once a week, but don't stop with the standards. To prepare anything from buckwheat to cousriz (a cross between couscous and rice), simply grind the whole dry raw or toasted whole or cracked kernels to a gritty powder and cook as you would commercial cream of wheat/rice cereal.

8. Flour without grinding: Substitute whole wheat (or other grain) berries for half of the flour in a pancake/waffle recipe. Process in a

blender with milk at high speed, fold in remaining ingredients, and bake off.

Buying, Storing, and Using

Grains are highly perishable because of their oil content. Keep them in the freezer in airtight bags to prevent insect infestation and spoilage or store in an airtight container in a cool pantry cupboard.

Proper measuring and preparation is the key to whole grain success. Take a look at this chart:

Grain (1 cup dry)	Cups of Water	Cooking Time	Yield
Barley	3	1–4 hours	3½ cups
Buckwheat (kasha)	2	15 minutes	2½ cups
Millet	3	45 minutes	3½ cups
Oats	2	30 minutes	3 cups
Quinoa	2¼	20 minutes	2 cups
Whole wheat			
Berries	3	2 hours	2⅔ cups
Bulgur	2	15–20 minutes	2½ cups
Cracked	2	25 minutes	2⅓ cups

Three Tips

◆ Grains can be baked pilaf style. Sauté aromatic vegetables (onions, garlic, carrots) and grains in oil or butter. Add liquid, bring to a boil. Cover. Bake in a medium-hot (350 degrees) oven until the liquid is absorbed. Pilafs can be easily reheated in the microwave.

◆ Quick-cooking grains (couscous, etc.) benefit from steaming. In fact, traditional North African couscous pots have an upper chamber to hold the tiny couscous grains over a simmering stew of meat and vegetables. Sometimes the steamed couscous is sautéed in oil with herbs.

◆ Buckwheat groats holds their shape better if mixed with a beaten egg and then sautéed briefly in a dry pan to separate the grains before adding boiling liquid to the pan.

Try these recipes:

Polenta Plus

> *2¹/₂ cups vegetable stock*
>
> *8 tablespoons un-degerminated polenta*
>
> *¹/₈ teaspoon salt substitute*
>
> *1 ounce Romano cheese (¹/₃ cup coarsely grated)*
>
> *Freshly ground black pepper to taste*

Bring stock to boil in covered pot. Stir in polenta slowly and cook for two minutes, until thickened. Season the polenta with low salt substitute and pepper and stir in cheese.

Makes two servings.

Serve hot with tossed green salad.

Variation: Add ¹/₄ cup oat or corn bran in place of cheese.
    Add ¹/₄ cup diced, cooked red or green bell pepper after cheese.

Four-Grains Tossup

> *¹/₄ cup quick-cooking barley*
>
> *¹/₄ cup whole grain rye*
>
> *¹/₄ cup kamut*
>
> *¹/₄ cup whole kasha (roasted cracked buckwheat groats)*
>
> *Stock or broth, as needed*
>
> *¹/₂ cup cucumber, peeled, seeded, and chopped*
>
> *Generous ¹/₄ cup each: chopped tomatoes, yellow pepper, red pepper, green onions*
>
> *3 tablespoons olive oil*
>
> *2 tablespoons red wine vinegar*
>
> *¹/₈ teaspoon pepper*
>
> *¹/₄ teaspoon salt substitute*
>
> *2 tablespoons Dijon mustard*

Cook grains individually in broth according to instructions. Cool, and then combine in large bowl. Add vegetables. Shake the dressing ingredients in jar and toss with the salad. Serve chilled or at room temperature.

Makes six servings.

Benefits healing zones: 2, 3, 7

Also see: Breakfast Foods, Rice, Diabetes, Hemorrhoids, Antioxidants, Vitamin E, Fatigue, Sprouts

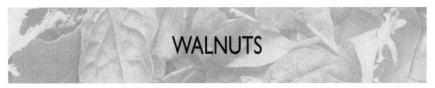

WALNUTS

Walnuts are seed money in your health bank. Actually native to Iran, the Greeks called them the fruit of the Persian tree, and it was believed that the gods feasted on them. In Rome, walnuts were strewn in the path of newlyweds, served stewed at the wedding feast, and sprinkled over the floor of the bedroom chamber as an offering to Jupiter. Originally a symbol of fertility, in time the walnut came to augur danger, misfortune, or unfaithfulness. In medieval times, the walnut because of its two-lobed resemblance to the human brain, was used to treat a wide range of mental illnesses.

BRAIN AND NERVE NIBBLE

Walnuts supply more vitamin B_6 than lemons, lima beans, or brown rice (vitamin B_6 is essential for the formation of body protein, hormonal balance and immune function) plus the B vitamins thiamine and folate for memory and concentration. Walnuts are the best food source of nerve-nourishing manganese. More nutrition in the nutshell: Walnuts have fewer calories (182) per ounce than pecans, filberts, or macadamias with twice the protein (49 grams per ounce).

HELP YOURSELF TO A HEART-BUILDING HANDFUL

Eating walnuts six times a week, conclude studies of the diets of Seventh Day Adventists, may lower your risk of heart attack and lengthen your life. The magic ingredient? Monosaturated fatty acids, which reduce cholesterol and vitamin E (walnuts are one of the 12 best nonanimal sources of this heart-protective antioxidant). Walnuts have less total fat than Brazil nuts (18 grams) and a smaller percentage of calories from fat (89%) than pine nuts, filberts, or macadamias.

FOLK CURE FOR THE SIDE EFFECTS OF A COLD OR THE FLU

According to legend, walnuts are a traditional medicine for a cold sore or fever blister. Just apply a salve of ground walnuts and cocoa butter to the area twice a day for four days.

Buying, Storing, and Using

◆ Shelled walnuts are highly perishable and should be refrigerated or frozen. Toasting improves flavor, but use a light hand since heating destroys vitamin B_6.

◆ Add chopped or crushed walnuts to fruit and vegetable salads, muffin or cake batters, stir-fries, and pilafs.

◆ Grind walnuts in a nut mill and use for a peanut butter alternative or supplement.

◆ Use chopped walnuts over steamed vegetables or grains or fold into whipped sweet potatoes.

◆ Walnuts add crunch and nutrition to hot and cold cereals.

◆ Don't fancy everyday English walnuts? try the distinctively flavored black walnuts, a favorite of American Indians 5,000 years ago. They provide more protein than regular walnuts plus omega-3 oils and iron and zinc.

Try this recipe:

Walnut Vinaigrette

1/3 cup fresh orange juice

1/4 cup walnut oil

2 tablespoons Dijon mustard

1/4 cup safflower oil

1 finely chopped shallot or 1 chopped green onion

3 tablespoons vinegar

2 tablespoons minced walnuts

Freshly ground pepper to taste

Combine all ingredients and beat with whisk until thoroughly blended. Refrigerate until ready to use.

Makes four servings.

Benefits healing zones: 2, 4, 6

Also see: Fatigue, Depression, Nuts, Coronary Heart Disease, Stress

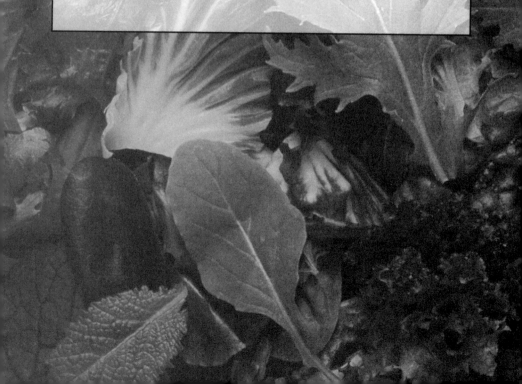

PART TWO

Common Health Problems and Their Food "Cures"

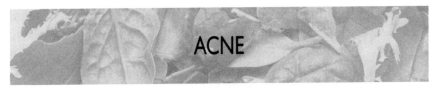

ACNE

Having a bad face day? You've got plenty of blemish-embarrassed company. Acne is America's #1 skin disorder (with psoriasis, seborrhea, eczema, dermatitis, dry skin, and broken capillaries syndrome not far behind). Acne occurs when the sebaceous (oil) glands secrete too much oil (sebum) . Dead skin then accumulates, plugging pores and preventing natural skin functions and allowing bacteria to build up and pimples to form. Other acne makers include food allergies, a fruit- and vegetable-deficient diet, dehydration, emotional stress, exposure to environmental pollution and overexposure to sunlight, faulty genes, oral contraceptive sensitivity, and hormonal imbalance. Fortunately, of all the causes, only three are beyond your control. For the remaining ones an improved diet is the most promising place to begin a face-your-face reform. Here are some internal and external food-based steps to improve acne.

ACNE MAKER-BREAKERS

1. Spot treat (don't squeeze or pinch) pimples, which can cause scarring. Use fast-fix herbal oil daily. Good choices: tea tree oil or aloe vera gel (which, says Varro Tyler, Ph.D., professor of pharmacognosy at Purdue University, inhibits the action of bradykinin, a pain-making peptide, and inhibits the formation of thromboxane, a chemical that blocks skin healing). Or apply this facial oil blend several times daily. Aromatherapy Blemish Blend: Mix jojoba oil, lavender oil, chamomile oil, and geranium oil.*

2. Increase your consumption of acne-antagonist foods (containing beta-carotene and vitamins A and E, zinc, chromium, selenium). Ten that are tops: sweet potatoes, leafy greens, apricots, wheat germ, beans, carrots, spinach, nutritional brewer's yeast, parsley, and apples.

3. Take a super healing skin dip: Two times a week or more, bathe your face and other affected parts in aromatherapy salts to reduce

---

* Available from aromatherapy suppliers, and health pharmacies (see Mail Order Sources.

the stress that triggers inflammation and to soothe and soften skin. Soak for 30 minutes. Switch to once-a-week maintenance dip when symptoms are under control.

4. Make a good antiacne facial and use it daily. Here are two:

   ◆ Combine one cake of dry baking yeast with enough lemon juice to produce a paste with cold-cream-like consistency. Apply evenly, and remove after 20 minutes with warm water.

   ◆ Powder ⅓ cup uncooked oats in blender. Add warm water (less than ⅓ cup) to consistency of paste. Apply to pimples and allow it to dry completely. (Hot or cold water can cause capillaries to break, so be sure to use warm water when you rinse off facial masks.)

5. Put fruits rich in glycolic and alphahydroxy acids on your menus for acne control. Best sources: apples, pears, berries, and cherries.

6. Avoid all salty, iodine-rich foods; refined carbohydrates; and foods that are fried or that contain acne-triggering trans-fatty acids (e.g., milk, margarine, shortening).

7. Avoid medications with bromide or iodide and greasy creams and cosmetics, and thoroughly cleanse your face with a sulfur-containing soap (an alternative is calendula soap) daily. An optional follow-up is lubrication with tea tree oil.

8. Build your omega-3 and EFA stores in three ways. A shortage of both is common among acne sufferers, says skin specialist Gustav Skreiner, M.D., of Graz, Austria. Salad, green juices, low fat dairy foods, and vegetable/nut oils—especially flaxseed oil—are the three best nonanimal sources of omega-3 EFAs.

See the useful charts on the following pages.

SKIN-DEEP TRIVIA

Did you know these interesting skin facts?

◆ Your skin is the largest organ of your body.

◆ You have an average of 17 square feet of skin.

◆ The total weight of your skin (from your forehead to your big toe) is 5 pounds (5% more or less of your body weight).

◆ By the time you reach age 70, you will have shed 40 pounds of dead skin.

SUPER HEALING BEAUTY
20 Top Herbs and Foods

	Astringent	Calmative	Cleansing	Cuts, Bruises, Skin, Massage	Eczema, Acne, Skin Disorders	Inflammation	Moisturizing Softening
Aloe			•	•	•	•	•
Almonds							•
Apricot							•
Arnica							•
Avocado							•
Chamomile	•		•	•	•	•	•
Cucumber	•	•		•			•
Dandelion			•				
Echinacea				•	•		
Eucalyptus	•		•				
Ginseng	•	•					•
Goldenseal	•				•		
Horsetail	•	•	•	•	•	•	
Lavender	•	•	•	•	•		•
Nettle	•		•				•
Papaya			•	•	•		•
Plantain			•	•	•	•	
Rosemary			•		•		
Sage	•	•	•		•		•
Witch Hazel			•	•	•	•	•

FACE VALUE VITAMINS AND MINERALS
The Five That Prevent the Five Most Common Skin Problems

Vitamin	Uses	Deficiency Symptoms	Sources (Nonanimal)
Vitamin A is for the production of new cells and for repair of mucous membranes. Depleted by stress and illness.	Antiaging, antioxidant, prevents dryness, fights acne.	Weakened immune system, dry skin, dandruff, night blindness, toxicity, acne.	Deep green and yellow vegetables, milk, eggs, cantaloupe.
Vitamin B is for building protein, cell generation and repair, nervous system health, and antistress. Helps liver make glycogen, which enables the skin to cleanse itself of dead cells.	Antistress, antioxidant, collagen building.	Premature aging of skin, tiredness, stress, scaling and cracking of the skin, dark circles under the eyes, tiny lines above the lips.	Whole grains, bananas, eggs, mushrooms potatoes, legumes, yogurt, brewer's yeast.
Vitamin C helps the body heal, builds and maintain collagen and elastin, resist infection and form pigment. Need increases with age. Important for metabolization of amino acids and activation of folic acid.	Detoxification, antiviral, antibacterial, builds collagen and elastin.	Premature aging of skin, broken capillaries, acne and psoriasis, bleeding gums, skin that bruises easily.	Citrus fruits, tomatoes, dark green and yellow vegetables, strawberries, cantaloupe, cabbage.
Vitamin E has the strongest healing ability of all the vitamins. Helps protect Vitamin A and other oils or fats from rancidity. Transports oxygen to cells.	Treats "liver spots," varicose veins, and premenstrual and menopausal symptoms.	Premature aging of skin, dry skin, clogged arteries, and veins.	Vegetable oils, fresh vegetables, wheat germ, nuts, legumes.
Zinc is the most important trace mineral for healthy skin. Combines with vitamin A for protein synthesis, for healing. Helps regulate oil glands and clear skin.	Aids with skin problems.	Dry skin, white spots under fingernails, slow metabolism.	Peas, nuts, beans, grains, brewer's yeast, dairy products.

See foods for healing zones: 1, 4, 6

Also see: **Herbs, Beta-carotene, Water, Stress, Allergies**

For more information about acne, call the Medical Information Line's Acne Hot Line at 1-900-230-2300.

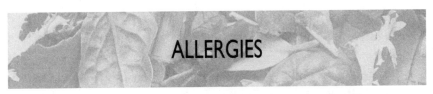

ALLERGIES

One of every two of us suffer from allergies, whose symptoms run the gamut from sneezing, hives, eczema, diahrrea, and constipation to anxiety, depression, eating disorders, and memory loss. If you'd like to stop being a statistic and reduce your dependence on the allergy drugs that may be interfering with your mental functioning, motor skills, and general well-being, there are a number of food-driven directions you can take.

FOUR STEPS TO RELIEF

First, know the enemy. The term *allergy* describes an altered physiological reaction to a substance that is often harmless. Although the exact cause isn't fully understood, susceptibility depends on heredity, hormone imbalance, emotional or environmental stress, toxic waste substances, and liver and gallbladder problems. The best method for coping with allergies is to seek treatment, avoid or reduce your exposure to your personal allergens, reduce physical and emotional stress, and heal your immune system.

NUTRIENTS FOR ALLERGY CONTROL

After identifying your sensitivities, the next step is to design yourself a defensive daily eating plan that accentuates the positive and minimizes the negative without sacrificing the essentials. Once you know your eating limits, help yourself to as many of the following sensitivity-reducing nutrients and the foods they're found in as you can, beginning with the flavonoids (such as quercetin, a potent antiallergen found in yellow onions, strawberries, and citrus fruits which, says Bastyn College Health Information Project's N.D. Wayne Mitchell, inhibits the release of histamines and other allergenic compounds).

- ◆ Vitamin B_6 (found in dark green and sweet peppers).

- ◆ Vitamin C (leafy greens, citrus fruits, melons) reduces blood histamine levels and chemical sensitivities.

- ◆ Bioflavonoids (melons, parsley, berries, citrus) potentiate the action of vitamin C.

- ◆ Yogurt, kefir, and cultured milk products reduce the burden of antigens in the digestive tract.

- ◆ Vitamin E (found in asparagus, nuts and seeds, and spinach) provides anithistamine activity.

- ◆ Molybdenum (found in cauliflower, spinach, and garlic).

- ◆ Flavonoids (found in oranges, grapes, and berries).

10 HERB TEAS THAT REDUCE HISTAMINES

Your next best bet: herbs and herb teas that reduce both seasonal and chronic allergy suffering. Two cloves of garlic a day (baked, juiced, or added crushed to salads and spreads) not only supply plenty of molybdenum for sinus decongestion but also improve digestion and work even better if you follow up with a cup of ginger root or astralagus tea with fresh lemon or lime juice 15 minutes before meals to enhance stomach acid secretion. (Bitter greens do the same if you're citrus-sensitive.)

Medicinal herbal teas that turn hay fever around (if they're not off limits) include eyebright, goldenrod, chamomile, and nettle. Drink three to four cups a day during the allergy season. Even better, green tea extends the effectiveness of vitamin C and reduces the likelihood of infection due to a stressed immune system.

Gargling with eyebright or ginger is a drug-free aid for an irritated throat. Chilled herbal tea bags are also good for reducing external inflammation. (Black tea contains tannic acid, an anti-inflmmatory astringent.)

When chronic food allergies are the problem, it's consoling to know that there's always a next best thing, a taste-alike you can substitute. For a list for your back pocket and fridge door, briefcase, or computer disk, see "Substitutes" (p. 191).

11 TIPS FOR ALLERGY SUPER HEALING

1. Be prepared for an allergy crisis with cysteine, an amino acid (at health food stores) that inactivates the insulin raised by a reaction and brings blood sugar levels back to normal. One gram helps, especially when taken with 3 grams (3,000 μg) of vitamin C.

2. Give your body an "allergic rest period now and then," advise clinical ecologists, and in six months you should be able to eat 50 to 70% of the foods you can't tolerate now.

3. What allergy test is best? The most popular method, the Four-Day Fast, has a 90% accuracy rate. The least effective (for food sensitivity) is the skin test, which pinpoints food problems only 20% of the time. If you suffer from chronic sinusitis, have your immune function tested. Half of all patients studied in one recent survey suffered from problems controllable with immunoglobulin.

4. Allergic to most common fruits? To satisfy your uncommon craving for jams and jellies, check stores for sapodilla scuppernong (an offbeat grape jelly from the South) or muscadine or jellies made from acerola (the Barbados cherry, rich in vitamin C), carissa (the Natal plum), and the pyracantha jelly of Texas or Hawaii's papaya preserves and guava jelly.

5. Barbiturates and tranquilizers are poorly tolerated by the allergic. If you can't sleep, maybe you need to restore your body's mineral balance. You can do that by simmering a small head of lettuce in one pint of water (or milk, which contains nature's tranquilizer amino acid, L-tryptophan) for 15 minutes. It makes a healthy sleep tonic and is rich in seven healing minerals, including calcium and iron.

6. Avoid smoke, paint, insect spray, moth balls, and even magic markers. Allergic symptoms from foods are often aggravated by chemical stress.

7. Are you allergic or aren't you? Ask your health pharmacy about Rescue Test, a service of the Institute for Biological Ecology, which allows you to monitor your physical and emotional reactions to suspected offenders that you ingest. The company promises a "50

% refund to any client if no relief of symptoms is recognized with-in three months following the tests."

8. Enzyme action: You can arrest an allergic food response—even eliminate it—by taking protein-digesting pancreatic enzymes with every meal. A good supplement should provide 300 to 400 µg of pancreas concentrate.

9. Avoid restaurants that use gas for cooking or illuminating. It often induces allergic attacks. Ditto sterno (i.e., canned heat).

10. Blue-green relief: Spirulina, a blue-green algae (seaweed) available in powdered form at health food stores, is rich in phenylalaline, an amino acid that helps suppress allergic symptoms, says the Association of Naturopathic Physicians. Stir a teaspoon into juice two to three times daily.

11. Allergies that aren't: Allergy-like reactions, says Dr. S. Allan Bock, pediatric allergist at the National Jewish Hospital Asthma Center in Denver, can have other causes. Three common ones: sensitivi-ty to a natural substance or a contaminant, such as penicillin in milk (from antibiotics given to cows) or contamination in seafood; enzyme deficiencies, such as insufficiency of lactase, the enzyme that digests milk sugar (lactose); and stress and emotion-al problems.

12 TOP MEALS-THAT-HEAL JUICES

What's the next quickest way (besides teas) to get healing? Get juicing. Here are the 12 top ingredients for juices, soups, or liquid meals that heal (any of the aforementioned teas may be added for healing plus): kale, spinach, collard greens, parsley, carrots, asparagus, cauliflower, garlic, oranges, cantaloupes, onions, berries.*

Besides edibles, exercise and alternative therapies (such as acu-pressure, body balancing, and shiatsu, which targets and helps alleviate organic problems that trigger hypersensitivity) can provide help for allergy sufferers. Here's an allergy sufferer's guide to safely getting phys-ical, from the Allergy Information Center.

---

* Avoid those to which you are sensitive or allergic.

Good	Bad	Maybe
Aerobics (indoor)	Hiking/climbing	Sailing
Swimming	Running	Fishing
Weight training	In-line skating	Wind surfing
Bowling	Horseback riding	Tennis
	Running (outdoors)	

Call the Allergy Information Center at 1-800-727-5400 for more information.

See foods for healing zones: **1, 3, 4, 6**

Also see: **Herbs, Vitamins, Leafy Greens, Juices, Ecology, Dairy Substitutes**

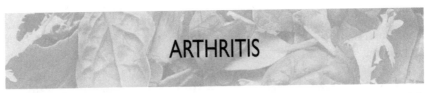

ARTHRITIS

According to a recent survey by the National Center for Health Statistics, there are more than 40 million Americans (one out of every eight) who suffer from arthritis, rheumatism, and gout (a form of arthritis), a 37% increase over the past decade. Counting related diseases such as bursitis, low back and shoulder pain, juvenile arthritis, lupus erythematosus, and scleroderma, the total figure is nearer 50 million.

ANATOMY OF AN ACHE

You don't have to be all that old to get arthritis (which is usually labeled a disorder of the elderly) or all that unfit—even runners run the risk. Arthritis pays no attention to age, although the older you get the likelier you are to be a victim. Only 5 to 7% of us between the ages of 17 and 44 are arthritic, for example, compared to 23% of us between 45 and 64, and 40% of us age 65 and over. Twice as many women as men are victims, and even children suffer from autoimmune disorders within the arthritis syndrome. Arthritis causes significant crippling in children under the age of 18—retarding growth, causing serious social or emotional problems, and can lead to severe kidney disease, blindness, or even death.

And arthritis shows no mercy where anatomy is concerned.

Just what is it that's out of order when you have this disorder? It could be any organ or body system. Most Americans do not realize that the diseases involved in arthritis may affect not merely bones and joints but also blood vessels, the kidneys, the skin, the eyes, and the brain, says the Arthritis and Health Resource Center in Wellesley, Massachusetts.

THE CRIPPLER WITH 100 NAMES

Nor is arthritis a simple disease. Osteoarthritis and rheumatoid arthritis, the two most commonly encountered forms, are only two of the approximately 100 conditions known collectively as rheumatic diseases, a term that encompasses such seemingly diverse conditions as tendinitis, hepatitis, gout, syphilis, diabetes mellitus, and multiple myeloma. For example, fibromyalgia or fibrositis—actually a soft-tissue rheumatic condition affecting three to six million Americans—is often misdiagnosed as chronic fatigue syndrome (previously known as Epstein-Barr virus syndrome). So is the debilitating bone disorder Paget's disease. Secondary osteoarthritis can occur from infections, disease, injury to a joint, the physical stress of obesity, or poor posture. Primary osteoarthritis (degenerative joint disease), says the Arthritis Foundation, affects almost everyone in midlife as a result of aging. Arthritis can also be activated by allergies. What's called Type I hypersensitivity, for example, expresses itself as cell inflammation in the joints within two hours of ingesting an offending food. The characteristic progression involves inflammation of membranes lining the joints, which can gradually erode cartilage and involve blood vessels, muscles, and other organs. A deficiency of hydrochloric acid can also be a contributing factor.

STEPS TO HEALING WHAT HURTS

While a true cure short of surgical replacement may be hard to find, there are plenty of effective ways you can get a handle on what hurts with your knife and fork—plus a little exercise to reduce the stress of this "wear-and-tear" disease. First, get professional testing to determine food allergies and identify if a hypochloric acid deficiency is present. Then follow these seven steps to healing.

More Histidines and Less Cake, Iron, and Eggplant

"Keep your histidine high and you could reduce the chances that your joints will be jumping, now or ever," says Dr. Donald A. Gerber, associate professor of medicine at Downstate Medical Center in New York. To prevent arthritis or relieve early symptoms, eat a lot of high histidine foods, Gerber advises. (Histidine, an essential amino acid, is characteristically low in arthritis sufferers.) This means more eggs, whole milk (unless you're a strict vegetarian), wheat germ, soybean foods, brown rice and whole grains, nutritional yeast, dried peas, and beans on the menu. And to eliminate pain, you'd be better off without baked goods.

"Maps of areas of the planet where gluten-high cereals are eaten correspond to areas where rheumatoid arthritis is most prevalent. The disease is least common where rice and corn (both low in gluten) are the basic cereals," says Dr. Raymond Shatin of the Alfred Hospital in Melbourne, Australia.

Other staple foods that may cause you to feel considerably more arthritic and less well are eggplant and other nightshade foods such as potatoes, tomatoes, and peppers. According to Dr. Norman F. Childers, a professor of horticulture at Rutgers University, the nightshade family of plants is often responsible for the aches and pains of arthritis. Nightshade-substitute foods include sweet potatoes, yams, corn, turnips, radishes, onions, cucumber, cauliflower, cabbage, lettuce, celery, melons, parsley, squash, artichokes, garlic, olives, and leafy greens. Relief often occurs in four to six weeks. But not if you keep popping those iron pills. Excess iron, especially from supplemental sources, is stored in various parts of the body—including the liver, spleen, and joints. In the joints, iron causes a chemical reaction that results in painful inflammation. "Unless it's absolutely necessary medically, arthritics should avoid taking iron supplements, advises Dr. Paul Bacon, professor of rheumatology at the University of Birmingham in England.

More Alfalfa and Less Refined Food

Trace elements that are in very short supply in the bodies of arthritis patients are zinc, manganese, molybdenum, chromium, tin, and aluminum," advises Dr. Carl Pfeiffer of Princeton New Jersey's Brain Bio Institute. Is it any surprise? "White sugar and white flour and every food made from them contain relatively huge amounts of carbohydrates, from which practically all of the B vitamins, the minerals, and trace minerals have been removed in the refining process," says Dr. Pfeiffer.'

Proper nutrition is essential for healing both rheumatoid arthritis, which results from insufficient fluids to keep the joints free from friction, and osteoarthritis, which causes a breakdown of cartilage that protects joints.

"Many arthritis patients eat too many sweets, fats and foods made from refined flour," explains noted nutritionist and rheumatology researcher Dr. Ruth Yale Long. In place of snacks, try alfalfa sprouts and alfalfa tea and liquid alfalfa (to fortify prepared dishes). Alfalfa is 18.9% protein and supplies the vitamins A, B complex, C, D, E, K, and U,* along with the minerals magnesium, phosphorus, sulfur, silicon, sodium, and potassium, several digestive enzymes, and chlorophyll, an antioxidant which speeds the healing process. Additional noninvasive anti-inflammatory healers are the homeopathic salts compounded from honey called Apis and bryonia, a salt derived from wild hops.

More B₅, Less Beef

Studies show that the dietary intake of patients with degenerative joint disease and rheumatoid arthritis is typically deficient in B-complex vitamins, especially pantothenic acid (B_5). Pantothenic acid reserves are often 50% lower than normal.

Prolonged stress can increase the nutritional requirements for vitamin B_5, and the adrenal glands which handle stress can become severely damaged. Good food sources of B_5 include soybeans, broccoli, and whole grains (which also provide a well-tolerated natural source of iron).

Reducing saturated fats by switching to a meat-free or semivegetarian diet that includes low or no fat dairy foods is also beneficial.

---

* Not a vitamin at all but a healing substance also found in cabbage juice that also benefits the ulcer-prone.

According to researchers at the Albany, New York, Medical School, arthritis-prone tissues produce large amounts of certain pain- and inflammation-promoting natural substances called prostaglandins. A diet low in meat, fatty fishes and cheeses, and poultry and high in EPA-rich polyunsaturated vegetable and nut oils often reduces stiffness, tenderness, and joint discomfort in a matter of weeks. For even greater relief, try raw vegetarian foods and juice fasting.

Less Grocery-Shelf Tea, More Garden-Patch Herbs

If you have arthritis or hope never to have it, take regular tea off your menu. Besides the bad-for-the-metabolism caffeine, regular teas are high in fluoride—a toxic metal (also found in many municipal water supplies). A high fluoride intake has been suggested as a possible cause of arthritis, warns the Preventative Medical Research Institute, and complete relief is often the result of abstaining from all regular tea drinks and fluorine food sources. (*Note:* The amount of fluoride you absorb varies with the strength of the leaf and brewing/steeping time. Brewing with fluoridated water doubles the dose.)

Teacup solutions: Try yucca and green teas. The first is an ancient healing herb used as food and medicine by desert Indians. The second is one of the two top sources of the antioxidant flavonoids.

Yucca saponin appears to have an indirect systemic effect on arthritis or collagen diseases, probably through enhancement of the enterocoelic flora, says the Herb Research Foundation. Green tea is rich in vitamin C and a major source of antioxidant flavonoids and polyphenols, which the National Cancer Institute is studying for their anti-cancer and immunity-boosting activities. Other arthritic-relief herbs to brew include nettle, sage, basil, rosemary—and cornsilk tea, a time-honored American Indian nostrum. A time-honored East Indian ayurvedic arthritic herb healer is Boswellia Serrata (look for it in cream form at health pharmacies).

Less Cortisone, More Celery

It may not beat cortisone, gold salts, and salicylate for fast action, but common, garden-variety celery is a lot softer and side-effect free.

According to the American Association of Naturopathic Physicians (AANP), nonsteroidal anti-inflammatory drugs (NSAIDs) can produce serious long-term side effects resulting in cartilage damage and sometimes bone loss.

Celery leaves are a top rated source of natural sodium; the stalk is high in potassium. The combination of these two organic substances appears to help dissolve inorganic calcium deposits characteristic in arthritis. Celery also contains chlorine, magnesium, sulfur, phosphorus, calcium, and vitamins A, B, C, and E. (A deficiency of these four vitamins is considered a contributing factor to the development of this autoimmune disease. A juice of equal parts celery and carrot provides an almost perfect mineral-balanced healing cocktail (see the recipes at the end of this section).

Forget Cocktails, Increase Copper, Boron, and Vitamins C and E

What caffeine and nightshades do, alcohol does in spades. Instead of coffee and cocktails, increase your intake of copper-rich and vitamin E foods, including apples, carrots, and ginger, plus the enzyme bromelin (found only in fresh pineapple); all have anti-inflammatory properties. Sulphur (found in cruciferous vegetables) is needed as part of the protein infrastructure of the joints.

Don't forget boron. According to researchers at the Royal Melbourne Hospital in Australia, "The indication is that boron is a safe and beneficial treatment of osteoarthritis and that further research is required." The best sources are unfermented green tea and apples. Five juice combinations that supply all seven nutrients: broccoli, green tea, and kale; kale, parsley, and spinach; spinach and carrots; carrot, ginger root, and pineapple; and cherry, apple, and blueberry.

For good measure, nibble on leafy dark greens tossed with toasted flax seeds. There is growing evidence that the vitamin C and omega-3 fatty acids that both contain (also in fish oil for nonvegetarians) reduce arthritic stiffness and pain.

Weight Training— and Hot Rice for Arthritis Relief

Another good defense against arthritis—now or later—is weight training, which builds strength and flexibility, which in turn improves the mobility of the joints. (Gentle stretching exercises, such as yoga asanas, also help.) Weight training also increases muscle tone, strength, and endurance.

Especially important is arthritis-specific exercise. For example, the muscles that govern the bending process are much stronger than the muscles that pull the other way, advise experts. Since most stiff joints are already bent, bending them still further may be the worst thing you can do. Instead, they should be exercised in other ways to strengthen the muscles that pull against the bending muscles. If shoulders and back are stiff, the best way to exercise these is to move the arms away from the body, to the side, and to lie face down on a bed for stretching the back. Sitting for long hours keeps the knees and hips bent, thereby making the bad joints which are already bent worse. When you can't get to the gym, treat your joints to "rice bag therapy." Fill a 7 × 11 inch sack with 1 cup of regular rice. Place in a microwave oven and heat on high for two to four minutes. Apply the sack to painful areas. The grains absorb and gradually release the heat in the form of a healing, moist heat.

Try these recipes:

Antioxidant Celery Tonic

Combine equal parts of freshly juiced celery and carrot juice.

For more vitamin C, add 1 teaspoon of powdered high-potency ascorbic acid (such as Ester C) or dilute with green tea.

Blue Ginger Beer

> *1 quart blueberries*
>
> *1 medium bunch red grapes*
>
> *1/4-inch slice ginger root*
>
> *Sparkling water or green tea*

Push blueberries through chopper, followed by grapes and ginger. Pour juice into ice-filled glass. Fill glass to top with sparkling water or tea.

For more guidance, call the Arthritis Hotline at 1-900-230-4800, extension 7121.

See foods for healing zones: 3, 5, 6

Also see: **Herbs, Juices, Vitamin C, Aspirin Alternatives, Cruciferous Vegetables, Celery, Antioxidants**

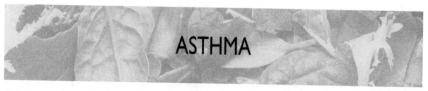

ASTHMA

Are you one of America's 15 million asthmatics? Asthma is defined as difficulty in breathing accompanied by sporadic wheezing caused by spasms of the bronchial tubes or a swelling of the mucous membranes. Asthma means shortness of breath, coughing, and mucus for most victims. Although allergens are the primary culprit, emotions and stress also play a part.

What are the best teacup solutions when you're wheezing? For openers, try chamomile (especially the super healing German varieties). One of its chief components, for example, is azulene,* a compound which offsets asthmatic attacks when three to four cupsful are drunk on a daily basis or when it is inhaled as a vapor and/or used as a back-of-the-throat spray to relieve choking sensations, says author John Heinerman. A second herbal tea is cherry bark, and a third is made with ginger root and lemon and is drunk one cup before meals and before bed. Another folk remedy with a track record is a tumbler full of freshly extracted endive/celery/carrot juice.

Even better, fill your mug with *ginkgo biloba,* the most widely prescribed phytopharmaceutical (healing herb) in the world, which improves capillary integrity, collagen formation, and helps maximize recovery from asthmatic inflammatory responses, says the Herb Research Foundation.

Foods rich in magnesium and calcium and vitamins B_6 and B_{12} (dark leafy greens, including kale and chard, yogurt, kefir, nuts, and seeds) are your next line of defense. All three promote relaxation of bronchial smooth muscle tissue, which in turn opens passages and facilitates normal breathing. B_6 is also a key coenzyme in the synthesizing of neurotransmitter chemicals such as serotonin, adrenaline and norepinephrine, needed for asthmatic relief. Magnesium reduces histamine response in allergy-related asthma.

---

* Which also works antiwheezing wonders with hay fever.

B_{12} hastens the body's overall recovery from asthma that is allergy related by blocking sulfite-induced bronchial spasms, says Mitchell Chavez, B.S.C.N., of the Alternative Medical Research Foundation.

Chili peppers, which can desensitize air passages to irritants, and onions and garlic, which contain an anti-inflammatory substance that blocks an asthma-triggering enzyme (leukotriene), are also helpful for asthmatics.

A vegetarian diet (preferably organic) eliminates the allergic/inflammatory reactions that the arachidonic acid in animal products often produces. Try eating fewer cereal grains and more fresh greens and noncitrus fruits.

What you don't eat is as important as what you do, since over 75% of children and 40% of adults suffering from asthma have some type of unrecognized food allergies that contribute to their condition. The worst offenders are eggs, citrus fruits, coffee, tea, alcohol, corn, wheat, dairy products,* and all chemical food additives, says nutritionist Allan Gaby, M.D.

The less salt the better. Excessive salt, which can increase the severity of an attack, is a factor in 90% of all asthma episodes, according to British researchers.

Besides professional help in identifying food allergies and other sensitivities, natural antiasthma therapies with a track record include homeopathic salts, and acupuncture (see Mail Order Sources).

Getting Help

◆ Call the Asthma Helpline at 1-800-230-1311.

◆ Write to the Asthma Information Center, P.O. Box 790, Springhouse, PA 19477-0790.

◆ Call the National Jewish Center for Immunology and Respiratory Medicine Information Services at 1-800-222-LUNG.

See foods for healing zones: **4, 3**

Also see: **Substitutes, Vegetarian Foods, Stress**

---

* Cheddar cheese, which contains tyromine, an amino acid that exerts an antiwheeze effect on breathing passages, may be an exception.

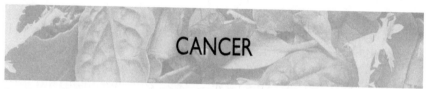

CANCER

Don't know beans about nutrition? It's worth boning up, and beans—which are rich in both fiber that lowers your risk of colon and rectal cancer and isoflavones (antioxidants) that reduce your risk of breast cancer—aren't a bad place to begin if you're defending yourself from America's second deadliest disease.

NUTRITIONAL SELF-DEFENSE IS 90% OF THE BATTLE

While cancer will affect two out of every five Americans by the year 2000, says Dr. Charles B. Simon, director of the Simone Cancer Center in Princeton, New Jersey, 80 to 90% of all cancers are related to nutritional factors (a high-animal-fat, high-cholesterol, low-fiber diet), lifestyle (tobacco smoking, excessive alcohol consumption) , the environment (chemical carcinogens, ozone, air pollution, industrial exposure), and self-induced drug abuse.

Sixty percent of all female cancer and 40% of all male cancer is related to what you eat and drink. The upside is that only 8 to 10% of all cancers are linked to factors beyond your control, like heredity—the rest is more or less your own doing including bad habits like smoking, alcohol, drugs, uncontrolled stress, and—above all—poor eating patterns.

A lot of common sense and a little commitment could save your life. Here are the only eight anticancer commandments you'll ever need.

1. Know the enemy. One third of all cancers can be prevented with a little know-how. The first step is to know how to spot the warning signals (and the sooner the better, since the risk increases with age):

   ◆ A lump or thickening in the breast

   ◆ A change in a wart or mole

   ◆ A sore that does not heal

   ◆ A change in bowel or bladder habits

- A persistent cough or hoarseness
- Constant indigestion or trouble swallowing
- Unusual bleeding or discharge

Know how to find a doctor who knows how to administer a comprehensive, cancer-detective, A-to-Z physical annually (see Mail Order Sources).

If you're already a cancer victim and want to improve your survival odds, consider integrating an alternative healing method into your treatment program such as acupressure, acupuncture, or *chi gong*, a traditional Oriental medical method of healing championed by David Eisenberg, M.D. of Harvard Medical School in Boston (see Mail Order Sources) and check with the American Holistic Medical Association.

2. Do a bad-habit inventory and do something about it. Reduce your use of all recreational drugs (including excessive caffeine, alcohol, and nicotine). Get your recreational high from a recreational sport or a new health modality like dance therapy, reiki, or creative visualization/meditation. If you must take drugs, follow your doctor's directions, ask your pharmacist about nutrient interaction, think twice about estrogens for conditions besides contraception, and avoid androgen steroids taken for any purported physical advantage or enhancement.

   If you can't stop smoking (or until you do), foods rich in antioxidants, especially elegiac acid (apples, cherries, berries, and nuts), can protect you from some of the harmful effects of polycyclic hydrocarbons and the 42 carcinogens in every cigarette. (Quitting adds almost two years to your life.)

   As for alcohol, according to the USDA Nutrition Research Center of Beltsville, Maryland, the equivalent of two mixed drinks a day can increase estrogen levels 7 to 32% during the menstrual cycle of healthy young women. Elevated estrogen puts you at increased risk of breast cancer.

3. Exchange fat for fiber. According to researchers at the Harvard School of Public Health who examined the diets of more than 7,000 men, those who consumed the most saturated fat and the least fiber were four times more likely to develop colon polyps (often a prelude to cancer) than those who ate diets high in fiber and low in fat.

A fatty treat is double trouble if it's fried or grilled, releasing carcinogenic pyrolosates. If you're not going to stop braking for beefsteak and butter, up your fiber to slow the risk and rate of certain cancers by as much as 30%.

Do what people do in Japan, where rice and complex carbohydrate vegetables are staples: An intake of 50 to 60 grams of unsoluble fiber a day (2½ times the American average) from bran, fruits, vegetables, and beans speeds up the amount of time food spends in the digestive tract, reducing exposure to carcinogens and binding to bile acids to prevent them from irritating stomach and colon walls. As a bonus, foods rich in fiber are usually rich in beta-carotene and other protective phytochemicals.

4. Get physical. The leaner you get, says Rose Frisch, a geneticist and associate professor emerita at the Harvard School of Public Health, the better use your body makes of nonpotent estrogen, the non-cancer-forming form of the female hormone. The more fat you have, the more storage space you provide for potent estrogen.

5. Stay in the RDA black. Nutritional deficiencies leave you wide open to autoimmune disorders, especially cancer. Vitamin K, for instance, which is similar in chemical structure to a potent chemotherapy drug, doxorubicin, and nontoxic in normal dietary intake, has demonstrated a selective toxin effect in human cancer studies. Vitamin A functions as an antioxidant in the form of beta-carotene and stimulates intercellular communication, which in turn encourages abnormal cells to convert their DNA material back to normal. Coincidentally, scientists find that vitamin A also lowers the recurrence of head and neck tumors in cancer patients. Many vitamins and minerals do double duty as anticancer antioxidants.

Another notable anticancer nutrient, found in sunflower seeds, wheat germ, oat flakes, granola, cheese, milk, and eggs, is the essential amino acid methionine. A methionine deficiency raises the risk of cancer, especially of the colon, and can lead to folic acid deficiency, which in turn increases your risk of developing cervical cancer, says Bernard Levin, M.D., at the M. D. Anderson Cancer Center of the University of Texas at Houston. (Folic acid is found in leafy greens, nuts, and seeds; see Mail Order Sources.)

If you suspect deficiencies your doctor hasn't uncovered, see a nutritionist.

6. Think antioxidants and vitamin A. Learn what they are and where these 100 or more cancer-combating compounds are found (see Antioxidants)—such as the isoflavones in soybeans, which reduce the risk of reproductive system cancer, and the beta-carotene in broccoli and carrots, which prevents cancers of the stomach, colon, lungs, and esophagus.

7. Don't overlook the uncommon healing power of common herbs. Topping the list is green tea, which contains the most potent natural antimutagen known (phenolic acid, also found in berries, plums, and apples), which can cause reductions in stomach cancer of up to 40%, say researchers at the National Cancer Institute of Japan and China.

   Even culinary herbs such as cumin, poppy seed, and basil appear to inhibit stomach cancer by boosting levels of an enzyme believed to block cancer in the digestive tract.

8. Know the hidden enemy. There is increasing evidence that exposure to low-level electromagnetic (ELM) radiation that is given off by power lines, electric blankets, video display terminals (VDTs), and even some electric clocks may trigger cancer. More than a dozen studies of men whose work exposed them to ELM radiation were found to have an increased incidence of leukemia, lymphoma, and brain cancer. At least two epidemiological studies show that a statistically high number of young victims of cancer lived near high-current electrical lines, and a study of New York State telephone workers by an epidemiologist at Johns Hopkins University showed that exposure to magnetic fields on a daily basis increased the risk of leukemia and other cancers. ELM radiation impairs the ability of T-lymphocyte cells—the infection fighters of the immune system—to combat cancer.

FIVE STEPS FOR SELF-DEFENSE

◆ Reduce (or eliminate) your use of electric blankets, heating pads, and heated waterbeds. At the very least, use a low-ELM-emission product.

◆ Keep at a 3-foot distance from all digital electronic devices, including TV receivers.

- Safety-proof your workplace: Never sit closer than 30 inches from the front, side, or back of your VDT.

- Keep informed and join a consumer activist group like the Fund for the Environment, and be part of the solution.

- Reduce your exposure to environmental carcinogens as well as prolonged exposure to toxic chemicals—including household cleaners, solvent, paint thinners, pesticides, fungicides, and other lawn and garden products. A University of Oregon study says that homemakers who are exposed to such dangers, are twice as likely to die from cancer as some office workers or the unemployed.

SEVEN WAYS TO CANCER-PROOF YOUR DIET IN SEVEN DAYS

Day One: What do the Japanese, Finnish, and America's Seventh Day Adventists eat that prevents tumors of the colon, the United States' #1 cancer? Plenty of pectin—a fruit and vegetable fiber that's more beneficial than bran. Today, have a pectin-rich snack before bedtime instead of low-fiber, high-fat pizza. The fruits richest in pectin are apples, pears, strawberries, plums, and tangerines.

Day Two: Think alternative protein. The purines in protein-rich foods raise your uric acid levels and lower your risk of cancer, but the fat raises the risk. Two soy foods with all of meat's protein but only one third of its calories and fat: tofu and tempeh, low-calorie meat substitutes that can be broiled or baked and sauced to taste like broiled chicken, veal, or beef. Have one for dinner or swap your lunchtime dairy milkshake for a cup of creamy tofu milk (at health food stores).

Day Three: Concentrate on reducing your exposure to sunlight, air pollution, and needless medications and reduce your cancer risk by 5%. Skip foods with artificial food colorings (one of the two major causes of lymph gland cancer), according to the government's Occupational Safety and Health Administration (OSHA) and you lower your risk of getting cancer even more. But don't desert dessert. Make Very Cherry Gelo: Heat 2 cups of fresh juiced or bottled cherry or cranberry juice, combine with two packages of plain gelatin (dissolved in 1 cup cold water). Mix well and chill until firm.

Day Four: Practice bad-habit control today and be a survivor. Thirty percent of all cancer deaths are linked to smoking. If you can't stop, switch to tobacco-free cigarettes filled with healthy dried herbs as a good *temporary* crutch. Or ask your doctor about nicotine chewing gum, which has a long-term success rate of 40% even for the heavily addicted. Herb teas that reduce the urge to smoke include calamus root, mullein, coltsfoot, and rosemary. End every day in the black with a cup of anticancer green tea (see Herbs).

Day Five: Don't brake for coffee. Take time out for a Carotene Cocktail: Add 1 teaspoon of real cream to 1 glass of carrot juice. "The cream helps the body absorb the beta-carotene, which inactivates the blocking shields on the surface of the cancer cells," according to world-famous cancer specialist Dr. Hans Nieper.

Day Six: Munch a bunch of cole slaw for lunch. Cabbage helps combat cancer of the lungs, colon, rectum, and stomach. If you hate cabbage, make friends with its milder relatives—watercress, white and red radish, and cauliflower. All are crucifer vegetables, which improve your body's output of tumor-inhibiting enzymes. After you grate them, make them with a low-fat soy mayo and season with a no-sodium Super Healing Salt (p. 276).

Day Seven: Today have Health Cappucino instead of coffee. Heavy regular coffee drinking is linked to cancer of the ovary, bladder, pancreas, and bowel. And drinking caffeinated tea with lemon juice in styrofoam cups causes polymers (carcinogens) to migrate from your cup to your bloodstream. Tea also contains potentially carcinogenic tannins. Sip something safer, rich in cancer-blocking calcium, in a china cup. Health Cappuccino: Put 1 tablespoon blackstrap molasses in a china cup, pour in 1 cup of soy or low-fat milk steamed until frothy. Sprinkle with grated or diced fig or nutmeg and soy lecithin granules.

Have one for the road, but make it H_2O. Alcohol is a greater cancer risk than nicotine. Six ounces of whiskey a day increases your cancer risk 15-fold (compared to a three-fold increase for pack-a-day smokers) . Water nourishes and mineralizes every one of the body's healing zones. For a treat, try the new immunity-boosting "H_2O plus" (purified, oxygenated, and potassium fortified).

Super Healing Hummus

> *½ cup lentils, rinsed*
>
> *3 cups water*
>
> *1 cup cooked chick peas*
>
> *2 cloves garlic, crushed*
>
> *1 teaspoon oregano*
>
> *¼ teaspoon each cumin and pepper*
>
> *Pinch cayenne*
>
> *4 teaspoons lemon juice*
>
> *2 tablespoons finely chopped parsley*
>
> *½ medium-sized tomato, finely chopped*
>
> *2 tablespoons olive oil*

Place the lentils and water in a saucepan and bring to a boil, then cover and cook over medium heat for 30 minutes. Drain, cool, and purée in food processor with remaining ingredients.

Optional: Stir in ¼ cup toasted sesame seeds before serving.

Use as a chip and vegetable dip or as a spread for bread or crackers.

See foods for healing zones: 1, 3, 4, 7, 9

Also see: Antioxidants, Betacarotene, Herbs, Vitamin C, Stress, Substitutes, Juices

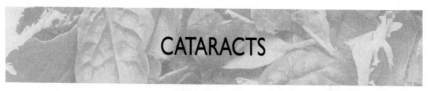

CATARACTS

Eat your spinach, carrots, and broccoli and reduce your risk of cataracts, the #1 cause of treatable blindness worldwide, say researchers at Harvard Medical School. In the United States, over a million cataract operations are performed each year. But Popeye's favorite snack can keep you from being part of that statistic.

FOUR STEPS TO CATARACT PREVENTION

According to a Harvard 10-year study, spinach, carrots, and broccoli are rich sources of antioxidant carotenes or pro-vitamin A, which is essential for the formation of visual purple (which, in turn, improves night vision). A high intake of spinach and other carotene-rich foods is consistently related to the lowest incidences of cataracts. In a 10-year study of more than 50,000 female nurses, Harvard researchers reported that women who ate large amounts of beta-carotene-rich vegetables significantly reduced their risk of developing cataracts—by up to 39%.

Stop Smoking—
Save Your Sight

The second step after stepping up your spinach intake is to say no to nicotine. In two Massachusetts studies, researchers from Harvard Medical School and Brigham and Women's Hospital in Boston found that men who smoked 20 or more cigarettes a day were twice as likely as nonsmokers to develop cataracts and that women who smoked heavily were 63% more likely to develop cataracts than nonsmokers. It's long been suspected that smoking increases your risk of cataracts and that the risk rises with the number of cigarettes smoked. In August 1992, the *Journal of the American Medical Association* published two studies (one involving 17,000 male physicians, the other 69,000 female nurses), both of which showed a strong association between cigarette smoking and cataracts, with the heaviest smokers running the greatest risk. In an accompanying editorial, Dr. Sheila West of the Johns Hopkins Hospital in Baltimore estimates that at least 20% of all cataracts could be attributed to smoking.

Eye injuries or steroid drugs can trigger cataracts at any age; diabetes or exposure to X-rays contributes to their formation. Senile cataracts are the most common form and to some degree affect most people over the age of 65. But cataracts are a degenerative condition in that the thickening and clouding of the eye's transparent lens often results from accumulated cell damage due to years of exposure to sunlight's ultraviolet rays. (Wearing sunglasses designated Z80.3 or prescription glasses with a UV-protective film lessens the risk of cataracts and slows their growth.)

The Five Better-Sight Nutrients

The third step is to follow a diet rich in vitamin C (which constitutes much of the ocular fluid), beta-carotene, vitamin E, selenium, and zinc. According to Allen Taylor, director of the Laboratory for Nutrition and Vision Research at the USDA Human Nutrition Center at Tufts University, antioxidants such as vitamin C could reduce the incidence of cataracts by 50%. Vitamin C accumulates in the eye in direct proportion to the amount consumed. Researchers also found that people getting 2 grams of vitamin C a day showed less of the oxidative damage that leads to cataracts.

The fourth step is to reduce your heavy metal levels (such as cadmium), which, says the Huxley Institute, are significantly higher in the lenses of cataract patients. The best corrective measure is a super healing cleansing diet (p. 355) preceded by or alternating with raw juice fasts.

LET THE LIGHT SHINE IN WITH BREWER'S YEAST AND BIOFLAVONOIDS

Researchers at the University of Georgia Hospital say that deficiencies of vitamins B and B_2 and iron (best source of all three is brewer's yeast) may be cataract culprits as well. Folk and naturopathic approaches include chamomile eyewashes and drops of the herbal extract bilberry taken internally (a berry rich in bioflavonoids that builds retinal health). a fresh green bean juice cocktail daily (add a beta-carotene- and C-rich red or yellow vegetable for added healing) is also beneficial.

Try this recipe:

Anticataract Cocktail

> *2 carrots, chopped (provides beta-carotene, zinc, vitamin E)*
>
> *$1/2$ head peeled garlic (B_1 and B_2, zinc, selenium)*
>
> *$1/2$ bunch parsley (C, beta-carotene)*
>
> *$1/2$ cup string beans, cooked (beta-carotene, E)*
>
> *6 leaves spinach (beta-carotene, B_1, E, iron)*
>
> *$1/4$ cup diced green pepper (optional) (C)*

Alternate ingredients and put through juicer. Dilute with 1 cup water. Sip during the day.

For tips from a pro, call the Medical Information Cataract Hotline at 1-900-230-4800, extension 4312.

See foods for healing zones: 8, 10

Also see: **Antioxidants, Berries, Juices, Vitamin C, Vision**

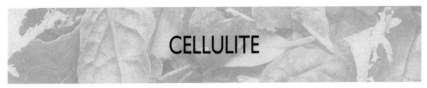

CELLULITE

Are you the victim of the 23-day-dead-cell syndrome? You are if you have cellulite—and you do if your dermis isn't doing what it was designed to do. In both cases, there's a solution—if you've got persistence and a properly stocked pantry.

According to California cosmetologist Zia Wesley-Hosford, "There is a 23-day cycle of birth, growth, and death that begins in the dermis, or lower layer of skin. When new cells are born, they are round and filled with fluid. As they make their way toward the surface of the skin, they lose their fluid, becoming elongated and flat. Once the cells reach the outer layer of the skin, they fall off as a result of washing or rubbing."

The dermis consists of collagen and elastin fibers that give skin its resiliency. Within these fibers are the glands that produce sebum, the body's moisturizer, plus sweat glands, blood vessels, hair follicles, and nerve endings. Each depends on a healthy epidermis to function properly. When a build-up of dead cells clogs the epidermis and sweat becomes trapped beneath the skin, you've got troubles.

What's not safe—or effective—for cellulite is surgery, warns Dwight Scarborough, assistant clinical professor of dermatology and medicine at Ohio State University Hospital in Columbus. "The amount of fat a woman has and where it's deposited is under genetic and hormonal control. ... It's possible that after removal of fat from one area [by liposuction], the body, still in need of energy reserves, will deposit that fat into other estrogen-sensitive tissues."

Here are the you-can-do-it-yourself facts:

1. Cellulite is an accumulation of trapped waste and water in the fatty areas of the body that gives skin a pock-marked appearance. Reducing these lumps and bumps takes work: massaging skin daily with natural vegetable oils such as safflower and rice, along with vitamin E, and then sloughing skin vigorously with natural granulated grains to increase circulation in tissues. The better your circulation, the more trapped water and toxins are released.

2. Toxic accumulation and fluid retention contribute to cellulite, but poor blood circulation causes a breakdown of the connective tissue between cells and ultimately creates a cellulite-promoting environment. Vigorous exercise three or four times a week along with

eight glasses of water every day improves circulation and helps create muscle tone and firm tissue. Many yoga postures also stimulate body organs.

3. Daily cleansing normalizes and balances skin. If your skin is on the dry side, cleansing stimulates the oil glands to work more efficiently. If it's oily, clogged pores will be unblocked and excess oil drained and controlled. Use soap lightly and only where needed (use glycerine bars made from pure olive oil).

4. Exfoliation draws out stubborn impurities and helps slough off the top layer of dead skin cells, keeping skin glowing and healthy. Use a loofah sponge or dry with a rough terry towel, or deep-pore cleanse with a full-body scrub using a natural abrasive such as sea salt, apricot kernel seeds, or almond meal mixed with yogurt or water. Massage entire body. Rinse off in the shower with warm water until skin is totally clean to increase blood flow in the tissues and stimulate glands to work more efficiently.

5. Moisturize to provide constant hydration to the skin. Cream or lotion prevents excessive evaporation of moisture from the skin's surface and also adds water. Apply just after washing. Best bets: products containing vitamin E (promotes healthy tissue), lecithin (keeps skin soft and supple), and aloe vera (soothes and protects).

6. Deep breathing/oxygenation helps purify the blood, rids the system of toxins, and burns cellulite-triggering waste in the connective tissue.

7. Nourish and replenish skin cells with proper nutrition. Healthy, youthful skin requires vitamins and minerals:

   ◆ Vitamin A for forming healthy skin cells and to enhance the skin's moisture level

   ◆ Vitamin D to nourish dry skin, especially during winter, when there is less natural sunlight

   ◆ Vitamin C to prevent wrinkles and hardening of the collagen in connective tissue

   ◆ Minerals that promote skin health, including calcium, magnesium, zinc, manganese, and potassium (see the recipes at the end of this section).

EIGHT CELLULITE-CONTROL TIPS

◆ Follow a low-fat (preferably vegetarian) diet, avoiding fried foods.

◆ Fill up on vegetables and green leafy greens.

◆ Emphasize high-fiber foods (beans, fruits, vegetables, and whole grains).

◆ Sharply limit salt and sugar.

◆ Sip a cellulite-control tea daily. The six best are bergamot, chamomile, eucalyptus, lemon, mint, and rosemary. (TIP: They can also be used as oils for aromatherapy healing.)

◆ MASSAGE TIPS: On the front, sides, and back of your body, use long, sweeping single strokes, always upward in the direction of the heart.

◆ To rid cellulite from tops of thighs and buttocks, massage upward in circular strokes.

◆ Shower or bathe in tepid water. Dry off with a thick towel and smooth on rich moisturizer.

Each of the following low-fat, low-calorie recipes rich in the eight nutrients that fight cellulite can be plugged into any healthy diet. Be sure to augment your diet and massage routine with 30 minutes of vigorous aerobic exercise daily.

Carrot-Parsnip Purée

2¹/₂ cups vegetable stock or broth
1¹/₂ cups carrots, finely diced
1¹/₂ cups parsnips, finely diced
2 tablespoons unsalted butter, softened to room temperature
2 tablespoons light brown sugar (or to taste)
Several grinds of black pepper
Minced parsley, as garnish

Preheat oven to 350 degrees. Place stock, carrots, and parsnips in saucepan and bring to boil. Reduce heat and simmer until tender, about 30 minutes.

Strain and drain well. Transfer to blender and process to a smooth purée. Add softened butter, sugar, and black pepper and blend well.

Pour into lightly buttered 1¹/₂ quart baking dish. Cover with foil and bake for 15 minutes. Remove foil, bake for five minutes more, and serve sprinkled with parsley.

Makes six to eight servings, 10 calories per tablespoon.

Four-Way Juicy Fruit Vinaigrette

Juice of half a lemon

¹/₄ cup raspberry or champagne vinegar

¹/₂ cup fresh raspberries

¹/₂ cup olive or sesame oil

Combine lemon juice and vinegar in a processor or blender. Add berries; purée until smooth. With machine running, add oil in a steady stream. Dress salads or drizzle on fruit or chicken or fish.

Makes about 1½ cups, 42 calories per tablespoon.

See foods that benefit healing zones: **1, 6, 8**

Also see: **Basic Dieting Facts and Advice, Herbs, Water, Juices**

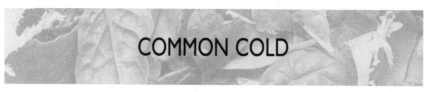

COMMON COLD

A cold is nothing to sneeze at. If you're average, you have three colds per year. What's good fruit-and-vegetable medicine if you're running off at the nose? Lemons, garlic, red and green peppers, and herb tea are all good for starters. All five are first-rate sources of the four anticold and flu antioxidants: vitamins C and A plus the carotene complex and flavonoids (including the bioflavonoid factor, or vitamin P) that energize your immune system and help detoxify your respiratory system.

PUT YOUR GREEN ON GREENS, NOT ANTIBIOTICS

Drugs are ineffectual in the long run and in the short run may do more harm than good: Symptoms such as nasal discharge are part of the body's defenses, so dosing yourself with drugs to dry up mucous membranes is a counterproductive inhibition of the body's efforts to defend itself. Instead, use apples, oranges, and bananas to make peace with your immune system.

NINE WAYS TO FIGHT 200 VIRUSES

The common cold can be triggered by any one of 200 common rhinoviruses (while only three of them are influenza makers). Fortunately, both colds and flu are self-limiting conditions that usually run their course in under two weeks depending on how battle-ready your immune system is.

If you're already running off at the nose, here are the nine best moves:

1. Stock the pantry. The 10 best rhinovirus terminators to unplug nasal passages and replace nutrients rapidly depleted by the stress of infection, says the American Society of Alternative Therapists, are garlic and onion, leafy greens, apples, apricots, beets, red and green peppers, citrus fruit, pineapple, and horseradish. Collectively they supply the vitamins A, B, C, and E, selenium, zinc, and bioflavonoids needed to fortify your immune system. All 10 can be converted into easy-to-swallow-and-digest soups, juices, and slushes.

2. Have an All-day Lemon Fizz: to shorten a cold's duration. Lemon's potent antioxidants include vitamin C, limenoids, and bioflavonoids. Dissolve 2 teaspoons baking soda in ½ cup boiling water, stir juice of half a lemon into cold water, and combine mixtures by pouring one into the other until fizzy. As alternative or augmentative therapy, sip a citrus-mint tea (lemon mint, orange mint, peppermint) with lime or lemon slices.

3. Soak your feet and clear your head. A 20-minute footbath may be the best way to clear a stuffed head, says the Therapeutic Foods Nutrition Council. It's even speedier coupled with hourly aromatherapy inhaling sessions. Best essential oils for fighting respiratory ills: cinnamon bark, thyme, lavender, and pine.

4. Garlic straight up, don't hold the onion. Garlic's antibiotic and decongestant capabilities can be accessed two ways: by eating two to four garlic cloves at the onset of infection, or by holding a peeled garlic clove between the teeth and cheek (without chewing or

swallowing) at regular round-the-clock intervals. To avoid garlic breath, soak cloves in yogurt or kefir or eat with parsley or fennel seed. Garlic and onion contain allicin, a compound that thwarts cold-causing bacteria. How to dish them up together? See the recipe for mock chicken soup at the end of this section.

5. 24-Skidoo: Have one or more round-the-clock cups of any of the 20 top cold-exorcising and decongesting teas: chamomile, dandelion, echinacea, elder, fenugreek, goldenseal, horehound, lemon grass, licorice root, mullein, peppermint, rose hip, rosemary, saffron, sage, sarsaparilla, savory, skullcap, slippery elm, or yarrow. Add fresh lemon juice or a teaspoon of dried, grated grapefruit peel to each cup of tea. For pain relief, use catnip, cayenne, ginger, or a combination of equal amounts of boneset and hyssop. To double decongestant action, have hot, light broths and clear soups, coupled with one full tumbler of plain water on the hour. Even better, use them with a homeopathic anticold and -flu tissue salt like allium cepa or pulsatilla (a wildflower derivative).

6. To clear nasal passages without drugs or the side-effects connected with commercial nasal sprays, use one or two drops of saline solution (¼ teaspoon salt in ½ cup warm water with ½ clove crushed garlic in each nostril). Repeat as needed, or inhale steam (with or without the addition of eucalyptus, chamomile, or ginger in tea leaf or liquid extract form) for 10 minutes twice daily.

7. A teaspoon of eucalyptus oil (held in the mouth for several minutes before swallowing) is said to slow the progress of a cold or any other viral infection. Ditto a broth made from Oriental mushrooms (shitake, reishi), laced if you like with grated horseradish (the cruciferous healer nobody knows about).*

8. Get juiced. The seven best healing quaffs for a healthy respiratory system: celery, carrot, pineapple, apple, watercress, leek, and citrus. Take your pick and dilute with fresh spring water.

9. Consider a hands-on therapy such as therapeutic massage or a spoon-up therapy using plain yogurt. Massaging the sore points at the base of your skull, the orbits of your eyes, and cheekbones with firm circular strokes opens the sinuses and relieves viral-related

---

* See Radishes.

headaches. Also, pressing the acupressure point at the base of the thumb relieves sinus congestion, says Robert Ullman, N.D. of Northwest Center for Homeopathic Medicine in Edmonds, Washington. Likewise, one cup of low-fat, live-culture yogurt a day causes a fivefold increase in gamma interferon, which boosts immunity.

If all else fails, try a little humor with your healing. Here are two gone (and best forgotten) remedies from stagecoach days:

Take some hot fried onions, put them in a flannel or woolen cloth, and bind to chest overnight. or put slices of raw onion on the soles of your feet (hold in place with woolen socks), go to sleep, and wake up infection- and fever-free.

Try these recipes for relief:

Cold Sufferer's Mock Chicken Soup

> *Handful of parsley, chopped*
> *2 onions, chopped*
> *3 carrots, chopped*
> *2 cloves garlic, crushed, peeled*
> *$^1/_4$ teaspoon anise seed (optional)*
> *$^1/_2$ teaspoon caraway seeds, crushed*
> *1 or 2 bay leaves*
> *1 teaspoon dill leaves or seeds, crushed*
> *1 tablespoon dried marjoram or 3 sprigs fresh peppercorns*
> *1 teaspoon sage*
> *$^1/_2$ cup white wine*
> *1 gallon water*
> *1 or 2 tablespoons olive or canola oil*
> *1 pound diced tempeh or hickory smoked or plain firm tofu*
> *1 tablespoon nutritional yeast (optional)*

Combine all ingredients (except tofu or tempeh) and bring to a boil quickly. Reduce heat and simmer, covered, for 45 minutes. Meanwhile, sauté diced tempeh/tofu in oil until lightly browned.

Remove vegetables; strain soup through sieve. Add vegetables to broth when ready.

Optional: Add 1 cup cooked brown rice or whole grain noodles before serving.

Variation: Substitute 1 or 2 cups cooked dried beans.

Also use in recipes for vegetable stock or broth or to dilute fresh juices.

Optional: Serve with the oyster cracker alternative (rice cake croutons), or break each round into quarters, or crush whole crackers.

Yield: Three to four servings.

Vitamin C Green Tea

> *2 teaspoons green tea leaves*
>
> *8 fresh mint leaves*
>
> *4 cups bottled water*
>
> *2 tablespoons natural sweetener*

Put 1 teaspoon tea and 4 mint leaves in teapot. Heat 1 cup water until hot, not boiling. Pour over leaves and steep for 5 minutes.

Strain into ice cube tray and freeze.

Brew remaining teaspoon tea and mint leaves with 2 cups hot water, and steep for 5 minutes. Cool. Serve sweetened, in chilled glasses over green tea cubes.

See foods for healing zones: 3, 6, 10

Also see: Herbs, Vitamin C, Juices, Antioxidants, Lemons, Oranges, Aspirin Alternatives, Water

CORONARY HEART DISEASE

In the next year, your heart will pump 1.5 million gallons of blood, and during your lifetime, it will pump the equivalent of enough liquid to fuel the tanks of an entire fleet of 2,100 Boeing 747 jet planes. Exercise keeps your heart pumping by keeping your entire cardiovascular system operating efficiently—taking in oxygen and delivering it to muscles and organs with a minimum of wear and tear.

And so does abstinence. According to researchers at the Jefferson Medical College in Philadelphia, alcohol is toxic to muscle cells, and the more you drink, the more your muscles deteriorate. The two heart-rending heart disorders that go with excessive drinking are myopathy and cardiomyopathy.*

Getting physical (i.e., exercising) won't get you far if your lifestyle includes smoking, alcohol abuse, or a diet high in unhealthy foods, especially fatty ones such as meat, cream, butter, and processed foods, which lead to unhealthy deposits of fat, cholesterol, fibrin, calcium, and cellular debris in the arteries (which narrows artery channels and reduces the flow of blood). The smartest nutritional self-defense is to consider 30% fat a high-fat diet, advises Aerobics and Fitness Association of America nutritionist Reg Jordan, and 10% fat a low-fat diet and see how low you can get.

The mortality rate from heart attack has dropped by half since 1960, but coronary heart disease (CHD) is still the leading killer of men and women in America, causing 500,000 deaths a year and affecting 20% of the population under age 65. Only 18% of us are free of the five major coronary risk factors—smoking, obesity, hypertension, diabetes, and lack of exercise, says the National Center for Health Statistics. A 23-year-long 1993 study by the President's Council on Physical Fitness found 26% fewer coronary disease deaths among physically active subjects and a 17% decrease in the risk of CHD. There are four risk factors you *can't* change: heredity (having a parent or sibling with CHD puts you at risk); race (African Americans are more vulnerable to hypertension and diabetes); age (55% of all heart attacks occur before age 65); and sex (men are a higher risk group than women until age 60). There is one factor you can work on: your biochemical shape.

Most of the risk factors connected with CHD can be countered by simple preventive measures, conclude 1992 coronary research studies at Harvard University—especially diet (a leafy green one is the best). According to both Dean Ornish, M.D., director of the Preventative Medicine Research Institute, and William Castelli, M.D., director of the celebrated Framingham Heart Study, the single most important way to prevent coronary disease and increase longevity is to "go on a vegetarian diet."

---

* Sixty-six million Americans suffer from some form of heart or blood vessel disease, and over 60 million are victims of high blood pressure.

Here are 10 ways to eat well and shape up your body's biggest muscle in only 10 days. But before you start, check out your cardiovascular awareness with this quiz.

Heart-Smart Quiz

1. Which oil is higher in health-promoting monounsaturated fat?

    (a) Canola oil

    (b) Olive oil

    (c) Sunflower oil

2. Ounce for ounce, meat, poultry, and most cheeses have about the same amount of cholesterol.

    (a) True

    (b) False

3. Oat bran is the only food that will lower blood fats.

    (a) True

    (b) False

4. Two percent milk contains

    (a) 2% fat calories

    (b) 17% fat calories

    (c) 37% fat calories

5. What biochemical risk factor linked to stress puts you at a greater than average risk of heart attack?

6. The three best sports for building cardiovascular fitness for life are swimming, bowling, and bicycling. True or false?

7. Which has more cholesterol?

    (a) Coconut oil

    (b) Mayonnaise

    (c) Lard

8. Why do you use the index and middle fingers instead of the thumb to take your pulse?

Answers:

1. (b). Olive oil has the highest percentage of monounsaturates, at 77%. Canola oil is close, at 62% monounsaturates; and sunflower oil has 20% monounsaturates. Ten to fifteen percent of your total daily calories should come from monounsaturated fat.

2. True. But most cheese has more saturated fat. Substitute low-fat and imitation cheeses (which have between 2 and 6 grams of fat per ounce) for natural, processed, and hard cheeses.

3. False. Although studies show that oat bran can lower blood cholesterol in some people, it is the soluble fiber in the oat bran that lowers blood cholesterol levels. Other sources of soluble fiber include whole grains, dried beans, and fresh fruits and vegetables.

4. (c).

5. An apple-shaped physique. According to Yale University researchers, women with apple-shaped (rather than pear-shaped) physiques accumulate fat around the abdomen in part because of an increased output of cortisol, which is linked to chronic, uncontrolled stress. Pear-shaped individuals whose excess weight appears at the hips and thighs produce less cortisol and score lower on stress tests.

6. False, says the President's Council on Physical Fitness. Jogging or brisk walking is better than bowling.

7. (c) Lard has 12 mg per tablespoon; mayonnaise has 8; coconut oil has none—but it is 92% saturated fat. Look for the new low-fat versions.

8. Because the thumb has a pulse of its own, and thus using the thumb could give you an inaccurate reading.

10-DAY HEART-HEALTHY NUTRITION

Day One

Change your oil. Most saturated fats raise cholesterol levels. Polyunsaturated fats lower cholesterol, but they reduce beneficial HDL cholesterol along with harmful LDL cholesterol. Monounsaturated fats reduce LDL cholesterol, apparently without affecting HDL levels, says the USDA. Stock them all, but think before you pour. Here's a scoreboard:

Column I: Cholesterol (mg/tbsp)
Column II: Saturated fat
Column III: Polyunsaturated fat: Linoleic acid
Column IV: Polyunsaturated fat: Omega-3 fatty acid
Column V: Monounsaturated fat

	I	II	III	IV	V
Canola oil	0	6%	26%	10%	58%
Safflower oil	0	9	78	trace	13
Sunflower oil	0	11	69	—	20
Corn oil	0	13	61	1	25
Olive oil	0	14	8	1	77
Soybean oil	0	15	54	7	24
Peanut oil	0	18	34	—	48
Cottonseed oil	0	27	54	—	19
Lard	12	41	11	1	47
Palm oil	0	51	10	—	39
Beef tallow	14	52	3	1	44
Butter	33	66	2	2	30
Palm kernel oil	0	81	2	—	11
Coconut oil	0	92	2	—	6

Source: United States Department of Agriculture.

Day Two

Have a chin-up and a chuckle. According to Dr. William Fry, a psychiatrist at Stanford University, laughing 100 times a day does your heart as much good as a 10-minute workout on a rowing machine. The everyday guffaw stimulates the production of hormones that increase heart rate and flow, says Fry.

Another way to treat your ticker right? Look for the new advanced formula form of the B vitamin niacin (B_3). In its standard form, niacin—the brain- and circulation-beneficial B vitamin that also reduces stress—can cause skin flushing, irritability, and gastrointestinal acidity. The secret of the new no-sweat formulation is the addition of guar, a grain- and fruit-derived fiber nine times more effective than bran. The new form is available in powder and tablets at health food stores.

Day Three

Know where the fat is at. A tablespoon of fat has almost triple the calories of a tablespoon of sugar, advises Washington DC's Center for Science in the Public Interest.

Start the day with a better breakfast that eliminates both fat and sugar: In place of high-fat, high-calorie butter and syrup, try these alternatives on your hotcakes. (1) Purée one-fourth cup each of nonfat yogurt, buttermilk, and all-fruit apricot preserves in a blender. (2) Purée the juice and pulp of two oranges with one-fourth cup maple syrup until smooth. (3) Put 1 cup frozen raspberries and one teaspoon honey in a small saucepan, and simmer for three to five minutes until reduced slightly.

Here are some more substitutes to health-proof your heart:

In place of	Substitute
2 tablespoons butter mixed with 1 tablesoon flour to thicken soups and sauces (7 grams fat)	Kudzu (2 tablespoons = 0 grams fat)
Dairy mayonnaise (1 tablespoon = 11 grams fat)	Tofu mayonnaise (1 tablespoon = 4 grams fat)
Sour cream (1 cup = 47 grams fat)	Low-fat yogurt (1 cup = 4.2 grams fat)
Cream cheese (1 tablespoon = 5.3 grams fat)	Kefir cream cheese (1 tablespoon = 3 grams fat)
After-dinner coffee with light cream (1 tablespoon = 2 grams fat)	Carob coffee with 2% soy milk (1 cup = 0 grams fat)
Chocolate syrup (2 tablespoons = 5.4 grams fat)	Carob or rice syrup 2 tablespoons = less than 1 gram fat)
⅓ large frozen pizza (17.3 grams fat)	⅓ large frozen pizza with soy cheese (2 grams fat)
Deluxe dairy ice cream (1 cup = 23.8 grams fat) (1 cup = 5 grams fat)	Dairy-free soy frozen dessert
Frozen lasagna with cheese (12 ounces = 15 grams fat)	Frozen lasagna with tofu filling (12 ounces = 8 grams fat)
All-beef hot dog (13 grams fat)	Tofu hot dog (5.4 grams fat)
Hamburger (3 ounces ground beef = 19.4 grams fat)	Natural grain and vegetable burger (11 grams fat)

Ingredients in right column are carried at all health food stores, or see Mail Order Sources.)

Day Four

Keep your hummus up and your homocysteine down. Heart disease is the #1 killer of women, striking one in three. (Today, breast cancer risk is one in eight.) Worse, a heart attack is twice as likely to be fatal for a woman as a man.

A key culprit for men as well as women? High levels of homocysteine, a naturally occurring amino acid that increases the risk of heart attack, say researchers at the Harvard School of Public Health in Boston. What reduces the risk? A diet high in folic acid and vitamin B_6. Best sources: hummus and other bean-based dishes, leafy greens, whole grains, and brewer's (nutritional) yeast.

Day Five

Have a happy day and get more vitamin A. According to heart specialist Dean Ornish of the University of California, San Francisco, cynical attitudes and hostile emotions can cause biological responses that trigger coronary disease, attract patches of cholesterol that block blood flow, and boost heart attack potential. To become the worry-free type you were meant to be, take a daily walk (preferably to and from work) or buy an antistress machine (two to try—Minds Eye Plus, 800-388-6345; Relaxmax, 216-749-1133).

To prevent stroke, up your beta-carotene A levels. Victims of stroke (the most common neurological disability in the United States) have less vitamin A in their bloodstreams and a lowered chance of recovery or survival than the betacarotene empowered. (Best sources—red, orange, and yellow fruits and vegetables.)

Day Six

An unbuttered diet is better. Thirty grams of fat a day is the limit set by the American Heart Association. Here are six ways to remove five or more grams of fat from your three squares a day and stay within the limits:

1. Freeze unsalted sticks of soy margarine and use in 1-gram-of-fat-or-less curls (peel off with swivel-bladed vegetable peeler), not 7-grams-of-fat pats.

2. Try salsa in place of cream and butter sauces.

3. Marinate meat in no-fat fruit juices. Grill meat, poultry, and fish before removing skin and trimming fat.

4. Substitute spinach or cabbage leaves for pastry in crepes, turnovers, and blintzes.

5. Use cocoa in place of chocolate in cooking. It's free of chocolate's cholesterol-raising cocoa butter. Even better, switch to low-fat, no-sugar carob powder.

6. Skip Danish and donuts and sip your decaf with this Healthy Heart Cake: Press one layer of any hot, high-fiber cooked cereal (such as oatmeal, cornmeal, or kasha) into a greased cake pan. Make a second layer with sliced fresh berries or bananas. Add a final layer of cereal, firmly pressing down on each layer as you add. Refrigerate until the "cake" is cool. Cut carefully into squares and eat plain or spread with 1 tablespoon low-fat cottage or cream cheese.

Day Seven

Get an omega-3 fatty-acids-friendly diet going. Eat fish two or three times a week and you're less likely to die prematurely of heart disease. The protective fats in fish, known as omega-3 fatty acids, may also thwart the spread of cancer, help prevent autoimmune diseases, and counter arthritis and hypertension. Best sources: trout, haddock, sardines, salmon, and mackerel.

Between meals, get physical enough to perspire. According to researchers at the VA Medical Center in Jackson, Mississippi, regular aerobic exercise, such as brisk walking, jogging, swimming, and bicycling, produces moderate reductions in blood pressure if you persist. (Isometric exercises and weight lifting, which are not aerobic, may even raise blood pressure in patients with hypertension.)

Don't stop for guacamole too often. The avocado is the only vegetable that supplies a measurable amount of fat (33 grams). For a heart-smart dip, purée cooked asparagus or green beans with parsley and yogurt.

Day Eight

What's good for your heart is good for your immune system. Three months on a low (30%) fat diet causes a typical increase in aggressive infection- and disease-fighting blood cells of 14%, says the American Heart Association. That means living low on hydrogenated fats.

Hydrogenated fats also destroy vitamin E in the body and speed up hardening of the arteries. Fat saturation can be as low as 5% or as high as 95%. Since you can't guess, read labels to protect your heart, and shop smart. The good news: Vitamin E is usually found in foods high in heart-protective polyunsaturated linoleic acid.

You can eliminate nondairy creamers, which are as fatty as whole cream, and make your own Nonhydrogenated Nondairy Creamer: Put equal parts of dry powdered milk (noninstant types are richer in nutrients) and powdered lecithin in a jar, and add just enough water to make a slurry mixture when shaken. Refrigerate. Use in place of cream, coffee lighteners, and whole milk. (Or simply stir plain, no-fat powdered milk into your daily decaf.)

Day Nine

Use a clear-conscience cheese with less than 9 grams of fat an ounce (that rules out cheddar but leaves mozzarella, Swiss, Gouda, Edam, and Brie). If your blood serum levels are 200 or under, a healthy fat intake is 120 mg daily—the amount in 4 ounces of processed cheese or three chocolate bars. Make that 110 mg if your reading is 200 to 240; and if your level is higher, your daily allowance should be 100 mg or less.

Processed cheese has 400 mg of sodium and almost 10 grams of fat per 1-ounce serving. Switch to an alternative such as Alpine Lace's 2% fat slices, or check your health food store for Soyco's yellow American slices, the sliced cheese alternative that's milk-, fat-, and cholesterol-free with one quarter the sodium of regular brands.

When the occasion calls for cake, start with tofu and make your own:

Un-Cheesecake

> 2 10$^{1}/_{2}$-ounce packages silken/firm tofu, drained
>
> $^{1}/_{2}$ cup honey
>
> 2 tablespoons plus 1 teaspoon lemon juice
>
> 1$^{1}/_{4}$ teaspoon vanilla
>
> 3 tablespoons soy oil
>
> 1 tablespoon plus 1 teaspoon lemon peel, shredded
>
> 1 8-inch graham cracker pie shell
>
> 1 cup ground nuts (optional)

In a food processor or blender, combine tofu, honey, lemon juice, vanilla, and vegetable oil. Whip on high for 1 minute. Add lemon peel. Whip on low for 30 seconds. Prepare graham cracker pie shell, using your favorite recipe. For added flavor, add 1 cup nuts to pie shell ingredients. Pour mixture into pie shell and bake in a preheated, 350-degree oven for 1 hour. Cool. Chill and serve.

Day Ten

Don't be a conehead. Twenty percent of the fat in our diets comes from cheese, ice cream, and milk. If you've got a sundae-kind-of-love you can't lick, switch to a tasty, healthier substitute.

Frozen Treat	Calories	Fat (g)
Frozen yogurt, soft-serve (all, flavors), 1/2 cup	115	3
Frozen yogurt bar (all flavors), 2.5 oz.	65	1
Glacé, 1/2 cup	98	1
Reduced-calorie "ice cream" (all flavors), 1/2 cup	95	2
Tofu-based dessert, hard (all flavors), 1/2 cup	220	13*
Tofu-based dessert, soft-serve (all flavors), 1/2 cup	158	8*

*All vegetable.

HEART-TO-HEART FACTS

Home is where the heart is. It's where the heart attack is, too. According to the Framingham Heart Study group in Framingham, Massachusetts, an average American child currently has one chance in three of having a major heart attack before reaching the age of 60. Here are eight more facts to take to heart:

◆ The heart is your body's biggest muscle and pumps in the vicinity of 4,000 gallons of blood daily.

◆ Your heart is at its biological best at age 26.

◆ The peak age for that age-old ill—the heart attack—is 45 and up.

◆ The alternate beating of the heart creates the pulse, which is felt anywhere artery crosses bone near the skin's surface.

◆ Your heart pumps enough blood each day to fill 85 bath tubs.

◆ Ten percenters: At the bottom 10% of the corporate echelon your risk of heart attack is five times that of those in the top 10%.

◆ 95 percenters: Once total fat levels drop below 25% of calories taken in, cholesterol deposition halts for 95% of all people.

BEATING HYPERTENSION
12 Better-Than-Sodium Salt Substitutes

Hypertension (high blood pressure) is one of the five risk factors for coronary heart disease which has a simple home-plate solution: sharply reduced sodium intake. The average American consumes 10 to 20 times more sodium than the body requires. The salting of foods, almost all foods, is done largely out of habit. "The amount of salt we eat is almost totally governed by culture customs and food habits … [and] no other animal in the world eats as much salt as man," says Assa Weinberg, M.D., author of *How to Live 365 Days a Year The Salt-Free Way.*

But the healthiest people with the lowest blood pressure stay healthy on diets with daily sodium levels of 800 mg or less. You can, too. Here are 12 home-made, low- or no-sodium solutions for your shakers using spices, herbs, and pepper.*

General Directions

In a seed/spice mill, electric blender, or with mortar and pestle, grind the dried ingredients until powdery. Stir in powdered ingredients. (Experiment with proportions to suit your taste.) Spoon into an empty

---

* The world's most important spice, indigenous to India and the Far East, pepper, was one of the earliest articles of commerce between the Orient and Europe. In the Middle Ages, rents, dowries, and taxes were frequently paid in peppercorns. Peppercorns are berries that grow on a vine. Green ones are young peppercorns that are pickled in brine or wine vinegar, frozen, or air dried. Black peppercorns are aged on the vine, harvested, and then dried. White peppercorns have had their black outside husks removed. The finest quality black peppercorns, darker and more pungent than any others sold, come from Tellicherry on the Malabar coast of India. Crushed Red Peppers and Powdered Cayenne (Red Pepper): These are botanically related to bell peppers rather than peppercorns. Both are very hot. Use sparingly. Szechuan or Chinese Brown Peppers: These are aromatic, unusual, and a good, spicy alternative to black pepper.

spice jar. Cap tightly and keep dry. Keeps for three to four months. These recipes make 6 tablespoons (except as noted otherwise).

Super Healing "Salt" #1

1 tablespoon black peppercorns

1 teaspoon cayenne or crushed red pepper flakes

2 tablespoons garlic flakes or powder

2 tablespoons onion flakes or powder

1 teaspoon soy lecithin granules (optional)

1 tablespoon dried oregano

1/2 teaspoon mustard seeds or 1/2 teaspoon mustard powder (optional)

Super Healing "Salt" #2

1 teaspoon thyme

1 teaspoon marjoram

1 teaspoon celery seeds

1 teaspoon garlic flakes or powder

1 teaspoon onion flakes or powder

1/4 teaspoon dry mustard

1/4 teaspoon cayenne or 1/2 teaspoon paprika

1/4 teaspoon lecithin granules (optional)

1/2 teaspoon ascorbic acid powder or crushed vitamin C tablet

Follow directions above. Makes 5 tablespoons.

Short-cut "Salt"

Mix together 4 parts onion powder, 2 parts paprika, 2 parts garlic powder, and 3 parts cayenne pepper.

Calcium "Salt"

1 cup blanched whole almonds*

2 tablespoons unsalted butter

1/2 teaspoon celery seed or onion flakes

---

* Almonds are a good nondairy calcium source.

Heat oven to 350 degrees. Spread almonds on a cookie sheet, dot with butter, and season with celery seed or onion flakes. Toast, stirring occasionally, until lightly browned (8 to 10 minutes).

Cool, grind in nut mill or blender. Use as a salt substitute, a flavor enhancer, or a salad sprinkle. Keeps in a cool pantry shelf. Makes about 1 cup.

Variation: Substitute walnuts, pecans, or cashews for almonds.

Lemon Pepper "Salt"

> *1 tablespoon dried grated lemon or lime peel*
>
> *2 tablespoons black peppercorns*
>
> *1 teaspoon finely grated dried ginger root (or ½ teaspoon nutmeg)*
>
> *2 teaspoons powdered seaweeds (such as kelp or dulse) (optional)*
>
> *1 teaspoon fennel or anise seed (optional)*

Pâté Maison "Salt"

> *½ tablespoon each powdered bay leaves, cloves, nutmeg, paprika, and thyme*
>
> *¾ teaspoon each basil, cinnamon, oregano, sage, and savory*
>
> *¼ cup white peppercorns*

What this traditional French spice mix does for pâté maison, pot roast, or stew, it can do for your next salad. It even makes a snack chip sprinkle.

Mushroom "Salt"

Buy dried mushrooms and grind in blender—with or without equal amounts of dried parsley or dried tarragon and a pinch of dried lemon peel. The most flavorful dried mushrooms are the Japanese (sweet, light, and delicate) and Chilean (mild with a fresh mushroom flavor).

Three-Seed No-Sodium "Salt"

> *2 cloves garlic*
>
> *2 teaspoons salt or substitute*
>
> *½ teaspoon pepper*
>
> *10 large basil leaves*
>
> *2 teaspoons sweet marjoram leaves or oregano*
>
> *4 teaspoons fennel or dill seeds*

1 teaspoon poppy seed

1 teaspoon celery seed

Put first 6 ingredients in blender and process for 2 minutes. Add poppy and celery seeds and blend until smooth.

Note: Did you know that poppy, dill, caraway, and celery seeds taste better freshly ground? You can have them that way in a hurry if you store them in a spare peppermill and grind just before serving a dish.

Pungent Pepper "Salt"

2 tablespoons freshly ground white pepper

1 tablespoon ground black pepper

$1/2$ teaspoon ground ginger and nutmeg

Pinch cloves

$1/2$ cup dried mixed vegetable flakes

Sesame Pepper "Salt"

$1/4$ cup roasted sesame seeds, ground

1 teaspoon freshly ground black or white pepper

Pinch lemon peel

Combine all ingredients. Makes about $1/4$ cup.

Variations: Use $1/4$ cup each sesame and poppy or sesame and sunflower seed. Use pinch red pepper flakes in place of peel.

Spicy Pepper Plus

Combine $1/4$ cup each black and white peppercorns and 2 tablespoons whole allspice berries and place in a pepper mill. Use in place of black peppercorns to season any dish. Makes approximately $1/2$ cup.

Mustard Seed Pepper

Replace the peppercorns in your peppermill with mustard seeds. Keep on stove or tabletop to grind over salads, eggs, and soups.

Can't shake the habit? If nothing but real salt will do, buy a rock-type, kosher style, or natural mineral salt that has been minimally processed and is additive free. Along with the sodium, you'll get trace minerals processed out of ordinary salt. Best bet is 100% sundried Grey Celtic salt (see Mail Order Sources). Keep it in a salt mill to grind as needed. This will help you reduce your salt intake.

Seasoning Without Salt: Four Tips

◆ Toss watercress or a bitter green such as arugula with your salad greens and you'll never miss the salt.

◆ Start from seed and grow your own French tarragon (the variety commonly sold in the United States is the less pungent Russian variety). Authentic *Artesmesia dracunculus* tarragon can be grown anywhere, including a sunny windowsill. Fanciers say it makes a superior salt and all-purpose seasoning.

◆ Add roasted peppers to a dish and you'll never miss the salt. Place red or green bell peppers cut in half on broiler rack. Broil, turning until all sides are blackened. Remove the blackened skins while warm; discard seeds and cut into strips. Cover with flavored vinegar. Use to season salt-free salads, casseroles, pasta dishes, meatloaves, etc.

◆ Other single-ingredient salt substitutes include lemon, ginger, hot peppers, garlic, browned onion, and fresh (not dried) strong flavored herbs or bitter herb and greens.

If you want to buy ingredients to make salt-free "salts," write to the following:

American Orsa, Inc.
75 N. State
Redmont, UT 84652
(Natural sundried salt)

Herb Gathering, Inc.
5742 Kenwood
Kansas City, MO 64110

Heirloom Seeds
Box 245
West Elizabeth, PA 15332

See foods for healing zone: 2

Also see: **Substitutes, Dairy Substitutes, Vegetarian Foods, Vitamin E, Antioxidants, Dieting**

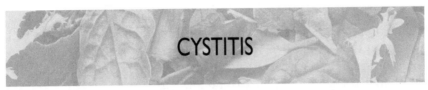

CYSTITIS

Cystitis? Maybe you should have had a B_8 (see recipe at the end of this section). Bladder infection (medically termed cystitis) is a condition in which the bladder is invaded by a microorganism that multiplies and causes inflammation. Women are more often victims than men. Symptoms include burning pain when urinating, abdominal pain, excessive and frequent urination, and odious or dark urine. Some studies indicate that chronic bladder infection can increase your risk of bladder cancer.

COCKTAIL A DAY TO RELIEF

Cranberries give more than symptomatic relief because of the hippunic acid they contain, which destroys the *E. coli* bacteria responsible for the release of ammonia. Cranberry juice actually coats the bacteria, preventing it from clinging to the urinary tract and, as a bonus, deodorizing the urine. One to two cranberry cocktails a day constitutes a healing dose. (A time-honored cystitis folk remedy recommends 1/2 cup of vitamin C-rich pomegranate juice mixed with 1 cup water twice daily.) Make the cocktail yourself by adding cranberry juice concentrate (1 to 2 tablespoons) to apple juice concentrate (1 quart).

Getting Juiced

In fact, your first line of defense is to increase *all* fluids, including cranberry juice, to 1 quart sipped round the clock to flush out invading bacteria, suggests the Pritikin Longevity Center of Santa Monica, California. (Enough is enough when your urine runs clear. As long as it's dark, you're still underdoing it.) Note that this liquid rule of thumb is true in nondisease states as well. Large amounts of liquids act as a painkiller for everyday aches and pains.

Second Line of Defense: Vitamin C

Juices rich in ascorbic acid counteract pain, speed healing, work as an antibiotic and cleanser, and increase the effectiveness of any prescribed medication you're taking. A thousand milligrams a day of vitamin C is the urine-acidifying dose level that retards bacterial growth. If that's too tall an order with juices alone, consider supplementing your juices with powdered C. (Vitamin C is most effective in the form of C plus zinc—another immune system antioxidant—ester-C, or vitamin C with either echinacea or astralagus—two potent immunity-boosting herbs.) Antimicrobial botanicals such as passion fruit, papaya, and pomegranate are also beneficial.

Salt-Cystitis Balancing Act

A third defense to consider is mineral deficiency. Are your sodium-potassium-magnesium and calcium levels in balance? Deviations of more than 1% can cause bladder and kidney dysfunction, advise researchers at the Office of Alternative Medicine (of the National Institutes of Health).

Juice-Fasting for Faster Healing

For faster healing and infection prevention, try this three-day cystitis-specific juice fast based on the 14 top cystitis-fighter foods.

Mix the following combinations (2 cups of each diluted with water) and sip 6 to 10 small cups a day.

- ♦ Cranberry juice (contains the "cranberry factor") plus pomegranate or papaya juice (source of antimicrobial agents)
- ♦ Kale, parsley, green pepper, and broccoli—sources of vitamin C
- ♦ Ginger root, parsley, garlic, and carrot—sources of zinc
- ♦ Carrots, collard greens, parsley, and spinach—sources of beta-carotene
- ♦ Cantaloupe, papaya, and lemon—sources of bioflavonoids.

TIP: Add 1 teaspoon of healing aloe vera gel to each quart of liquid as a juice booster. (See Juices for more tips, p. 104).

Directions: Dice, chop, or crush ingredients (cranberries should be cooked and cooled before juicing), use in 1-to-1 or 1:2:3 ratios; dilute with water (see Juices for more tips).

TEAS FOR SUPER HEALING

Better-bladder teas include the antimicrobial herbs goldenseal, comfrey, and juniper berry, which all exert a disinfectant effect on the urinary tract (as do cranberries). The American Indian Rx is corn-silk tea: Steep corn silk in 3 cups of boiled water for five minutes. Strain and sip round the clock. (Or use corn-silk extract from the health food store; 15 drops of extract to 1 cup of hot water.)

Try these bladder-beneficial juice recipes:

B_8 Cystitis Pitcher*

> 2 cups cranberry juice, unsweetened
>
> 1 cup pomegranate juice
>
> Fresh papaya, cantaloupe, 1 cup cubed
>
> 1/4 cup lemon juice
>
> 1 tablespoon ginger juice

Juice papaya and melons, put in blender with remaining ingredients, and liquefy until smooth. Add 6 to 8 ice cubes. Liquefy again, and decant into frosted pitcher. Sip 4 to 6 servings daily.

Variation: For shortcut B-4 juicer: Omit any four ingredients and follow general directions.

Papaya 2% (a no-fat fruit milk)

> 1 very ripe peeled and seeded papaya, chopped
>
> Water to cover
>
> 1 teaspoon honey or natural sugar substitute (optional)

Liquefy fruit and water in blender. Taste, sweeten if desired, or, to thicken, use less liquid; to thin, add more papaya. Use as a no-lactose, no-fat milk substitute.

Variations: Use passion fruit in place of papaya. Substitute lettuce for water for added calcium and vitamins.

Three-Citrus Crush

Juice one small peeled tangerine (by hand or electric juicer) and half a small peeled grapefruit. Combine juices with two to three cracked ice cubes in a blender. Liquefy until frothy. Add 1/2 teaspoon fresh lemon juice for fresher flavor and more bioflavonoids.

---

* Contains beta-carotene, the bioflavonoid complex, vitamin C, zinc, and four antimicrobial nutrients.

Variations: Substitute a peeled tangelo or orange for tangerine. Use one quarter of a peeled pink grapefruit or pommelo for white grapefruit.

Shortcut Crush: Substitute ¼ cup presqueezed or reconstituted orange juice and ½ cup unsweetened grapefruit juice.

Also see: Berries, Beta-carotene, Herbs, Juices, Vitamin C

For more information, call the American Information Line's Cystitis Hotline at 1-900-230-4800, extension, 6311.

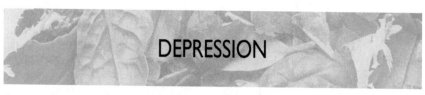

DEPRESSION

One in three of us feels depressed at least one day of the month, according to the National Foundation for Depression. Symptoms run the gamut from sleepless nights to suicidal reveries.

Genetic and metabolic factors aside, if you've got the garden-variety blues, chances are that your mind just doesn't like what your body is feeding it. Here are a few corrective measures for managing your bad moods with good foods and natural therapies.

1. A greens-free life can make you blue—so can a shortage of tryptophan-rich soybeans, fruits, and dairy foods or a deficiency of the B-complex nutrients B_{12}, folate, and thiamine or too little vitamin A (which protects the adrenal from stress).

   According to researchers at Rush-Presbyterian/St. Luke's Medical Center in Chicago, a severe deficiency in some amino acids, such as phenylalanine (PHE), may also contribute to depression. Poor nutrition exacerbates depression and anxiety, and it's the last thing an individual suffering from psychological distress can afford to ignore.

2. Eat the right foods in the right amounts. A small amount of protein without carbohydrate can be good (a small egg salad sandwich—without the bread—energizes the brain), while large amounts of protein create lethargy (a large steak followed by cheesecake). And while a 50/50 protein:carbohydrate snack (tofu/grains) creates calm and focus, make that no-fiber carbohy-

drates (a frosted Danish) and your brain chemistry reverts to its drowsy mode. For a quick pick-me-up, snack on no-protein complex carbohydrates such as whole grain crackers, dry granola, or cold pasta salad.

3. Aromatize and ionize. Both electric ionizers and aromatherapy, studies indicate, have the power to impact serotonin levels and other neurotransmitters in the brain that influence mood and even improve cognitive function, says Eric Braverman, M.D., of the Princeton, New Jersey, Wellness Center, especially if depression is triggered by indoor/outdoor pollution. Best red-light aromatherapy scents for the blues: basil, sage, rosewood, and lemon.

4. Eat a detoxifying diet: Elevated lead (seen in a variety of syndromes, including bulimia and lupus), copper, mercury (often caused by faulty dental fillings), and cadmium levels (common in smokers and even victims of second-hand smoke) can cause depression. Blood and hair tests can measure the damage, and a good diet fortified with antioxidant-rich onions and garlic can do damage control.

5. Let the sunshine in. If you're sad, not glad, you could be a victim of seasonal-affective disorder (SAD)—a weather-related immune-system-suppressing type of depression that triggers sadness, fatigue, and increased appetite, especially during the short, dark days of winter. Solution? Increased exposure to natural sunlight or regular full-spectrum light treatment. Full-spectrum lighting, the type that most closely resembles sunlight, appears to improve mood, learning, and overall behavior, according to psychologist Warren E. Hathaway. For a referral to the nearest SAD treatment center, call 212-960-5714.

6. Try an herbal mood-booster cup of tea. Three-thumbs-up candidates from herbalist Daniel Mowry are ginkgo, a vasodilatory plant medicine which also improves alertness/concentration and memory; Siberian ginseng, an adaptogen botanical that stimulates the adrenal and pituitary glands, increases resistance to stress, and improves circulation to the brain; and gotu kola, an antidepressive herbal used in India to improve memory and longevity and build mental stamina. (For best results, combine with the herbs damiama and skullcap.)

7. Try respiratory therapy. How you breathe is related to how you feel, and repressed breathing produces depressed thinking. Talk to an

exercise therapist or your doctor for a brush-up lesson on diaphragmatic breathing and practice it two to five minutes every hour until it becomes a habit.

8. Beef up your vitamin B$_1$ and magnesium. Thiamine is essential for the conversion of carbohydrates, glucose, and glycogen (two brain sugars), while magnesium activates the ATP (adenosine triphosphate) energy cycle that plays a role in transmission of nerve impulses. Good sources of both are whole grains and dried beans.

9. Watch your cholesterol. According to the National Foundation for Depressive Illness, a rapid rise in cholesterol can lead to slowed metabolism in the region of the brain that regulates mood.

10. Talk it up, walk it off. According to Brian L. G. Morgan, Ph.D., assistant professor, Institute of Human Nutrition, Columbia-Presbyterian Medical Center in New York City, race-walking or running for 30 minutes three days a week can make a substantial dent in your depression. Success therapies 2 and 3 are meditation and biofeedback. As an added benefit, weight-bearing exercise helps the body make better use of protein and calcium, two nutrients which the stress of feeling down eats up.

11. Take a homeopathic multi—not a diazepam. There are 50 serious side effects associated with even short-term use of tranquilizing drugs such as Valium (diazepam), reveal studies by Robert M. Carney, Ph.D., and associates at Washington University School of Medicine in St. Louis. A just-as-effective safe-not-sorry substitute formula made from flowers and herbs that also reduces rapid heartbeat, insomnia, restlessness, and other bad-mood byproducts includes *Cicuta virosa* (4×), *Asa foetida* (3×), *Ignatia* (4×), *Gaultheria* (4×), *Staphysagria* (4×), *Corydalis form.* (3×), *Sumbulua* (3×), *Hyoscyamus* (3×), and *Avena sativa* (1×). Check with your local health pharmacy.

12. Last but not least, have a family-sized dose of vitamin C (1 gram), which is rapidly depleted under stress, says Carl C. Pfeiffer of the Brain-Bio Center in Princeton, New Jersey. This can get you up when you're down. (For best results, get your C half from food, half from a natural bioactive* supplement, and wash it down with vitamin-C-activating green tea.)

---

*For a change-of-pace source of vitamin C, try the homeopathic ascorbic acid called aconite.

Try this recipe:

Good Cheer Rice Pudding

> *3 cups 1% milk or soy milk*
> *¹/₂ cup Arboria or brown rice*
> *¹/₄ cup firmly packed maple or date sugar*
> *¹/₄ cup dried cranberries*
> *¹/₂ cup mixed dried fruits*
> *¹/₄ cup dried sour cherries*
> *Pinch cinnamon*

Preheat oven to 300 degrees. Oil baking dish.

Pour milk into a 1-quart saucepan and warm over medium heat. Pour milk into baking dish and stir in remaining ingredients. Bake for one hour, stirring once, until rice is tender and milk is absorbed. Cool to almost room temperature before serving, with or without whipped low-fat no-dairy cream (see Dairy Substitutes).

Makes six servings.

See foods for healing zones: 8, 4

Also see: Herbs, Vitamin C, Stress, Leafy Greens

For more information, contact the National Foundation for Depressive Illness, P.O. Box 2257, New York, NY 10116, 800-248-4344.

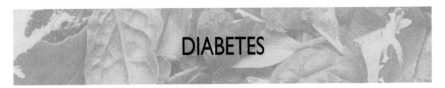

DIABETES

Diabetes, the #7 killer in the United States, is largely a knife-and-fork disease. In fact, diabetes is not one but a cluster of metabolic disorders which women are twice as likely to develop as men. The two main risk factors? Genetic predisposition and overweight (and anything that contributes to obesity contributes to the onset of insulin resistance, says the American Diabetes Association, or ADA). The older you get, the greater the risk. Complications, which are numerous and serious after you reach 40, include foot ulcers, heart disease, and circulatory abnormalities.

Life's eleven big commandments if you're one of America's 14 million sufferers, according to the ADA, are to

1. Sharply reduce sugar intake (sugars impair glucose tolerance and increase both cholesterol and uric acid levels) as well as moderating your total carbohydrate intake.

2. Maintain normal cholesterol and triglyceride levels, and keep your weight on an even keel.

3. Follow a no-more-than-30%-of-calories-from-fat diet, and if you're overweight, follow an M.D.-supervised weight-loss regimen. Ninety percent of all diabetics (insulin dependent) are overweight or obese, says the C. Everett Koop Foundation.

Beyond that, here are 11 insulin-sparing success tricks:

1. Keep it simple but complex. A diet of up to 70% simply prepared (preferably raw) complex carbohydrate foods is the key to diabetes control, says Dr. James Anderson, originator of the HCF Diabetes Control Diet. As a bonus, such foods (whole grains, raw fruits and vegetables, dried beans) provide blood-sugar-stabilizing fiber.

2. Use your bean and cut your insulin needs by up to 40% because beans produce a graduated rise in blood sugar, and thus a lowered need for glucose-control insulin (says the Preventative Medicine Research Institute. Legumes also create more insulin receptor sites on cells, studies indicate, reducing the amount of free-circulating insulin in the bloodstream. Best of the bunch? Soybeans (second only to peanuts among foods that promote a healthy blood-sugar response).

3. Build up your biotin reserves. Recent Japanese research studies indicate that this B-complex nutrient is useful in both normalizing blood-sugar levels and enhancing the effectiveness of insulin-stimulating medication.

4. Use flower power—especially if you're addicted to carbohydrates (as many diabetics are). In flower-essence healing, the spiritual component (essence of the flowers) is second to the physical component (the agent, flowers). The healing element is the vibration pattern of the species of flower used and how it is experienced psychically. Flower essences* are therapeutic for both mental and emotional

---

* The essence is in liquid form at health food stores and herb pharmacies.

states, helping your body back to a natural balance of mental and physical energy. A good beginner's essence is Star Tulip.

5. Pamper your pancreas with chromium-rich snacks. Chromium is an insulin-sparing trace mineral which, indicates USDA research, the typical American diet is low in. Best sources: grapes and nutritional yeast. (Nonvegetarian sources include ham and shellfish).

6. Up your fenugreek. According to Zacharia Madar of the Agriculture Department at Hebrew University in Israel, diabetes is rare among Yemenite Jews because of their high consumption of the bitter herb fenugreek, which can help reduce glucose levels by 15 to 18%. To enhance palatability, soak, boil, and liquefy the seeds and then use them to fortify soups and sauces and vegetable shakes.

7. Get into the garlic, onion, and oil habit. Allicin-carrier foods, especially garlic and onion, have significant sugar-lowering action. And linoleic acid (often deficient in diabetics) is critical for the healing of the glands and circulatory system. Best sources: olive, canola, and safflower oils.

8. Increase your inositol and magnesium intake with leafy greens, garlic, soy milk, and tofu, which speed healing of diabutic neuropathy and improve the pancreas's response to insulin. Best juices for the job: parsley, kale, spinach, and garlic.

9. Cook with herbs and spices. Among the baker's dozen that quadruple insulin's ability to metabolize glucose, according to researcher Richard Anderson, Ph.D., of the Beltsville Human Nutrition Research Center, are oregano, sage, cinnamon, cloves, turmeric, and sweet bay. And the two best diabetes-specific herbs for tea? Raspberry and strawberry leaf.

10. Become the vegetarian or ultramoderate meat eater you were meant to be to reduce sharply your risk of diabetes, advise directors of the Diabetes Treatment Program at the Bircher Benner Clinic in Switzerland. While you're upping your raw fruit and vegetable intake, be on the lookout for bitter melon (balsam pear)—a tropical fruit used extensively in complementary medicine for diabetes control.

11. Work out. According to William J. Evans, Ph.D., director, Noll Laboratory for Human Performance Research at Pennsylvania State University, aerobic exercise dramatically boosts levels of the protein GLUT 4, that helps clear glucose from the blood and puts a brake on blood sugar. It enhances insulin sensitivity, diminishes

insulin needs, improves glucose tolerance, and even accelerates weight loss. other studies indicate that strength training can improve insulin sensitivity by 33% in 12 weeks.

Try this recipe:

Insulin Relief Pitcher

> *1 bunch parsley or watercress*
>
> *2 garlic cloves*
>
> *4 or 5 carrots, greens removed*
>
> *2 stalks celery or ¹/₂ cup cubed celeriac*
>
> *6 broccoli florets*
>
> *1 or 2 tablespoons nutritional or brewer's yeast*

Bunch up parsley and push through chopper, alternating with garlic, carrots, broccoli, celery, or substitute.

Stir in yeast.

Optional: Add 1 teaspoon aloe vera to boost healing power.

Makes four servings.

See foods for healing zones: 6, 7, 8

Also see: Basic Dieting Facts and Advice, Vegetarian Foods, Beans, Juices, Herbs, Sweeteners, Vitamin E

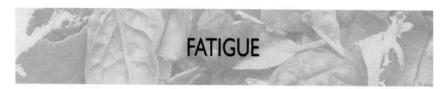

FATIGUE

Sir Thomas Powell Buxton, the English social reformer, once remarked, "The longer I live, the more deeply I am convinced that that which makes the difference between one man and another—between the weak and the powerful, the great and the insignificant—is energy."

If you don't have a tiger or two in your tank, there are plenty of reasons your wagon could be dragging. Take heart. Fatigue has up to 50 different causes and probably as many nutrition solutions, according to Dr. Harry Johnson of Houston's Life Extension Foundation. The good news is that only 5% of all fatigue victims require professional help.* "The rest of us," says Dr.Johnson, "are suffering from a combination of bad habits, inferior menus and poor mental attitudes."

Once you've eliminated anemia, allergy, PMS, CFS (Chronic Fatigue Syndrome), and thyroid imbalance, here are nine solutions.

1. Eat small, frequent meals and take vitamins B and C to beat fatigue. Eating small whole-food snacks (rather than breaking three times a day for large meals) stabilizes energy levels and facilitates digestion. Whole foods perform another service. According to the Toxicology and Human Nutrition Institute in Zurich, Switzerland, deficiency of vitamins B_1, B_2, B_6, and C can cause a 10% decrease in stamina and a 20% decrease in endurance. These four fatigue-fighting nutrients aid the body in its use of fatty acids, which account for 60% of your physical energy. Best sources: low-fat cheese, nondairy milk, soybeans, and whole fruits.

   To give those Bs and Cs a boost, add magnesium and potassium. A deficiency in these two minerals causes you to have tremendous fatigue. Your muscles may feel soft, flabby, and you may experience muscle pain and poor reflexes. Putting more milk, potatoes, dark leafy greens, raw nuts, and kelp (the peppery multinutrient salt substitute from the sea) on the menu should help, along with plenty of the fruits and vegetables shown in the following chart:

TOP FATIGUE-FIGHTING FRUITS
(Magnesium, potassium/vitamin C providers)

bananas	grapefruit	oranges	strawberries	blueberries
prunes	melons	raisins	dates	papaya
apples	mangoes	apricots		

TOP FATIGUE-FIGHTING VEGETABLES

beets	carrots	potatoes	sweet potatoes	turnips
dried beans	pumpkin	squash (all types)		

TIP: All of these can be juiced for liquid empowerment and seasoned with a pinch of rosemary or borage.

2. Skip the bearclaws and get boron. Despite their reputation as energizers, sugar, and even whole milk, can trigger ups and downs of
   insulin, the little-engine-that-could hormone that channels the
   sugar in foods into the body's cells for energy. Regular dairy milk
   is loaded with petrochemicals, pesticides, and growth hormone
   residues which interfere with the body's energy cycle. If you're carbohydrate sensitive or glucose intolerant, you need to think protein first and carbohydrate second (and keep fat—another energy
   defuser—low). A hard-boiled egg, 2 ounces of nondairy skim milk,
   3 ounces of tofu, and a boron-rich apple (not apple pie) are good
   snack bets.

   Boron, a trace mineral that improves the body's retention of calcium, also synchronizes brain functions and improves alertness,
   according to Forrest Nielsen, director of the USDA's Grand Forks
   Human Nutrition Research Center in North Dakota. As little as 1
   mg a day (the amount in two large apples or four carrots) does the
   trick.

3. Take tea and see. Switch from coffee or regular tea (which stimulate the adrenal glands to mobilize glycogen in the short run but
   contribute to glandular fatigue in the long run) to occasional cups
   of a grassroots, noncaffeinated stimulant such as Mu Huang or
   Mormon's tea, two herbal precursors of the body's adrenalin-
   boosting chemical, ephedrine. Or try ginseng, a blood tonic with
   a centuries-old track record that improves both stress tolerance
   and energy. Better, look into the American Indian Herb
   Company's "Clear Thinking Tea," a 17-ingredient alertness brew
   available at most health food stores.

4. Don't take fatigue lying down. Continual inactivity can lead to
   muscular atrophy and a loss of strength and endurance. Worse, it
   sets negative metabolic processes in motion that lead to slowed
   circulation, loss of muscle strength, diminished bone density, and
   a weakened immune system. Any form of regular exercise within
   your limits that increases your heartbeat—a bike ride, swim, or
   even a 20-minute simulated cross-country walk in your bedroom—has the effect of pushing back fatigue limits. Vigorously
   done, it produces a "feel-good" training effect that lasts six to seven
   hours in the well-conditioned body (30 minutes even in one that's
   not) because your brain receives an oxygen pick-me-up as your
   heartbeat rises. What simple mini-exercise works best? Try jump-

ing rope or quick-stepping with a soap box or stool. One five-minute workout a day is the equivalent of one set of tennis or nine holes of golf, says the President's Council on Fitness and Sports. Second best aerobic indoor upper: marching in place. If you've got a soap box or a step stool, add quick-stepping.

5. Take an oxygen break or breathe backwards. A technique called Breathplay restores energy by improving respiration up to 25%. It also lowers heart rate and blood pressure. The key is to turn the active and passive phases of breathing upside down. Here's how: Instead of sucking air in and letting it out, push the air out, then let it back in. Next, breathe in steps: Progressively flatten your stomach as you breathe out, and think of each breath as a footstep. The rhythm should be odd-numbered (three outbreaths followed by two inbreaths). Done twice daily, results are usually apparent within 10 days.

   If backward breathing doesn't give you your second wind, consider an oxygen cocktail. Oxygen helps your body cells fight off chemical toxins and disease-causing microbes, say ecologists. Oxygen inhibits the proliferation of harmful (anaerobic) microorganisms by destroying harmful bacteria, viruses, and fungi. Best of all, it's a brain perk and it's available in supplement form at better health pharmacies and also in treatment form from certified naturopaths.

6. Don't pop pills: pour rice oil. Two thirds of the 150 most commonly prescribed drugs—especially antidepressants, hormones, and anti-hypertension medications—can cause chronic fatigue, says the National Pharmaceutical Association. OTC uppers, such as diet pills and alertness aids, often contain more caffeine than coffee. Try a little rice bran oil, which contains ferulic acid bound to a plant sterol molecule that acts as a natural steroid in the body. Studies indicate that ferulic acid may be as potent an antioxidant as vitamin E and increases the autonomic nervous system's epinephrine levels. Twice-a-week cold brown rice salads or rice milk frozen desserts are other sources.

7. Energize with color, acupressure, or massage. Seventy-five percent of the sense stimuli we receive daily is visual, says the German Academy of Color Sciences in Bonn, Germany. Black, blue, and green are the commonest energy defusers. The three top colors to work into your work and home environment to wake up your ner-

vous system, says the academy, are yellow, orange, and red—in that order.

Alternative? An herbal energy massage to banish job burnout in 15 minutes for less than $25 an hour. Or try this acupressure upper: Hold the right ear lobe between your thumb and forefinger. Now very gently tug downward, then upward, and then sideways. Tug gently in all directions for a few moments, then repeat with the left ear lobe.

8. Sleep in, add a nap. or lift weights. Experiment with your night-time sleep pattern until you find one that produces the daytime energy you're after, adding or subtracting gradually from your usual six, seven, or eight hours of pillow time. When you can nod off 30 minutes after you bed down for the night (and wake up feel-ing refreshed), you've found the magic number.

   Weight training is another energizer. According to studies by Rebecca D. Brown, a professor of physical-education at Keene State College in New Hampshire, and Joyce M. Harrison, a professor of physical education at Brigham Young University, 12 weeks of weight training can improve posture, strength, and self-confidence and eliminate those two enemies of energy—anxiety and depres-sion. Twelve weeks should give you the lift you're looking for.

9. Take the aromatherapeutic waters or energize homeopathically. Herbal baths that are naturally therapeutic for fatigue include spearmint and apple cider vinegar. Use 1 cup as an all-over rub-down, then add 1 cup to bath water and soak 20 minutes or more.

   Two good sniff-for-life aromatherapy oils: spearmint and clove buds. Or take the homeopathic salt kali phosphoriciem through-out the day until your mood lifts.

Whatever your strategy, this quick-energy shake should maximize results.

Fatigue Fighter's Fruit Smoothie

> *2 ripe bananas or ¹/₂ mango*
> *8 strawberries*
> *1¹/₂ cups unsweetened cranberry-apple juice, chilled*

2 tablespoons instant rice milk powder (or instant skimmed dairy powder) or vitamin-fortified protein powder

Peel bananas or mango and place in blender container with strawberries, juice, and powder. Blend just until smooth and frothy. Chill and sip.

Variations: For added vitamins B and C and energy minerals, add 1 or 2 teaspoons nutritional yeast. or see juice boosters (Juices, p. 104). Or substitute any of the "fatigue-fighting fruits" for berries or bananas.

See foods for healing zones: 3, 6, 8

Also see: Depression, Bananas, Vitamin B, Herbs, Sweeteners, Substitutes, Dairy Substitutes

For more information, call the Chronic Fatigue Hotline at 1-800-866-0599.

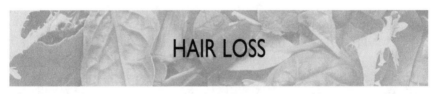

HAIR LOSS

Hair loss is higher on America's list of high anxieties than aging says the 1993 Trends Research Institute Study. Women are 15% more likely to be victims of hair-scare phobia. But hair loss is normal, temporary, and reversible in 90% of all cases, advises the government's Division of Cosmetology. Maybe you can't take it with you, but there's plenty you can do to keep a better grip on what you've got while you've got it.

First, the facts:

◆ There are two types of hair loss: loss from the roots, which is permanent; and breakage without the root, a common condition that is reversible with attention to causes, including stress, illness, (especially childbirth, thyroid disorders and autoimmune disease) and poor nutrition. A maximum loss of 100 hairs a day is normal.

If you're shedding more, check with a licensed trichologist or beautician or your family doctor. The best way to decide if hair loss is normal or excessive? Keep a hair-loss diary. Brush hair twice daily at the same time for two weeks. Collect and count hairs lost and place in a dated envelope. An average loss of 30 to 100 hairs daily is normal. Otherwise, consult a qualified specialist.

◆ Stress of all kinds causes hair loss, thinning, and recession. And physical or psychological tensions cause a condition called "telogen efflusion," in which the percentage of hair at rest increases by about 10%. The good news? When stress is resolved, normal growth returns.

◆ The #2 cause of excessive hair loss is poor health, especially conditions such as rheumatoid arthritis, flu or other infections, or overactive/underactive thyroid.

◆ Hair loss caused by injury or illness is deceptive and often doesn't become noticeable until a few months after the trauma, says dermatologist Michael Kalman, M.D., of Mount Sinai School of Medicine.

◆ Dieting is a major fallout maker, especially very-low-calorie, low-protein, and fruit-only regimes, says the American Dietetic Society. Vegetarians who are not careful to combine protein foods in large enough amounts often suffer protein deficiency fallout. Diets which omit a basic food group or fall below 1,000 calories a day for sustained periods also starve the hair.

◆ The commonest nutritional deficiencies leading to hair loss are iron, vitamin B complex, protein, and folic acid, which is supplied by the B-complex vitamins in most raw fruits and vegetables (see the recipes at the end of this section).

◆ Medications that can trigger temporary hair loss include anticoagulants and betablockers (heart drugs), antiarthritis medications, and antidepressants, says the National Nutritional Foods Association (NNFA). Ask your doctor about alternatives or new lower "mini" doses.

◆ Three hair abusers: excessive brushing or brushing when hair is wet; blow drying hair at high temperatures; and traction hair loss (a condition resulting from day-to-day stressing of the hair shaft through use of tight rollers, elastic bands, barrettes, braiding, hot waves, and permanents). Take an occasional "hair break" from these rituals to allow hair to recover. Brush smart—30 to 50 gentle strokes a day does the job. Blow dry only at low temps, and avoid wearing yank-and-tug hair styles, advises the Hair Dressers Council.

◆ Three women-only causes of hair loss: pregnancy, excessive menstrual flow (causing a loss of iron), and contraceptives. Women already predisposed to thinning hair by heredity are most susceptible.

HANG-ONTO-YOUR-HAIR HINTS

◆ To turn on "turned off hair," apply a rich conditioner before bed and comb it through to the ends, tuck under a plastic cap, and shampoo in the morning.

◆ Use less cream rinse and more conditioning. Rinses weigh your hair down and cause stress; conditioners coat the hair shaft, adding thickness.

◆ Cut your hair if it's thinning. Try a slicked-down style or move your part around for a less-is-more look.

◆ Lighten up. You've got nothing to gain by worrying about hair loss or a receding hairline. But you've got plenty to gain by improving your diet. Here's how, says the National Hairdressers and Cosmetologists Association:

◆ Feed your hair daily. The top hair-raisers are foods rich in vitamin A, B-complex vitamins, vitamin E, and iron. Found in protein (nonanimal, preferably): dried beans, high-protein grains, and soy foods, including tofu and tempeh.

◆ Eat fresh fruit, two servings daily. Try one new fruit-in-season per week for variety.

◆ Eat green salads made with lettuce, spinach, kale, collards, turnips, parsley, and watercress.

◆ Eat fresh vegetables, raw or lightly steamed and lightly seasoned.

◆ Eat whole grains: two servings whole grain breads or cereals plus six to eight glasses of pure water daily.

◆ Avoid whole milk, white bread, deep- or pan-fried foods, high-fat soft and hard cheeses, and chocolate and salt (hidden in many processed foods); all are hair-health robbers. Use real butter and polyunsaturated oils sparingly.

The effects of a balanced and varied diet should be apparent in your hair within six weeks.

◆ Don't become a "carbohydrate anorexic." "This is particularly common," says Philip Kingsley, "in younger weight watchers. The cause is almost total abstinence from complex carbohydrates— whole grain breads, fresh fruits, and vegetables. Hair follicles are especially sensitive to this form of starvation because carbohydrates provide the nutrients needed for proper follicle function. Prolonged deficiency progressively disturbs the hair cycle, and after that hair loses its luster and strength, and eventually the hair itself is lost."

◆ Up your garlic. Garlic, says the American Association of Nutritional Consultants, is rich in the hair-growth minerals iron and zinc and improves absorption of that A-1 hair vitamin, B complex. A garlic scalp massage (use a raw sliced bulb on scalp, shampoo out after 30 minutes) stimulates scalp circulation, says herbalist Jeanne Rose.

◆ Unhealthy hair is associated with high levels of androgens and high cholesterol. Mushrooms and legumes (lentils, peas, and soybeans) are antiandrogens and anticholesterol foods to include in your diet.

Here are two fast and healthy whole meals—to toss and pour—to give you a headstart on healthy hair:

Headstart Whole Meal Salad

> *3 cups washed, dried, torn or cut lettuce (combine two or three types, such as loose leaf plus Romaine or escarole)*
>
> *4 pitted diced olives*
>
> *1 small ripe tomato, diced*
>
> *1 hard-cooked egg, sliced, or 2 squares firm diced tofu*
>
> *$^1/_4$ cup thinly sliced cucumber or radish*
>
> *$^1/_2$ cup cooked dried beans*
>
> *4 paper-thin slices low-fat Swiss cheese*

Toss all ingredients. Combine with any low-fat, high-protein salad dressing.

Thick Shake for Thinning Hair

¹/₄ cup cranberry juice

1 cup apple juice

Medium ripe banana

¹/₂ cup diced celery

1 cup plain yogurt or calorie-reduced sour cream or tofu

Purée all ingredients in blender. Add 2 crushed ice cubes. Process again until thick, smooth, and frothy.

Makes three to four servings.

See foods for healing zones: 1, 6

Also see: Stress, Basic Dieting Facts and Advice, PMS, Leafy Greens, Vitamin B, Vitamin E

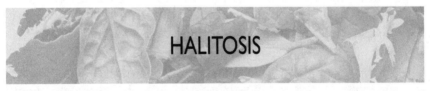

HALITOSIS

Are you getting as much out of your mouth as you're putting in? Not if you have halitosis, and 25 million of us do. But you can nip bad breath in the tastebuds if you know the reasons and the remedy, and you will with this nine-step program for halting halitosis.

1. Respiratory Disease. Uppermost on the list of malodorous mouth-makers are upper respiratory infections (a stuffy nose promotes mouth breathing), and where there's postnasal drip, sinusitis, and allergies, there's bound to be oral odor.

2. Bad food, bad breath. Food is the culprit in 90% of all cases of halitosis, says Mel Rosenberg, Ph.D., microbiologist at the School of

Dental Medicine at Tel Aviv University. All refined carbohydrates (especially sticky ones)—and especially sugar—increase odor-causing bacteria. Switch to protein-rich snacks which increase saliva, especially foods high in vitamins A and C and the bioflavonoids complex to strengthen gum tissue. Reach for cubes of aged cheese (cheddar, Swiss, and Monterey) for dessert rather than cookies and cake.

3. Avoid high-fat and sulphurous foods. Both garlic and onion and fatty foods like butter and some cheeses* secrete aromatic substances that are exhaled after metabolizing. But note that garlic is not effective or detectable until a full 24 hours after entering the bloodstream and thus is little affected by after-meal brushing or rinsing. Rx? Chew raw parsley or mint, which follow the same metabolic route as allicin-containing foods and thus will be releasing their neutralizing powers via the lungs simultaneously.

4. Mouth-drying medications. Antianxiety drugs, antihistamines, diuretics, and decongestants and certain illnesses themselves (diabetes, ulcerations of the stomach or intestines, and any serious metabolic disorder) all interfere with hydrochloric acid essential to normal digestion and the normal flow of the slightly acidic saliva that suppresses bacteria. Ask your doctor about artificial saliva if you're a medication long-termer.

5. Life changes. Fluctuations in hormones that characterize pregnancy, menopause, and puberty also disturb normal mouth pH levels, Another artificial-saliva-to-the rescue situation.

6. Fasting. If you're one of the 33% of all Americans who skip meals, or if you abstain from food and drink for extended periods, saliva production slows and mouth bacteria multiply, causing dry mouth or day-long "morning breath." Get back on the three-squares track to prevent bad breath.

7. High anxiety. Nervous stomach? Dry mouth? Beware a mouth gone bad in the bargain. When stress goes up, saliva production goes down and stomach acid increases.

8. Food intolerance. Bad breath is sometimes the result of enzyme deficiencies, especially problems with digesting sulphurous amino

---

* Aged cheeses are an exception.

acid foods. Try a garlic-onion-broccoli-turnip-cauliflower elimination diet.

9. Nicotine. Ninety-nine percent of all smokers have some degree of halitosis, says Dr. Israel Kleinberg, chairman of oral biology and pathology at the State University of New York at Stony Brook, because nicotine disturbs the chemistry of the stomach and the SSH levels of the saliva. Cut out or cut back on smoking.

Final Tips

1. Minimize your use of mouthwash. According to the Academy of General Dentistry, habitual use of antiseptic mouthwashes with high levels of alcohol (18 to 26%) has been linked to oral and throat cancer and can cause intoxication if swallowed or used excessively. Long-term use can also conceal signs of serious gum disease. If you must rinse, ask your doctor about a chlorhexine-containing brand (by prescription only) or make your own green gargle and mouthwash: Mix a teaspoon of chopped fresh parsley, a tablespoon of lemon or lime juice, and 6 ounces of papaya or pineapple juice. Rinse as needed. This is a fast-fix alternative to liquid chlorophyll diluted with water.

2. Minimize (or eliminate) your use of sulphurous-source products—garlic, onion,* red meat, coffee, tobacco, pineapple—and allicin-source foods (garlic, onion); and combine cabbage/broccoli and other cruciferous vegetables with aroma-reducing ingredients such as parsley, mint, and yogurt).

3. Don't cut carbohydrates from your diet. Eliminating raw fruits, vegetables, and starches can cause a negative shift in bacterial balance. The no-no bacteria are the ones that flourish on a high-protein diet. To improve your oral flora, eat buttermilk or active culture yogurts that counterbalance odor-making oral bacteria.

4. Brush your tongue. Best tools for dislodging odor-making bacteria are a tongue scraper (from your dentist) or a soft-bristled brush (or even the edge of a teaspoon). Make this a twice-a-day ritual. While you're at it, scrub the walls of your mouth, too.

---

* Coating these foods in yogurt or kefir before eating helps reduce after-odor.

5. Make your mouth water. Eat on schedule to prevent mouth dehydration. Snack on high-fiber, saliva-stimulating, teeth-scrubber foods and keep well watered.

6. Carry seedy snacks like fennel and anise and celery seeds, which contain breath-freshening oils that also aid digestion.

7. Excessive jawing or open-mouthed sleeping (the largest build-up of oral bacteria occurs while sleeping) lets oral bacteria do their dirty work. Periodontal diseases and improperly cleaned bridge-work or broken fillings also allow dead cells and bacteria on the gums to flourish (flossing and special cleaning devices help).

8. Last but not least, if you're halitosis prone, get first-hand guidance from an oral hygienist. If all else fails, talk to a halitosis pro. (There are four centers devoted to this specialty in the United States. Ask your dentist, or contact the American Dental Association at 1-800-283-4089.)

See foods for healing zones: **3, 4, 6, 7**

Also see: **Vitamin C, Water, Stress, Parsley, Allergies**

HEMORRHOIDS

Hemorrhoids (a.k.a. piles) may not be as common as the common cold, but they come close. One third of the general population has them at any given time. They start early—most victims are in their twenties when they first get them, although often symptoms such as rectal pain and itching, bleeding, and blood in stools don't appear until the thirties—and they persist. Over 50% of the 50-plus population is affected. The primary culprit? Low-fiber, high-refined-carbohydrate diets that produce chronic constipation and unnaturally hard stools which trigger, in turn, abdominal straining and pressure. The latter cause venous overload and pelvic congestion, weakening the veins and producing the swelling (which is actually just varicose veins in the anal area).

Take-control measures begin with bran and a better diet and end (if you're serious about prevention and control) with a weight-stabilizing exercise program. Here's how.

1. Get your diet up to high-fiber speed by including one or more vegetables and fruits in every meal and one to two servings of whole grains (crackers, bread, sugar-free cookies, sugar-free cake). Supplement each meal with 1 tablespoon of oat, wheat, corn, or rice bran.

2. Don't sit when you can walk, run, or climb. Don't make a habit of fast foods or refined foods rich in no-fiber white flour and sugar. And downplay chile peppers, curry, and all inflammatory spices in your healing plans.

3. Get juiced daily. Have an A.M. and P.M. juice rich in anticlotting, anti-inflammatory nutrients. Best choices: cantaloupe, garlic, onion, ginger, and berries.

4. Have a hemorrhoid-healing snack rich in zinc vitamin E and beta-carotene once or twice a day. Three foods that supply all three: carrot or pumpkin bread, whole grain vegetable crackers, fruit-and-nut trail mix.

5. Whet your appetite before meals with bromelain, a digestive enzyme found only in fresh pineapple that promotes the breakdown of fibrin and prevents formation of blood clots.

6. Have berries, not banana splits. Dark berries (black and blue berries, cherries, currants, etc.) supply two antioxidant pigments that strengthen venous walls and improve vascular muscle tone. Beta-carotene-rich cantaloupe also promotes posterior healing.

7. Consider bulking compounds, which are easier to assimilate than wheat germ: natural fiber supplements such as psyllium seed husks and guar gum, for example, which have the ability to attract water and form a gelatinous mass and can significantly reduce bleeding, pain, pruritis, and improve bowel habits over the short term.

8. Topical aids such as suppositories, ointments, and anorectal pads are only band-aids but, used temporarily, may speed healing. Look

for products containing witch hazel (Hamamelis water), cod liver oil, cocoa butter, balsam, zinc oxide, live yeast cell derivatives, and allantoin.

9. Drink up. Water is the purest of all bowel lubricants and the best of all natural hemorrhoidal preventatives.

Try this recipe:

Hemorrhoid Healing Smoothie

¹/₄ pineapple, with skin

¹/₂ cup melon cubes

¹/₄-inch slice ginger root

2 green tea ice cubes (optional)

Push pineapple through chopper with melon and ginger. Add to blender with ice cubes and process until smooth and frothy.

See foods for healing zones: 2, 7, 8

Also see: **Indigestion, Juices, Stress, Berries, Ginger, Whole Grains, Water**

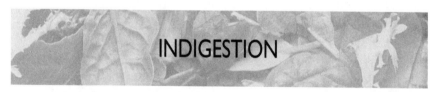

INDIGESTION

Are you practicing regular random acts of kindness for your digestive tract? If not, you're probably paying the price with some kind of gut reaction in the form of flatulence, heartburn, nausea, fatigue, constipation, diarrhea, hemorrhoids, colitis, IBS, ulcers, even halitosis and impaired immune function.

The intestinal lining has the highest rate of cell turnover in the body, so you need to treat it right. Undigested foods stay undigested, producing enzyme deficiencies and toxic byproducts that block absorption of nutrients. Malabsorption lays the groundwork for anemia, obesity, allergies and a host of degenerative ills. On the other hand, a finely tuned digestive system is the key to no-fault elimination, which is critical to smoothly operating body chemistry.

What are the top six stressors when your digestion's off track?* Stress, irregular eating patterns, inadequate nutrition (a low in fiber, high in refined foods diet), drugs (including excess amounts of aspirin and other analgesics), alcohol abuse, and smoking (which can trigger ulcers because nicotine inhibits production of the fatty acid prostaglandin needed to protect the stomach lining).

Here are five rules of order that make for orderly digestion:

1. Take it slow and keep it small. Six modestly proportioned snacks beats three big, hastily eaten square meals a day.

2. Eat by the clock (but only when your appetite's up).

3. Drink before or after, but not during, meals (but make it tepid and nonacid if you do; fluids interfere with the absorption of solids).

4. Limit digestion-disruptive drugs, especially excessive laxatives. If you must take some, take only as directed to prevent damage to stomach lining.

5. Break for fresh fruit between meals to tone digestion, improve energy, and normalize elimination.

When digestive function stalls, there are plenty of grassroots panaceas. Take your pick:

1. Have an antispasmodic tea. Herbs that soothe the digestive tract tissue include angelica, balm, caraway, chamomile, comfrey, marjoram, spearmint and peppermint, oregano, pennyroyal, savory, and thyme.

2. Put eugenol or anethole in your postdinner cup. A natural substance that gets digestive enzymes moving again, eugenol is found in allspice (chew ½ a teaspoon of whole berries well, then down with tea). Cloves are a secondary source of eugenol. Or try anethole, another substance that promotes normal digestion and is found in anise seed.

---

* People with type A blood are likely to be deficient in digestive enzymes, advises Corey Reimick of the National College of Naturopathic Medicine.

3. Turn a leafy green for relief. Dandelion greens and turmeric powder (a common ingredient in curry is a second source), says the Herb Research Foundation, secrete a substance that triggers the flow of bile, a critical step in the digestion progress.

4. Try premeal indigestion prevention. Both dill and fennel seed contain an antifoaming substance said to block the formation of intestinal gas and inhibit the growth of bacteria that attack the intestinal tract. They may even help prevent infectious diarrhea.

5. Get plop-plop, fizz-fizz relief from four time-honored herb and spice stomach settlers: catnip; cinnamon (eat the powdered bark or the aromatherapeutic oil); gentian, an herb with a 4,000 year track record; or ginger, a root which contains enzyme-like substances that help break down hard-to-digest proteins.

6. Prevent or speed the healing of ulcers or IBS with peppermint oil or licorice extract, which, studies suggest, provides better-than-Tagamet™ protection against duodenal ulcer relapses and relief of irritable bowel syndrome.

7. Pop a papaya or a red pepper. Papaya supplies the protein-digesting substance called papain along with other enzymes that digest starches. Red pepper in vegetable or supplement form triggers saliva flow and decreases the production of stomach acids.

Try this recipe:

3 Little Peppers (The bicarb alternative)

> 3 red or yellow bell peppers: roasted; stemmed, cored, seeded
> 2 teaspoons crushed dill
> 1/2 teaspoon olive oil
> 2 teaspoons fresh lemon juice
> Freshly ground pepper to taste
> 2 teaspoons chopped Italian parsley
> Optional 1/2 teaspoon majoram or oregano

Coarsely chop the peppers and place them in a food processor or blender with the dill. Process until coursely combined. Stir in parsley and dried herbs. Use as a dip or vegetable "jam" on crackers.

Yield: 2/3 cup.

See foods for healing zones: 7, 8

Also see: Peppers, Herbs, Leafy Greens, Hemorrhoids, Ulcers

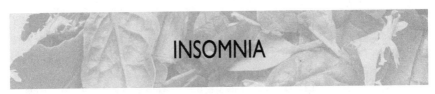

INSOMNIA

Did you know the following facts about insomnia?

- King Louis XIV slept each night in a different one of his 413 beds.
- Trees sleep to get relief from sunlight.
- The world's record for going without sleep—276 hours—was set in 1964.
- Taresthesia is when your foot goes to sleep.
- Talking in your sleep is called somniloquy. Kids do it more than grownups.
- Zebras in a herd never sleep all at the same time. One always stands guard.
- Sleeping pills account for one third of all drug-related deaths.
- One out of six sleepers is capable of waking spontaneously at a given hour.
- The fear of going to sleep is called hypnophobia.
- It takes an average of 20 minutes to fall asleep, while 60 minutes is not uncommon, and a few of us even do it in less than seven minutes.
- Smokers dream less than nonsmokers.
- Famous artists and writers who had nightmares regularly: Richard Wagner, Nathaniel Hawthorne, Goya, Mark Twain, Edgar Allan Poe, and Robert Louis Stevenson. (*Dr. Jekyll and Mr. Hyde* was based on a nightmare goes the legend.)
- Riding a motorcycle burns three times as many calories as counting sheep.
- Sleeping pill users have a 50 percent higher mortality rate than nonusers.

The ancient Egyptians described lying in bed unable to sleep as a living hell. Insomnia, says Pennsylvania Dutch folklore, is the sure sign of a troubled conscience, while nightmares and the like mean that a vengeful witch has crossed your path somewhere along the line.

Insomnia is a fact of our night life. Sixty million Americans, or one out of every three of us, have trouble making the switch from day to night. Sooner or later, one out of every two of us develops a nocturnal difficulty. While married women complain about it the most, insomnia is no respecter of age or marital status. A recent Institute of Mental Health study revealed that 46 percent of all teenagers suffer from insomnia and 5 percent sleep-walk.

To find a solution, you need to know which type of sleeplessness you suffer from, says the National Sleep Foundation. The three basic types of insomnia are as follows:

Type A: When you can't fall asleep within 30 to 45 minutes

Type B: When you get less than five or six hours of total sleep time

Type C: When you spend more than 30 to 60 minutes awake during the night.

Actually, says the National Commission on Sleep Disorder Research (NCSDR), there are five types of insomniacs (six if you count so-called pansomniacs, who suffer from all five forms of sleeplessness):

1. Initardia: The inability to fall asleep. Rx? Get up one hour earlier every day for one week. The time it takes to fall asleep is related to the number of hours you've been awake. If seven days later you're still having trouble, set your alarm back an additional hour. Once you begin sleeping better, start lengthening your sleep span, adding 15 minutes a week either in the morning or at night.

2. Scurzomnia: Waking up for no apparent reason after a short sleep and not being able to go back to sleep. Don't take a nap, but do get in some vigorous exercise before 4 P.M. and delay bedtime one hour. When you wake up, stay in bed at least 30 minutes, and then get up and get going again.

3. Hyperlixia: Excessively light sleep. Eliminate naps. When you wake up at night, after 30 minutes of not sleeping, get up and stay up until you're sleepy. Add daytime exercise and limit your liquid intake after 5 P.M.

4. Pleisomnia: Constantly broken sleep. Don't stay in bed more than 30 minutes when you wake up. Sit up, do something until you're sleepy, and then go back to bed. Set your alarm one hour earlier and get out of bed promptly. After one week, if you haven't shown

improvement, subtract another hour. When you find yourself waking less often, restore lost sleep time by moving the alarm ahead 15 minutes each week.

5. Insomnia turbula: Sleep characterized by recurring nightmares. Don't eat, drink, or watch TV in bed. Bed should be a place for sleep, maybe sex, but nothing else, says Dr. Charles P. Pollak, who heads the Sleep-Wake Disorders Center at the Westchester Division of the New York Hospital-Cornell Medical Center.

WHY INSOMNIA?

There are at least 100 reasons why we don't nod off on schedule. For starters:

1. Sickness: Victims of serious disorders such as asthma, angina pectoris, migraine headaches, arthritis, cancer, and pulmonary disease, as well as "restless leg syndrome" (vague discomforting sensation in the legs relieved only by rising) are all notorious poor sleepers, along with the depressed.

2. Bad habits: Nicotine is a notorious offender. Studies by the Sleep Research and Treatment Center at Pennsylvania State University conclude that smoking increases the nervous system's production of the chemical called catecholamines and that while coffee drinkers may develop a tolerance to caffeine, no such tolerance for nicotine appears to be present for smokers. Alcohol, caffeine, and pills of any kind (from amphetamines to antihistamines to aluminum-containing antacids) should be avoided. Sleeping pills work in the short run but lose their sleep-inducing potency after two weeks and then begin to reduce sleep, says the American Association of Nutritional Consultants, because they contain aluminum, a toxic metal that the body stores and that can cause disturbed sleep patterns.

3. Age: Advancing age is another major factor in insomnia. The older you are, the lighter and less continuously you sleep, the more often you get up to urinate, and the more sleep-disruptive side effects you suffer from medications. The ability to sleep soundly begins to decline after age 20.

4. Timing: You could be missing out on a good night's sleep because you're bedding down at a bad time. According to Martin C. Moore-

Ede, M.D., Ph.D., professor of physiology at Harvard Medical School, and other researchers at the Sleep Research Center at Stanford University, subjects who went to sleep when their body temperatures were lowest slept an average of 7.8 hours. Those who went to sleep at or just past the body's high point averaged 14.4 hours and got a poorer quality sleep. (The body's lowest temperatures are usually reached between 6 P.M. and 4 A.M.) To make matters worse, it takes four to six weeks of sufficient sleep to recover fully from prolonged sleep deprivation.

THE BIG THREE SLEEP DISORDERS

According to the NCSDR, the three commonest non-life-threatening sleep disorders are as follows:

- ◆ Snoring: One out of every eight of us snores. Men of all ages do it more than women.* Snorers may sleep very soundly; it's their bed-fellows who are kept awake. Snoring results from the blocking of an air passage during sleep. The noise is caused by the vibration of the soft palate as the lungs struggle to take in a diverted current of air. The primary culprits are excessive fatty tissue in the throat, large tonsils or nasal deformities (such as a deviated septum). Drinking before bed tends to increase snoring, as does sleeping on your back because your tongue blocks your airway. To correct, stack up pillows to keep your head propped. Or tie a hard ball around your waist or sew it to your pajamas so you'll roll onto your side as soon as you shift into the prime snoring position of sleeping on your back.

- ◆ Sleep-walking: Kids between five and 15 do it the most, and researchers believe there may be a hereditary predisposition to take to your feet in the night. On the other hand, neither this nor sleeptalking is a health hazard unless it is extremely frequent. To prevent accidents, block off stairs and lock windows and doors.

- ◆ Leg movements (nocturnal myoclonus): Some 15 to 20% of sleep problems originate in the lower limbs. Sufferers jerk their legs just

* Children under the age of 10 may snore because of enlarged tonsils and adenoids. Teenagers and young adults rarely snore, but after age 30 the incidence of snoring climbs from 10% to as high as 30%.

as they're about to fall asleep. Others involuntarily kick their legs in the night—waking themselves and their partners. Doctors don't know why. Antistress exercises before retiring often help.

BEYOND INSOMNIA

Sleep problems don't stop with insomnia. In fact, daytime sleepiness sends many more Americans to sleep clinics than nighttime insomnia. Half of all patients who seek help complain about the daytime "drowsies." As much as 45% of all daytime sufferers are victims of nighttime obstructive sleep apnea (a potentially fatal disorder characterized by frequent bouts of interrupted breathing); in 25% of the cases drowsiness is caused by narcolepsy (a disabling inherited disorder of the brain's sleep-wake controls in which the victim is overcome by attacks of irresistible sleepiness throughout the day); while the remaining complaints are linked to nervous-system abnormalities.

There's also hyperinsomnia, the tendency to sleep too much, which commonly affects pregnant women and teenage girls prior to the onset of regular menstruation. There's even something called "pseudoinsomnia." Commonly, sufferers are sleepers who overestimate the time they spend in bed before falling asleep or getting back to sleep. Under sleep laboratory conditions, pseudoinsomniacs turn out to be sleeping normal lengths of time. They just don't wake up feeling rested because of some abnormality in their sleep pattern.

GETTING YOUR ZZZZZ'S
Nutritional and Drug-Free Techniques

If you've reevaluated your sleep position (the best one is the semifetal) and upgraded your mattress, pillows, and sleep environment and you're still not nodding off, here are some nutrition-based tips for inducing 40 winks.

◆ The early American settlers filled their cups with red bergamot tea and pennyroyal tea to induce sleep.

◆ Eighteenth-century German herbalists prescribed infusions of ground anise and honey in a cup of warm milk before bed.

◆ Cowslip and lemon balm leaves were brewed for a bedtime tea in Dickens's day.

- American Indians anointed the forehead of nonsleepers with hot lemon juice. According to the English herbalist Maude Gerard, woodruff leaves in wine or mulled apple cider with a few cloves and a stick of cinnamon provide that elusive Zzzzz factor too.

- Sleep researchers in La Tour-de-Peilz, Switzerland, serve steaming cups of valerian. (British doctors during World War II used tinctures of the herb to calm the shattered nerves of bombing raid victims.) In a recent U.S. study of 128 sleep-troubled men and women, valerian produced significant improvements in sleep quality, most notably among poor and irregular sleepers. Valerian does not affect dream recall or cause the morning-after drowsiness, as prescription sleeping pills and OTC sleep aids do.

- If you're out of herbs, hot lemonade, orangeade, and grapefruit juice are also sleepers which provide carbohydrates to lull you to sleep by promoting the release of sleep-inducing chemicals in the brain, according to Richard J. Wurtman, M.D., and John D. Fernstrom, Ph.D., Massachusetts Institute of Technology researchers.

- Baby yourself. Try finger cradling, advises naturopath Jane Guiltinan, chief medical officer at the Natural Health Clinic of Bastyr College in Seattle. Hold the thumb of one hand by wrapping the other hand so gently around that you can still slip the thumb in and out. Hold this thumb three to five minutes, then repeat with your index finger, and so on. There is an emotion related to each finger—from worry to perfectionism to anger—and people tend to fall asleep while holding the finger that represents their target, goes the theory. If you have a lot of anger and frustration, You'll fall asleep holding your middle finger.

- Milk's power to cloud minds comes from the generous amounts of a tranquilizing amino acid called tryptophan which it contains. Amino acids are the building blocks of all protein, and tryptophan is found in all protein foods such as cheese, meat, and poultry. Dairy products such as milk also contain fat, another sleep-promoting factor. Better yet, add a teaspoon of the B-vitamin booster, Brewer's yeast (flakes or powder), to a cup of Postum™ or Ovaltine® made with skim milk before bed.

- The ordinary apple may be a food to sleep on. Romantic novelist Alexander Dumas, who is said to have fathered 50 children and who wrote hundreds of novels during his insomnia-filled nights, was ordered by his physician to eat an apple every day at 7 o'clock under the Arc de Triomphe. (An apple, like other common fruits, is high in sleep-promoting carbohydrates.)

Herbs are a sleeper aromatherapy as well. Best botanical choices for 40 winks: chamomile, basil, lavender, and cedarwood.

See foods for healing zones: **4, 5, 6**

Also see: **Herbs, Lemons, Stress**

KIDNEY STONES

The kidneys continuously filter 500 gallons of blood in 24 hours. The waste and surplus nutrients filtered by the kidneys are in solution (urine). In one in 10 Americans, minerals combine with other elements in the urine to form stones, and once a stone forms, the risk of recurrence is 20 to 50% within 10 years. The most common type is calcium oxalate, composed of calcium and oxalic acid. Some stones are formed when calcium is combined with uric acid or phosphates. A stone can be large or minute, and the trouble begins when a small stone breaks off and moves down the urinary tract, causing severe abdominal pain, blood in the urine, and other symptoms such as nausea and vomiting.

No single piece of advice is appropriate for all stone sufferers; treatment should be individualized. Calcium is only one dietary factor that may affect stone formation. But foods rich in oxalates (especially leafy greens such as spinach, collards, and beet greens) as well as chocolate, peanuts, rhubarb, tea, and berries are generally to be avoided. Stone formers are advised to eat less animal protein (high-protein intake increases the excretion of calcium in the urine) and more potassium-rich foods (a good twofer source: nectarines) and to drink plenty of fluids.

The common treatment for stones is surgery, which can cause scar tissue and lead to other problems. A holistic approach that prevents the creation of stones includes a change of lifestyle and a fruits-and-vegetables diet high in fiber, low in salt, and high in herbs that help prevent stones from forming, or help dissolve, and eliminate them.

MILK
A Culprit?

Researchers from Harvard now challenge this traditional advice, suggesting that a low calcium intake actually increases the risk of kidney stones. According to the Harvard study, published in the *New England Journal of Medicine,* data from a study of 45,000 male health professionals, ranging in age from 40 to 75, who had no history of kidney stones and who consumed a calcium-rich diet (containing more calcium than four glasses of milk a day) had a nearly 50% *lower* risk of developing kidney stones during the next four years than men who consumed little calcium (less calcium than two glasses of milk a day).

HERBS THAT FIGHT STONE FORMATION

As for the preventive and curative herbs, a formula combining gravel root, hydrangera, marshmallow, and lobelia is effective since these botanicals are powerful toners for the urinary system and widely used in kidney and bladder disorders. Gravel root is also used to treat gallstones, rheumatism, and gout.

Three More Better-by-Botanicals Approaches

- ◆ Try tea and white birch tree oil, a traditional remedial for kidney stones and urinary infections, says the British Medical Herb Association.

- ◆ Apple cider vinegar (1 teaspoon to 6 ounces water) cocktails and almond-barley milk (barley water liquefied with crushed raw almonds) are also time-tested nostrums.

- ◆ Rice bran (about one third of an ounce twice a day for a month or longer), according to Japanese investigators, is an effective preventive by helping reduce calcium in the urine. The phytic acid in the rice bran blocks the intestinal absorption of unwanted calcium, preventing formation of stones.

If there is a high uric acid level, ½ pound of fresh cherries (because of their alkaline nature) helps reduce pain.

The following charts will help you fight kidney stones nutritionally.

HIGH-POTASSTUM FOODS: 12-BEST BETS

Food	Portion	% RDA
Potato, baked	1 (approx. 7 oz.)	23
Prune juice	8 fl. oz.	19
Peaches, dried	5 halves (approx. 2 oz.)	17
Avocado	½ (approx. 3 oz.)	16
Nonfat yogurt	1 cup	15
Seedless raisins	½ cup	14
Carrot juice	6 fl. oz.	14
Apricots, dried	10 halves	13
Cantaloupe, cubed	1 cup	13
Lima beans, boiled	½ cup	13
Orange juice	8 fl. oz.	12
Banana	1 (approx. 4 oz.)	12

NON-OXALATE CALCIUM COUNTER

Food	Calcium (mg)
Lactaid™ calcium-fortified nonfat milk (1 cup)	580
Yogurt, nonfat, plain (1 cup)	500
Swiss cheese (1 oz.)	272
Tofu (3 oz.)	150
Turnip greens (½ cup cooked, chopped)	99
Bok choy (½ cup cooked)	79
Orange (1 medium)	52
Pinto beans (½ cup cooked)	41
Broccoli (½ cup cooked, chopped)	36
Sweet potato, baked (1 medium)	32

See foods for healing zone: **7**

Also see: **Water, Herbs, Cystitis, Dairy Substitutes, Juices, Substitutes, Rice**

For more information, call the Kidney Stone Hot Line at 1-900-230-4800, extension 6314.

LOW BLOOD PRESSURE

What's the best prescription for low blood pressure (hypotension)? High-protein salads, oatmeal, and sweet potatoes couldn't hurt.

Chronic hypotension—usually diagnosed when blood pressure checked while the patient reclines shows a 20-point drop in the upper systolic pressure when rechecked a minute later while the patient is standing—can be caused by anemia, diabetic nerve damage, low blood sugar, an underactive thyroid, and/or malnutrition. The commonest form (called orthostatic hypotension) is accompanied by temporary dizziness. Hypotension can also occur as a reaction to viral infections, influenza, antidepressive or antihypertensive medication. Other symptoms of hypotension include headache, fatigue, weakness, and fainting, which reduce blood pressure and blood volume due to dehydration.

Diet is often the number 1 culprit since nutritional deficiencies can cause the walls of blood vessels to lose their elasticity and expand. Fewer nutrients are able to penetrate the tissues in this state, causing the characteristic lightheadedness.

DIETARY IMPROVEMENTS THAT REVERSE HYPOTENSION

A high-protein diet with plenty of leafy green vegetables, soy foods, and wheat germ can help restore arterial elasticity, stimulate the adrenal glands, and normalize the blood pressure. Bell peppers, brewer's yeast, cabbage-type vegetables, citrus fruits, sweet potatoes, tomatoes, and grains are other good get-better solutions. Small, frequent meals throughout the day also prevent low blood pressure by preventing hypoglycemia. Foods rich in vitamins B, C, and E (parsley, garlic, onion, and whole grains) are especially restorative. Remedial drinks include beet, parsley, and bell pepper juice, and dandelion, ginger, and scullcap tea.

Acupressure massage by a professional therapist can also help normalize blood pressure levels.

For more information call the Blood Pressure Hotline at 1-900-230-4800.

Try this recipe:

Hypotension Control Soup

¹/₂ cup onion, chopped

4 large tart apples, cored and chopped

4 large tomatoes, seeded, chopped

5 stalks of celery, chopped

3 tablespoons unsalted butter or 3 tablespoons olive oil

2 tablespoons dry sherry (optional)

4 cups broth

fresh pepper to taste

Sauté onions in butter or oil until soft and translucent. Add apples, tomatoes, celery, and sherry. Cover and simmer for 5 minutes. Add broth and simmer for 25 minutes longer. Cool and strain vegetables, reserving liquid. Purée vegetables and remove any skins that remain by passing through a food sieve. Add purée to liquid in deep saucepot. Season and serve hot or cold with whole grain crackers or breadsticks.

See foods for healing zones: 2, 3

Also see: Coronary Heart Disease, Juices, Herbs, Vitamins B, C, and E

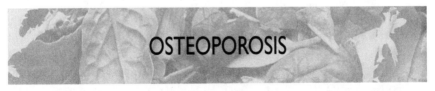

OSTEOPOROSIS

Osteoporosis, which affects 25 million of us (one out of two women will eventually be victims*), is a disease with or without one of the two commonest tipoff symptoms—leg and back pain—in which bone mass decreases below the level necessary for health. It is most common in women between the ages of 35 and 50, and loss is greatest in the spine, hips and ribs.

---

*Breast cancer, by contrast, affects one in nine women.

The good news is that a change of lifestyle is the #1 way to change the prognosis.

Caucasian and Asian females with slender ectomorphic body types are at greatest risk, as are women who go through early menopause or who are insulin-dependent diabetics. Bad habits that deprive the body of the primary mineral and nonmineral components of bone are the other primary risk factors—along with too little exercise and too much smoking, excess alcohol, caffeine, and salt (sodium interferes with calcium retention). The higher your salt intake, the greater your calcium requirement and vice versa. On a low-salt, low-protein diet, for example, 500 mg does the job.

The second piece of good news is that just an hour of moderate weight-bearing exercise three times a week can help halt or even reverse bone loss when bolstered by a healing diet high in all the other bone-building nutrients (calcium depletion is the culprit in only 25% of all cases of osteoporosis). That's not all; here are eight more tips for prevention, control, and reversal:

1. Raise your calcium and lower your protein and phosphorus intake. High-protein intake can trigger a loss of minerals, especially calcium, an alkaline nutrient released to neutralize the acidity of amino acids and excreted in the urine says the Physician Committee for Responsible Medicine. Animal proteins can double that loss since they are higher in the sulphur-containing aminos as well as a second calcium thief*—phosphorus (also found in white bread and soda drinks). Forty-five grams of high-quality protein daily is adequate. As for calcium, the numbers to remember are 1,000 before menopause and 1,500 after. For most people, bones are constantly undergoing a process of remodeling as calcium flows in and out of them. Although 98% of calcium is stored in bones, the nerves, the muscles, and the heart rely on calcium to function properly. When other body systems run short, they steal from the bones.

2. Change your milk ways. Here's how to get calcium without milk.

---

* According to a recent University of Florida study involving 150 vegetariam and non-vegetarian women aged 25-65, vegetarians had much greater bone density and less calcium excretion in their urine.

16 NONMILK CALCIUM SOURCES

	Calcium (mg)
Fruits	
Figs, dried, 2	54
Orange, 1 medium	56
Papaya, 1 cup	50
Raspberries, 1 cup	27
Grains	
English muffin, 1	92
Nuts	
Almonds, ½ oz.	38
Hazelnuts, ½ oz.	38
Seafood	
Clams, 60 oz.	200
Salmon; canned, with bones, 3½ ozs.	354
Syrups	
Molasses, blackstrap, 1 tbsp.	116
Vegetables	
Collard greens, ½ cup	152
Dandelion greens, 3½ ozs.	187
Kale, 3½ ozs.	134
Mustard greens, ½ cup	183
Turnip greens, ½ cup	138
Water	
Hard water, 1 qt.	350

Conversion of vitamin D to its biologically active form is dependent on the presence of magnesium, which also plays a mediating role in hormone secretion and leads to higher levels of calcium in the blood. Leafy greens, nuts and seeds, and egg yolks and sunshine are good, reliable sources of vitamin D.

3. Increase collagen boosters. Zinc, copper, vitamin A, and vitamin C are all involved in collagen synthesis, which forms about 95% of the organic bone matrix. (The body's efficiency in absorbing vitamin C appears to decrease with age, and osteoporosis can result from deficiency of this vitamin especially when zinc and copper are in short supply—which they are in the typical American diet.)

4. Eat your greens and grains. Leafy greens and whole grains are the best and contain the four trace elements boron, manganese, strontium, and silica, which play a critical role in shaping the skeletal infrastructure that is not yet fully understood.

5. Improve your homecysteine metabolism. This compound, derived from the breakdown of the amino acid methionene, is potentially toxic. If not neutralized by adequate levels of B_1, B_{12}, and folic acid, it can interfere with collagen formation. Best sources: soy foods, raw fruits, and vegetables.

6. Have a vitamin K day. Vitamin K has historically been used to help with blood clotting. Researchers are now discovering that vitamin K can be more important in the prevention of osteoporosis than calcium. Vitamin K plays an important role in converting bone protein (osteocalcin) from an inactive to active form, allowing the osteocalcin molecule—the major noncollagen protein found in bones—to join with calcium and maintain it within the bone structure. Vitamin K also helps reduce the loss of calcium, helping the body utilize it more effectively. Food sources include leafy vegetables, broccoli, spinach, and green tea.

7. Be a temperate pill taker. Long-term use of prescription medication such as corticosteroids, thyroid hormones, anticoagulants, as well as OTC antacids containing aluminum and diuretics also endanger your body's calcium reserves.

8. If you're at risk, avail yourself of the early warning strategy known as the Dex A bone-density scan, a painless, noninvasive, high-tech X-ray procedure that detects bone loss of as little as 1%. Ask your physician for referral to a Dex A facility nearby, or call the National Osteoporosis Foundation at 202-223-2226.

Try the following recipe:

Super Healing Posset

Note: A posset is an eggnog-like drink used as a meal to promote healing.

> *1 quart low-fat dairy or nondairy milk*
>
> *1¹/₄ cups dry white alcohol-free wine*
>
> *¹/₄ cup natural sugar*
>
> *¹/₄ lemon, juiced*
>
> *¹/₂ teaspoon ground ginger*
>
> *¹/₄ teaspoon freshly grated nutmeg*

Heat milk in large saucepan to just below boiling. Add wine; remove from heat. Strain through cheesecloth-lined sieve.

Add sugar and lemon, ginger, and nutmeg. Stir until sugar dissolves. Cool. Serve warm.

See foods for healing zones: 5, 9, 6

Also see: Dairy Substitutes, Substitutes, Soy Foods, Leafy Greens, Vitamin K

PMS AND MENOPAUSE

Menopause, a physiological phenomenon of indeterminate length marking the end of menstruation in a woman's life, and PMS (premenstrual syndrome), a condition of emotional and physical turbulence occurring regularly two weeks before the onset of the menses, are both characterized as periods of hormonal decrease or imbalance which respond well to dietary intervention.

THE END OF FERTILITY
Know the Symptoms

During menopause, production of estrogen and progesterone decrease and fertility ends. While there continues to be some marginal production of estrogen, most of the hormone activity is supplied during and following menopause by estrone, one or three members of the estrogen group which is formed from andnostenedione, a male hormone precurser. Eighty percent of all women are affected. The pituitary gland and the hypothalamus are also affected, explaining the wide range of symptoms including everything from hot flashes, cravings, and weight gain to increased blood pressure, fatigue, acne, and urinary tract infections.

PMS
Not One But Three Conditions

PMS, which is experienced by half of all premenopausal women, is divided into four symptomatic categories: anxiety, craving, depression, and hyperhydratic complaints (physical edemic complaints).

There are no miracles, but there are measures you can take to keep your physical and emotional stability.

EIGHT STEPS TO PMS AND MENOPAUSE CONTROL

1. Doubling your calcium intake (if it's well above 60 mg daily) can reduce PMS-related pain and mood disturbances and edema by half. Best bets: dairy or dairyfree yogurt, buttermilk, kefir.

2. Eat more foods containing vitamins A, E, D, and B, suggest studies by the University of Health Sciences in Bethesda, Maryland. A diet rich in source foods such as bright orange and red vegetables, nuts and seeds, and whole grains is the key to reduced mood swings, anxiety, weight gain, headache, fatigue, and depression. To benefit the most, reduce or eliminate your use of coffee, chocolate, sugar, and alcohol.

3. Take tea and see. Best PMS alleviators: black currant, raspberry leaf, and ginger or peppermint (for nausea) or a sarsaparilla, licorice, or wild yam tea. Best menopause antidote: black or blue cobash tea.

4. Reduce sodium and put some diuretic power into your daily juices. Best choices: asparagus, celery, and dandelion leaf.

5. Cold tubs and constitutionals: PMS-ers who exercise longer and harder usually rid their bodies of edema and produce more painkilling endorphins, say researchers at Hahnena University in

Philadelphia. A good folk remedy for hot flashes is a foot bath in 6 inches of cold water for five minutes, followed by a brisk walk.

6. Wild yam and chaseberry. The world's most widely used herb for PMS has been employed since the eighteenth century to treat menstrual complaints and childbirth-problems. The active super healing substance is diosgenin, which mimics progesterone, reduces sodium and fluid retention, and even heals osteoporosis, without-the side-effects of synthetic hormones, which include an increased risk of breast cancer. Both are taken daily first thing in the morning on an empty stomach.

7. Full-spectrum lighting can lift PMS-caused depression if your biological body clock is imbalanced. Check with your neighborhood naturopathic or homeopathic physician.

8. Downsize your meals and defeat low blood sugar. Six small carbohydrate-rich meals (every three hours) reduce hypoglycemic symptoms by stabilizing glucose and progesterone levels in the blood says Katherine Dalton, M.D., who coined the term for premenstrual syndrome.

For more help, dial PMS Access line at (800) 222-4PMS

See foods for healing zones: **5, 6, 8, 9**

Also see: **Herbs, Juices, Basic Dieting Facts and Advice, Fatigue, Depression**

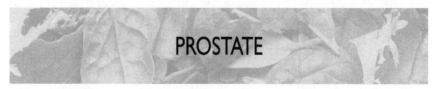

PROSTATE

The prostate is the size of a walnut but sometimes a seedbed of trouble. It is located below the bladder and surrounding the urethra and manufactures the sperm-carrying fluid in the male body. Nearly 60% of men between age 40 and 59 sufferer from one of the three types of prostate impairment: prostatitis (a bacteria or virus caused infection), enlargement (a.k.a. benign hyperplasia, or BPH, caused by hormonal changes), and cancer. The prostate is the most common site for cancer in men and the second most common cause of male cancer deaths. The lifetime risk of getting prostate cancer is 10%, and for 25% of those cases it proves fatal.

Symptoms reflecting some form of prostate impairment include an irresistible urge to urinate and difficulty in emptying the bladder. Untreated, such symptoms can lead to the retention of urine in the blood (uremia).

The good news is that you can prevent, heal, and even reverse the progress of all three forms of prostate trouble if you're on the right lifestyle track and if you're eating the right prostate-control foods. Here's a guide.

1. Add asparagus to your vegetable juice. Asparagine, the alkaloid in fresh asparagus, is healing for prostate disorders. Best daily juice combos: raw asparagus, carrot, and cucumber; asparagus, onion, and corn; or asparagus, watermelon, and ginger, another BPH beater. Best juice booster: slippery elm powder or nutritional yeast.

2. Pamper your prostate with a handful of pumpkin seeds daily. They're rich in prostate-healing nutrients including zinc, magnesium, phosphorus, iron, calcium, protein, and unsaturated fatty acids along with vitamins A and B_1. Pump more vitamin A/betacarotene-rich pumpkin into your diet along with deep orange vegetables such as squash and sweet potatoes, which the National Cancer Institute calls the best cancer-risk-reducing foods: ½ to 2½ cups daily is the dose that does it.

3. Explore the zinc link. The male gland which manufactures prostatic fluid and semen contains the body's greatest concentration of zinc. Mild deficiency can cause low sperm count, a major cause of male sterility. Zinc is also involved in the metabolism of testosterone, the male hormone responsible for sex drive and prevention of prostate gland enlargement. For maximum benefits, take your zinc with selenium- and vitamin-E-rich foods. Nuts, seeds, wheat germ, and nutritional yeast provide all three.

4. Inventory your bad habits and your good. Coffee, alcohol, and stress are prostate irritants. So is a high-animal-fat diet, which is linked to flawed testosterone metabolism. So is excessive or intense jog-

ging, which causes the bladder to impact the prostate negatively. Discuss your exercise choices with your physician to be safe.

5. Explore herbs and pollen. Extracts from the African evergreen tree, *Tygeum africanum*, promotes healing of BPH. So does flower pollen (use with caution if you have environmental allergies). Borage oil may also be beneficial. Both are available as tinctures, tablets, and teas.

6. Up your acidophilus and down your sugar. Liquid acidophilus or dairy or soy yogurts containing the live culture protect the prostate and promote prostatic healing. Avoiding sugar also improves your prospects.

7. Try self-help prostatic massage: Lie on your back on a flat surface. Place the sole of one foot against the other to create a bow. Keeping soles together, extend legs as far as possible and then bring as close as possible to chest. Repeat this massage-from-the-inside-out exercise 10 times each morning and night. The second best physical treatment is a sitz bath each night (three minutes at 55 to 75 degrees Fahrenheit).

8. Have a cup of saw palmetto tea. Dozens of clinical studies since the 1980s indicate that this indigenous-to-Florida, 63%-free-of-fatty-acids herb contains a number of hormone-imbalance-correcting substances, including carotenes, glucoside, and betasitosterol (the synthetic drug Proscar was derived from saw palmetto). Saw palmetto is available as a concentrated extract or tea or in whole dried berry form. Other good prostate-control teas: Watermelon seed and cornsilk, which work as kidney and bladder purifiers.

9. Minimize your prolactin with plenty of vitamin B_6. Clinical studies indicate that increased B_6 (found in soy foods, natural cheeses, and asparagus) can decrease high levels of prolactin, the hormone responsible for increasing the testosterone that leads to abnormal prostatic cell activity.

10. Perk up your diet with protease inhibitors. Increased consumption of seed foods and dried beans can lower your prostate cancer risk or reverse its progress and even protect you from coronary heart disease as a bonus, say researchers at John Hopkins University School of Medicine. Best inhibitor bets: rice, corn, and soybeans.

See foods for healing zones: 6, 9

Also see: Cancer, Beans, Soybeans, Beta-carotene, Herbs, Nuts, Asparagus, Sweetener

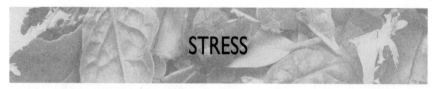

STRESS

Do long traffic lights make you see red? Do snail's-pace salespeople get your adrenaline up? Do you often feel hostile, annoyed, wired, impatient? If you answered yes to two or more of these questions, the world is pushing your stress buttons. And that's not good. Being what psychologists call a "hot reactor" is hazardous to your nervous system, your heart, your immune response, and your nutritional well-being.

According to the American Academy of Family Physicians, stress-related symptoms account for over two thirds of patients' visits and rank among the nation's leading killers (heart disease, cancer, accidental injuries, and suicides).

Stress is inevitable, but reacting to it isn't. Flying off the handle raises your blood pressure, increases your heartbeat, stimulates the overproduction of adrenaline, interrupts digestion, and depletes your system of major vitamins (such as B-complex and C). Worse, "production of disease is related to the way in which your body reacts to stress over long periods of time," advises the late Dr. Hans Selye, Czechoslovakian stress research pioneer. "Our stress levels may even decide how many colds we get in any given year, how many accidents we have, or how prone we are to cancer."

LOWERING STRESS, RAISING IMMUNITY

Studies of stress began more than 40 years ago, when researchers noted an increase in adrenal-gland activity and a decrease in immune-system response following physical stress. In one study of the development of infectious mononucleosis in a class of West Point cadets, cadets were screened to see if their blood contained the antibody to the disease caused by Epstein-Barr virus.* Those without the antibody were classified as susceptible. About one fifth of the susceptible cadets became infected each year, but only one quarter of those developed disease symptoms. Researchers reported that cadets who described their fathers as overachievers were more likely to develop symptoms. Those who

---

* Chronic Fatigue Syndrome.

developed the strongest symptoms were usually the ones who wanted a military career the most but who performed poorly academically because they perceived themselves as being under the greatest stress.

Other studies have revealed that sleep deprivation, bereavement, and depression can trigger a lowered immune response says the Better Sleep Institute.

GOOD STRESS

Fortunately, there is such a thing as good stress. Good stress is what motivates you to move on, stimulates you to work for positive change, and fosters success and self-esteem. The three tell-tale characteristics of good stress are as follows:

- You feel in control of your life, able to deal with problems, find solutions, and bring about change.
- You have friends in whom you confide, and this leads to a sense of well-being.
- You have resilience and an ability to look at life's troubles as challenges, not threats.

Anyone can improve his or her stress-handler's savvy and turn negative stress into positive energy. Changing your perspective on the stress around you and controlling your reaction to stress you can't avoid can keep you in control and help you keep your health. The following quick quiz may reveal a few of your personal hidden stress buttons. Give yourself a score of 1 for each situation or factor that triggers stress for you.

1. Being told to do something you were just about to do, or don't want to do
2. Unsupportive friends, coworkers, and family
3. Getting a telephone busy signal or being held up at a traffic light
4. Listening to long-winded speeches, sermons, and talks
5. Being interrupted when you're saying something important
6. Being given a bad suggestion or a wrong direction
7. Having to deal with at least two or more crises every day
8. Trying to get along with a boss (or spouse or lover mate) who expects too much

9. Knowing someone is staring at you

10. Having your train of thought interrupted

11. Standing in line at the deli, market, or movies

12. Having to wait for a table at a restaurant

13. Coworker who urges you to order something fattening or have seconds when you're dieting

14. Lifeless handshakes and grumpy salespeople

15. People who wear colors that clash; mirrors or pictures that are crooked

16. Having people hug, kiss, or pat you on the back unexpectedly

Scoring:

4 or less: Excellent. Your stress level is on a healthy keel.

5 to 8: Fair.

9 to 16: You need to learn a few stress-blocking tricks.

ANTISTRESS TIPS

1. Is it time to make time for that Wednesday-night-at-the-flicks-with-a-friend habit that work or compulsive behavior has squeezed out of your life?

2. Take up a tranquilizing hobby (knitting, raising an indoor or outdoor herb garden, writing to a shut-in or imprisoned pen pal*).

3. Get a pet. A cat or dog is one of the best of all stress reducers. According to Dr. Suzanne Megahan, a professor of psychology at Fordham University in New York City, "Pets provide a release for pent-up tensions, comfort in times of sorrow or stress, and friendship with no ulterior motives." Better yet, make it an act of charity; adopt from the local shelter. Even better, become a foster pet parent. To open your home to stray dogs and cats who

---

* To be matched up with people behind bars who need people, write Prison Fellowship, Box 17500, Washington, DC 20041-0500.

need a temporary home, check with PAWS, the ASPCA, or your local shelter.

4. Start a garden. Working with plants offers positive pay-offs—it melts away stress and anxiety and it gives you a sense of purpose, commitment, and control.

5. Unwind with a new relaxation technique—guided meditation. Or look into reduced environmental stimulation therapy (REST), or flotation relaxation therapy, which stimulates the theta presleep state and reduces stress levels dramatically while improving your learning skills. For further information, call the Flotation Association at 916-432-3794.

6. Have a daily laugh. According to Joel Goodman of the Humor Project in Saratoga Springs, New York, looking for humor in life's daily tensions and problems can relieve stress. Make humor a building block in your life by creating your own laughter first-aid kit filled with favorite cartoons clipped from magazines, a joke book, a classic comedy movie (a Chaplin one-reeler, Laurel and Hardy short, or a Disney cartoon compilation), or a taped monologue by your favorite stand-up comic—anything that helps you snap back when you feel like snapping.

7. Stress-proof your diet. The foods we use to battle stress are often the ones that get us deeper in stress debt, say experts. The worst nutritional stress inducers are sugary desserts and snacks, caffeinated coffee and tea and colas, salty snacks, high-fat foods, alcoholic drinks, and additive- and preservative-laced prepared foods (frozen dinners, dessert mixes, etc.), which overstimulate the nervous system and deplete essential nutrients.

Concentrate on stress-buster foods that supply protein, B-complex vitamins, magnesium, calcium, and vitamin C (yogurt and fruits, grain-fruit salads, low-fat grilled cheese on whole grain crackers, tofu-stuffed tomatoes, leafy green salads with reduced-fat creamy dressings).

For more help or referrals to a stress-reduction pro, write to the American Foundation for Counseling and Development, P.O. Box 9888, Alexandria, VA 22304.

***See foods for healing zones:* All**

***Also see:* 12 Diet Tips, Substitutes, Insomnia, Vitamin B, Vitamin C**

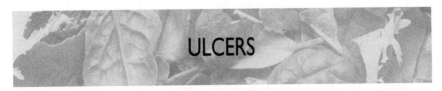

ULCERS

One in 10 of us is at risk of an ulcer sooner or later. A proneness to intestinal or stomach infections increases the odds, as does alcohol, nicotine, overuse of aspirin, and fatty and inflammatory foods and drinks, especially all types of coffee. Additional risk factors are food allergy and unrelieved stress.

There are two main types of ulcers: the gastric, which occurs in the lining of the stomach, often produces no symptoms, accounts for 15% of all cases, and is often caused directly by the wrong drugs and food, and the peptic or duodenal, which may affect the esophagus, doudenum, lower stomach, or small intestine. Both gastric and peptic ulcers flare up when acids irritate ulcerated areas, causing spasms. Gnawing pain, nausea, retching, and black stools indicate a bleeding ulcer. Bleeding ulcers also occur when the ulcer corrodes a blood vessel. Excess bleeding can cause anemia and lower blood pressure.

Peptic ulcers occur four times more often in men than women and four to five times more often than clinically evident gastric ulcers. Victims of duodenal ulcers have twice as many parietal cells in their stomachs, which secrete more hydrochloric acid, and many secrete more acid in general. Gastric ulcers have clinical aspects similar to those of duodenal ulcers but occur in the lining of the stomach.

Both types of ulcers are believed to occur when the digestive enzyme pepsin and stomach acids damage the gastrointestinal lining. Normally, an adequate supply of protective factors prevents this.

In general, to relieve an ulcer is to feed it (if it's gastric) or to starve it (if it's peptic). Antiulcer drugs, which are among the costliest of all prescribed medications with the highest relapse rate (92%) and numerous side-effects (including liver disfunction and kidney stones) are a typical second choice. But an adequate supply of protective factors in your diet can get your gastrointestinal tract back on track in a matter of weeks.

PREVENTION AND RELIEF
Nine Steps

1. Eat small, frequent meals; chew food well to ensure maximum mixing with enzymes that protect stomach lining; and drink between meals to keep the digestive function on track.

2. Keep cabbage juice on tap. In one study, 92% of all cabbage-drinking ulcer patients were cured in three weeks.

3. Eliminate food allergies. In one clinical study, 98% of ulcer patients showed lower and upper repiratory tract allergy disease. Food allergy is also consistent with a high recurrence rate of ulcers. (TIP: Ulcers will persist when all other offending foods are eliminated.)

4. Avoid the six top acid producers: coffee (even decaf); black tea; colas; and fried, acidic (citrus, vinegar), and sugary foods. Use carbonated drinks in moderation and spicy foods rarely, if at all.

5. Stop smoking. Nicotine increases ulcer frequency, decreases response to therapy, and, in combination with aspirin (which damages stomach lining and can trigger ulcer formation), is twice as risky.

6. Switch from dairy milk to cultured milk products such as yogurt or to nondairy foods. Despite the folk wisdom, milk actually stimulates acid production and doubles the trouble if there is underlying lactose intolerance or dairy allergy.

7. Use ulcer-healing juice boosters: aloe vera juice before meals and before bedtime; 1 teasponn of olive oil with meals; and 1 teaspoon chlorophyll liquid or powder with food or juice two times daily.

8. Take the six top antiulcer super healing nutrients: vitamins A, B, C, and E and calcium and magnesium. Best sources: citrus fruits, raw leafy greens, nuts and seeds, whole grains, cereals, and dried beans.

9. life. Get regular exercise, and use aromatherapy oils (5 to 10 drops in 4 ounces vegetable oil gently massaged over abdomen daily) such as chamomile, lemon, rose, and jasmine. These can calm, soothe, and speed healing.

See foods for healing zones: 7, 6 , 4

Also see: **Juices, Stress, Indigestion, Dairy Substitutes, Allergies**

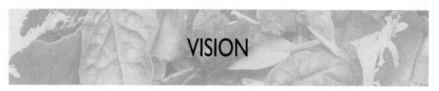

VISION

Setting your sights on good ocular health? Don't neglect canola oil and carrots. Beta-carotene (carrots) and vitamin E (canola oil) are two of the 12 or more nutrients critical to 20/20 vision and prevention of cataracts, macular degeneration, glaucoma, keratitis and infection.

SO NEAR, SO FAR

The two most common visual impairments are near- and far-sightedness. You need glasses when the curve in your cornea is misshapen—too steep in nearsightedness and too flat in farsightedness. With astigmatism, the shape of the cornea is completely irregular. The cornea's job is to focus light and send it through the lens to the retina, where it strikes a series of rods and cones, which transform the light into nerve impulses and send them to the brain. Defects in the cornea bend light the wrong way, focusing it away from the retina and distorting vision, just as oddly shaped mirrors bend reflections. Glasses compensate for the defect.

The third most common vision problem occurs after age 35 and is called presbyopia, a form of far-sightedness which results in a change in the eye's lens, the focusing mechanism situated just behind the pupil which directs light to the retina on the back of the eyeball. Like other parts of the body, the lens constantly creates new cells. But in the eye these new cells also lay down new fibers that eventually add to the lens's density. The lens becomes more and more compressed and has less and less elasticity.

Also common is dry eye syndrome. As with presbyopia, the treatment is frequent use of OTC artificial tears, a mild saline solution. Dryness can also cause redness, but unlike artificial tears, medicated drops contain drugs that tighten blood vessels and can create a cycle of dependency; occasionally, they actually induce glaucoma. Eye exercises (discussed later) supplemented by a careful diet can be remedial.

NOURISHING YOUR EYES

Here are 11 options for improving your optic verve.

1. Mirror, mirror. Puffiness around the eyes can be a symptom of allergies, sinus infection, or even kidney or heart disorders. If you've ruled these out, consider product sensitivity. To test for adverse reaction, take a make-up fast. Then begin using your usual cosmetics one at a time, one day at a time. To prevent flare-ups, switch to a natural organic, nonallergenic alternative.

2. Rx for red, tired eyes. Soak cotton balls in lukewarm herbal tea. Place balls on eyes and rest for 10 minutes to help relax eye muscles. (Chamomile is the traditional eye soother.) Or bathe eyes with 1 teaspoon of salt in 2½ cups of cold boiled water. Or soak cotton pads in milk, witch hazel, or just plain ice water, or use an eyecup. Another Rx is to place slices of fresh cucumber over eyelids to cool and soothe. Or press a cool teaspoon (hollow side facing down) very lightly over one closed eye for a few minutes and repeat on opposite eye. Also, sleeping with the head elevated helps reduce A.M. puffiness.

3. Exercise your eyes. First exercise: Holding a pencil or pen or finger 10 to 12 inches from face, focus on tip, then look into distance. Or focus on some nearby point or object outside, then on one far away. Repeat. Second exercise: Open eyes as wide as possible; shut eyes as tightly as possible, count slowly to six. Open eyes and relax while counting slowly to three. Third exercise: Lie on back with knees bent and feet flat on the floor. Close eyes, cover lightly with hands. Concentrate on breathing, allowing it to become slower and deeper. Uncover eyes, but keep closed and keep breathing deeply. Cover again and continue breathing. Repeat five to 10 times. Stay relaxed.

4. Perfect your 1-2-3 removal technique. When you have a foreign object in your eye, first, blink to induce watering (don't rub lids). Second, open upper lid with finger and thumb. Third, gently pull up and down until the upper lid covers the lower lid, and hold to encourage lubrication. This helps to dislodge the invading particle. If you can't remove the particle or if it is glass or metal, see a doctor immediately.

5. Be a conscientious contact wearer. Contact lenses can be another risk factor. More than 30 million of us wear them, but half of us make one or more ocular mistakes—including inadequate cleaning (do not use homemade saline solutions) and infrequent

removal of extended-wear lenses—which can lead to corneal ulcers and serious infections (such as acanthamoeba keratitis, which is similar to herpes simplex but largely resistant to treatment).

6. Just say no to unnecessary medication and yes to zinc. Long-term use of tranquilizers, sedatives, birth control pills, and recreational drugs like alcohol can destroy the chemical balance inside body cells and reduce oxygen to the retina. The highest concentration of zinc in the body is in the macula, located at the center of the retina. Deficiencies of this mineral (found in whole grains, nuts and seeds) can lead to gradual vision diminishment and even complete blindness.

7. Drink your orange juice. The closely related macula and retina require vitamin C concentrations 20 times higher than the bloodstream. Together with beta-carotene and vitamin E, abundant vitamin C source foods on a meal-to-meal basis help protect you from cataracts and degeneration of the inner eye. Two snacks that provide all three: leafy green salads and nut- and fruit-type cereals.

8. Limit your sun exposure. At least one quarter of all cataracts are the result of extensive ultraviolet radiation. Snow and waterskiing and sunbathing are the worst offenders. Look for UV-absorbing lenses that filter out 99% of rays. Best choice—gray, which reduces glare best and distorts least. Next best tint choices: green and brown. Polarrep™ and double gradient lenses are also good protective picks. Limit your indoor sunbathing as well. Excessive exposure to sunlamp radiation can cause keratitis, or inflammation of the cornea.

9. Don't smoke, and junk the junk food. According to Dr. Morgan B. Raiford, founder of the Atlanta Eye Clinic of the Atlanta Hospital and Medical Center, the greatest cause of blindness in America is clogged-up blood vessels, and "empty calories of refined sugar in thousands of food products are a major contributor to blood vessel deterioration." Likewise, nicotine causes contraction of ocular blood vessels.

10. Don't be a sight-for-sore-eyes beauty. Avoid lash-building mascaras that can migrate into the eye, creating redness and irritation. False eyelash glue is another offender. Avoid applying creams

on or around the eye area, and remove makeup with gentle strokes and a cotton pad, using lotion, not soap and water. Keep eyeliner outside of lashes to prevent irritation of the lipid pores on the lid itself.

11. Last but not least, consider for your sight balanced, full-spectrum, natural-sunlight-simulating fluorescent light bulbs. According to oral biologists, natural light improves visual acuity, reduces fatigue and stress, and even improves your body's absorption of calcium.

See foods for healing zones: 8, 10

Also see: Cataracts, Oranges, Vitamin C

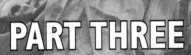

PART THREE

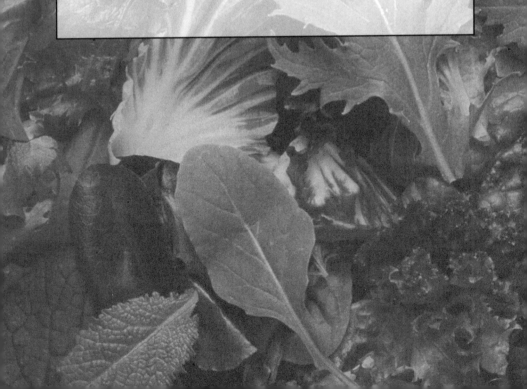

Super Healing Nutrition in Action

SUPER HEALING NUTRITION SCOREBOARD
10 Mind-Body Healing Zones

Certain disorders are specific to certain of the body's war zones, while other disorders affect more than a single organ or system (cancer or stress, for example). Likewise, there are specific healing foods rich in specific nutrients that can heal, prevent, or change the course of those health disorders. The numbers in this chart, which appear throughout the text, indicate the healing zone(s) which is health enhanced or likeliest to be healed by that particular fruit, nut, vegetable, or legume.

Zone 1: Dermal (integumentary) system (psoriasis, eczema, acne, cancer, and the related disorders)

Zone 2: Cardiovascular (arteriosclerosis, angina, vascular disorders, hypertension, coronary heart disease)

Zone 3: Immune system (AIDS/HIV, cancer, viral, bacterial and fungal infections)

Zone 4: Respiratory (allergies, asthma, bacterial and viral infections, bronchitis, pneumonia)

Zone 5: Musculoskeletal system (arthritis, osteoporosis, dental disorders, muscular dystrophy)

Zone 6: Endocrinal (PMS, hypoglycemia, diabetes, menopause, chronic fatigue syndrome)

Zone 7: Digestive/urinary/excretory (cancer, ulcers, gallstones, colitis, stress, cystitis, hepatitis, and kidney stones)

Zone 8: Neuropsychological (muscular dystrophy, hyperactivity, stress, depression, insomnia)

Zone 9: Reproductive (infertility, impotence, PMS, menopause, cancer)

Zone 10: Sensory (glaucoma, cataracts, tinnitus, vertigo)

10 STEPS TO 10 TARGET ZONE SUPER HEALING

Now that you know your greens, grains, beans, and berries ABCs, what is the next step? A super healing plan of action that includes not only a diet, meals, and menus but a 10-step plan for super healing health.

1. Know your target healing zones. Balanced eating is to nutrition what cross-training is to exercise. It covers all the bases, leaving none of the body's target healing zones undefended in the same way that a variegated fitness regimen leaves none of the body's muscle groups unexercised.

2. Is your body in biochemical balance for free radical control? (This is called biological ionization in nutritional biochemistry.) It's easier than it sounds because there's a one-size-fits-all equation that can help prevent formation of disease-generating free radicals. It's a 6.4 pH reading in your urine—the state indicating, says the American Association of Nutritional Consultants, that your body is in homeostatic balance. Free radicals can multiply rapidly when the urine pH strays too far from the ideal—becoming either too acid or too alkaline. There are approximately 10 quadrillion human cells and one hundred quadrillion healthy bacterial cells in a ratio of 1 to 10 to keep the pH at a balance of 6.4 and to feed us with various nutrients. When the balance is upset, free radicals invade the body, compromising the immune system and producing disease unless defender cells—which super healing foods help your body manufacture—intervene. Antibodies and drugs are indiscriminate killers that exterminate billions of healthy cells along with disease promoters, unbalancing your 10-zone health in the process.

If you've got a good more-alkaline-than-acid diet going, abundant in fruits and vegetables, all you need to do to maintain the inner balancing act is to have your family doctor do a urine pH reading or check with your pharmacist for a do-it-yourself kit.

3. Keep slim and trim by knowing your resting metabolic rate (RMR) to calculate your caloric needs. Your *resting metabolic rate,* unlike your pH, is not a one-for-all figure. It's based on body weight, and the following calculation will yield your ideal, more or less.

    a. Convert your current weight to kilograms by dividing by 2.2.

    b. Multiply kilograms by the RMR factor (1.0 for men and 0.9 for women due to the fact that the formula was first used for men and rates must be adapted for the female metabolism).

    c. Multiply by 24 (the number of calories per kilogram required to maintain basic metabolic function).

Meeting your own purely personal caloric needs is important because it prevents your metabolism from shifting into a "starvation mode," which triggers biochemical imbalance and ill health.

4. Normalize your weight. Thinner is better than fatter for a long, healthy life, say progressive health professionals, and this means 15 pounds below what the Metropolitan Life tables (the most commonly consulted guide) consider ideal. Normalizing your weight improves your circulation and promotes a better assimilation of antioxidants.

The #1 way to get a grip on your girth is to reduce your intake of fat. Not only does an ounce of fat have more than double the calories of protein or carbohydrate, but fat oxidation does not respond rapidly to increases in fat intake. The best way to fight fat is to become a vegetarian.

5. Lift your spirits. A principle of both orthodox and nontraditional religious disciplines is that affirmative attitudes and emotions are essential to the holistic healing process. Studies reveal that negative feelings such as depression release the toxic enzyme cathypain, which, along with free radicals, compromises immune system responses and functions. Exercise can allay negative emotions, so take up a realistic personalized long-range fitness plan. A pro at the nearest YMCA, health club, or parks and recreation department can be your guide.

6. Drink up for faster healing. Water is the oldest of all natural medicines. H_2O can decrease or increase muscle tone, reduce pain, generate energy, improve digestion and elimination, and dissolve and remove the free radicals that trigger disease and speed the aging process. Water down an hour before or after meals, not during, which dilutes antioxidants. Juicing daily (with an occasional juice fast) is liquid health-keeping strategy #2.

7. Get bad habit control. A diet that protects you from diseases and ill health won't do you as much good if you smoke, drink, or indulge in recreational drugs.

8. Sign up for wind-down therapy and stress control. You need eight hours (give or take an hour) of sleep daily to restore vitality. Your body clock runs on a circadian rhythm cycle, and the more you deviate from the asleep-by-11-awake-by-7 model, the greater you get into stress debt and the greater your need for stress intervention in the form of meditation, yoga, shiatsu, reiki, or similar therapies—anything that causes a rise in your interleukin-1 levels, a disease-fighting chain reaction. But give your choice some deliberation time or that biofeedback might backfire. "The brain has an influence over blood chemistry," says William H. Keppel, M.D., study leader and psychiatrist at Providence Medical Center in Portland, Oregon. Being relaxed isn't just about being dormant; it's actually about stimulating certain parts of the brain, and not everyone responds well to the same relaxation techniques.

9. Factor in faith and fitness. Keeping a firm foot on some spiritual path can make the difference between sickness or health.

10. Study the Super Healing Nutrition Diet (p. 355) and then choose the variation that is appropriate and get healing. With a little fine-tuning you can switch from one to the other as your needs change so you are always within eating distance of a meal that will heal.

THE SUPER HEALING NUTRITION PYRAMID

The Super Healing Nutrition Pyramid is a prevention-oriented adaptation of the USDA's *The Official Food Guide Pyramid,* created by the U.S. Department of Agriculture, and *The Traditional Healthy Mediterranean Diet Pyramid,* developed and endorsed in 1994 by Harvard School of Public Health and the World Health Organization.

The former (the USDA pyramid) is a direct descendant of the now outdated four food groups concept and recommends a variety of chiefly fruits, vegetables, breads, and other starches and allows small amounts of fats, oils, and sweets, with two to three daily servings from both the meat and dairy groups, from which most of the dietary fat is derived. The latter is based on the traditional eating style of southern Italy, Crete, and Greece, where chronic disease rates are low and life expectancies are high. Most of the fat comes from olive oil, with small portions of cheese or yogurt daily, plus bread, grains, fruits and vegetables, beans and potatoes, and fish and poultry in modest amounts. Even an occasional glass of wine is allowed to help lower heart disease risk. An easy-does-it fitness program is advised.

The Super Healing Nutrition Pyramid, by contrast, reflects not only a shift in our what's-healthy paradigm but in our daily meal patterns, which are evolving from three-squares-a-day to what futurists call a "formalized grazing pattern" of five small meals a day, which research suggests is much healthier. In the following 6-food-group Super Healing Pyramid, fruits and vegetables are combined into a single (and the most sizable) food group (four to five servings of each daily), followed quantitatively by the whole grains, pasta, and cereal group; dried beans, legumes, and soy foods; nuts, seeds, and oils. Low-fat dairy and a final optional group—fish and poultry (5% fat or less—occupy the top (and smallest) group of the pyramid.

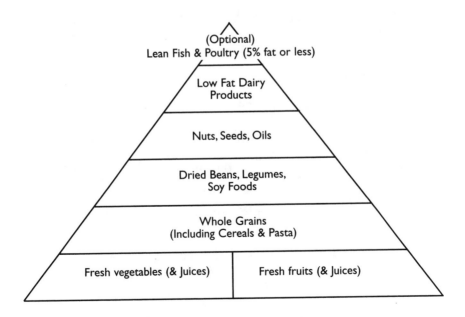

BASIC DIETING FACTS AND ADVICE

Consider the following diet facts:

- There are more than 28,000 diets on public record.
- Pickles were Cleopatra's favorite diet food.
- If you live 80 years, you will have used up a total of 90 million calories per each pound of body weight.
- If you tip the scales, the chances of your offspring following suit is 40%. (If both parents are heavyweights, the odds increase to 80%.)
- You have to stand around for five to six hours to burn 500 calories.
- It takes 15 minutes of running to burn the calories in one fast-food sandwich.
- Fat men and thin women have the most stable marriages. (Husky females and economy-sized males have the shakiest.)
- The average National Football League lineman weigh 260 pounds.
- A 15-minute strip-tease burns 36 calories.
- AC/DC calories: If all the energy to keep the fat of the land fat were turned into electricity, it would keep Boston, Chicago, San Francisco and Washington, DC plugged in for a week.
- A laugh burns the calories in half a stick of gum.
- Per capita consumption of our favorite get-fat food, butter, is 5 pounds (margarine, 11).
- The human body contains enough fat to make seven bars of soap.
- A 150-pound man gains 3 pounds twice as fast as a 50-pound boy.
- Three kisses a day burn 3 pounds a year.
- Riding a motorcycle burns three times as many calories as sleeping.
- The world's thinnest people are called cachexias. Cachexia—a kind of anorexia—causes victims to lose 65% or more of their total body weight.

- A 160-pound person burns about 285 calories in a 3-mile, hour-long walk.

- Planetary corpulence: If you weigh 100 pounds on earth, you'll weigh 264 pounds on Jupiter.

- The world's most caloric dessert is an "ice cream" called Natloda eaten by Alaska's Ten'a Indians. A batch includes 1 pound of bear, 1 pound of moose tallow, and 2 cups seal oil.

- Children are 20 to 30% heavier today than they were 100 years ago (and 10% taller).

- Readers losers: It takes 1 calorie to read 650 words.

- Sixty-five percent of the U.S. population starts a new diet at least once a year.

- Pigging out? Wait until March 1; that's National Pig Day, according to Chase's Calendar of Annual Events.

- One out of every 20 U.S. secretaries eats a full 650-calorie meal at noon, says the U.S. Commerce Department.

- Where calories don't count: It takes 7,000 calories a day to survive in the Antarctic without an outside source of heat.

- West Virginia has the most fat people; Utah has the fewest.

- Chewing the fat: Pure animal fat is the world's most caloric food (930 calories per 3.5 ounces).

- Waisting away: A tape measure is a good emergency scale—an additional ¾ inch at the waist, hips, or abdomen means 5 new pounds.

- The average American eats 10 tons of food in the course of a lifetime.

- To estimate the weight of your skin, divide your weight by 6.

- Calorie counting in the chocolate capitals: Belgium and Luxemburg consume more calories per day per capita than any country in the world—3,645. The lowest caloric intake is in Ghana (930).

Did you know that the quickest way to lose weight is to move to a mountaintop on the equator and run eastward? Fortunately, with 48 million of us trying to win at the losing game, there are less drastic ways to get into fighting trim.

In a nutshell, a diet like the Super Healing Nutrition Diet or any other slow, safe, balanced, physician-approved weight-loss plan that takes account of your personal likes, dislikes, sensitivities, and bio-chemical idiosyncrasies will do the trick, *if* you add a nutrition-support-ive, expert-approved fitness regime tailored to your likes, dislikes, and physical abilities (check with a health club, YMCA, personal trainer, or parks and recreation director) and balance the two with some mind-soul, stretching discipline. It will pay dividends. Being overfed and undernourished by more than 30% increases your risk of hypertension and diabetes in the next three years by more than 50%, says the Harvard School of Public Health.

If you're between 25 and 34 years old, weight gains of 20% (an average of 31 pounds) are typical, says the Department of Health and Human Services. The good news? You're in for a just as inevitable weight dip after age 55.

Downsizing has a big upside: It can lower your risk of every major disease and increase your lifespan, but losing weight has sizable risks if you take shortcuts, warns the Society of Bariatric Physicians (SBP). Diet drugs are an example: The $370 million we spend on them annually buy us nothing but trouble. The major active ingredient in most OTC diet pills is phenylpropanolamine, a chemical that raises norepinephrine levels in the blood, causing the release of increased amounts of norepi-nephrine in the brain, which in turn leads to feelings of agitation and anxiety along with a temporary reduction in appetite. Caffeine is anoth-er common ingredient in diet drugs. Both have a high potential for abuse, says the SBP. Side-effects include insomnia, depression, agita-tion, dizziness, tremors, headaches, dry mouth, constipation, confusion, hypertension, palpitations, hallucinations, and hyperstimulation of the central nervous system, says Peter D. Vash, M.D., M.P.H., an endocri-nologist and internist on the faculty of UCLA Medical Center. And that's only the start. There are 111 other diet drug ingredients that also get the red light from the FDA, including alcohol, saccharin, and guar gum (a soluble fiber that swells when wet and has been indicated in 17 cases of esophageal obstruction; according to the FDA, ten dieters have died) . At the very least, studies indicate that such drugs alone are only marginal-ly effective in promoting weight loss.

A crutch can be a secondary help if it's nutritional supplements to a good diet and a sound exercise program. Here are nine of the vitamin, mineral, and herbal alternatives that the Nutrition and Herb Trade

Association and the Holistic Resources Association call winners. (Note: Healthy weight loss is gradual. Plan on one to three weeks to see a 2- to 4-pound loss, and check with your physician before starting any supplement-based diet.)

1. Zinc, vitamin C, and tyrosine help curb both calorie intake and appetite. Look for foods and supplements containing vitamin B$_6$, a diuretic; kelp, a thyroid regulator; lecithin, which helps eliminate fatty tissue from the blood; and cider vinegar, which cleanses the digestive system.

2. GTF chromium, an essential trace mineral that helps synthesize cholesterol and other fatty lipids, lowers the desire for fat and sugar, accelerates carbohydrate metabolism, and spurs calorie burning. A good same-results supplement is chromium picolinate, a more biologically active form of this organic yeast derivative; 200 µg a day does the job. (Food sources: nutritional yeast, corn and corn oil, wheat germ.)

3. Lipotropics are natural substances that break down and liquefy fats in the digestive system. A winning combination should contain all or most of these: lecithin, inositol, choline, and the amino acid methionine. Look for an all-in-one combination, or combine separate powders into a power formula of your own. (Food sources: soybeans, soy milk, tofu, tempeh, lecithin granules, and liquid.)

4. Combinations of the amino acids arginine, ornithine, and lysine trigger human growth hormone secretions that cause fat cells to be burned and muscle to be built, while DL-carnitine regulates the amount of fat carried into the nucleus of a cell for more rapid burnoff and conversion into energy. To enhance the effect further, add vitamins B$_6$ and C. (Food sources: milk, cheese, eggs, soybeans.)

5. Fat-digesting enzymes: Partial digestion of high-fat foods leads to overeating and causes sluggish metabolism and fats that accumulate in the body's fat cells. Digestive enzymes like lipase and betaine break down foods more completely, giving you an appetite-regulating sensation of satiety. Fat-digesting enzymes may also include any of the lipotropic ingredients. (Food sources: pineapple, papaya.)

6. Teas and tinctures: California herbalist and nutritionist Christopher Hobbs's four favorite herb teas for losers are cayenne, gentian, butternut bark, and ginger. Take after meals and use in combination for best results. Tinctures are available for nontea drinkers. Saw

palmetto also helps control appetite, says herbal researcher Daniel B. Mowrey, Ph.D.

7. *Plantain, Gymnena silvestra and seaweeds:* The first two are herbs that balance the body's sugar chemistry and reduce the craving for sugar. For increased effectiveness, add GTF chromium. Seaweeds such as spirulina, kelp, and bladder wrack supply iodine crucial to the health of the thyroid gland, the body's thermostat for the normal burning of fats, plus bonus amounts of energy-elevating proteins, beta-carotene, GLA (gamma linolenic acid), iron, and B vitamins.

8. Fiber, which absorbs liquids, provides that feeling of not-another-bite fullness that depresses appetite and supplies the bulk needed for healthy digestion and elimination essential to weight loss. Best food sources: all *sea vegetables* as well as high roughage natural foods like dark leafy greens, celery, and parsley (which doubles as a diuretic, normalizing sodium-potassium levels).

9. Last but not least, get juiced. According to Yale University researcher Judith Rodin, eating a piece of fruit or drinking a 15-ounce glass of fruit juice 30 to 45 minutes before a meal satisfies the body's craving for calories and makes you eat less. Juicy fruit participants in the study not only cut calories by 40% but also reduced their fat intake.

12 DIET TIPS

1. Are you fit or fat? Read between the lines on the bathroom scales. If you've gained 10 pounds, it could mean you've lost 5 pounds of muscle and gained 15 pounds of fat. So you're really 20 pounds in the red. Or a loss of 6 pounds after a month of workouts may mean you've added 3 pounds of muscle and lost 9 pounds of fat, giving you a net improvement in body composition of 12 pounds. The moral: Never diet without a four- to six-times-a-week exercise routine.

2. Walk off calories and lower your risk of heart disease. How? Simply by multiplying your weight by 1.8 and burning off that many calories in exercise each day. If you weigh 180 pounds, you can burn off 324 calories a day just by walking for an hour.

3. Get a second opinion—from your inner self—on hunger pangs. Before you dip another chip, ask yourself how hungry you really are on

a scale from 1 to 10—1 representing a growling stomach and 10 representing eaten-past-your-stop full. Lift a fork only when your hunger rates a 1 or 2; stop when you get to 5.

4. Good chip bowl substitute: a pound of fresh sweet cherries buried in chipped-ice—served for snacks, desserts, and appetizers,

5. To lose a pound of fat a week, you need to get rid of 500 calories a day. Best way? Cut your intake by 250 calories (as simple as giving up soda) and burn off another 250 calories with exercise (take an easy 2½-mile walk).

6. Ten foods with less than 10 calories: ½ cup cabbage (7); one stalk celery (7); one large maraschino cherry (10); six raw cucumber slices (7); three leaves of iceberg lettuce (6); two large leaves of loose-leaf lettuce (9); one tablespoon chopped parsley (7); one medium green boiled pepper (10); four small raw radishes (7); five sprigs raw watercress (10).

7. Five hours of weekly aerobic activity (plus a reformed diet) will bring your cholesterol blood sugar readings, blood pressure, and weight down in five weeks, says the Palo Alto Medical Foundation.

8. A snack that satisfies your hunger for 80 minutes at noon satisfies only half as long at 6 P.M. says the Georgia State University Department of Psychology.

9. Two ways to lose 4 pounds in 12 months: Skip 30 potato chips or one donut a week.

10. Where the fat is at: 15% of your total weight is skin; 7 to 9% is blood; the rest is your fault. Mild obesity is 10 to 20% above ideal weight, moderate is 20 to 30% above; 30% and up is red-light heavyweight. But remember, any weight table is a gross simplification of a complex problem.

11. If you're over 40, a healthy weight gain is ½ to 1 pound each year, says the American Heart Association.

12. Beat the exercise blahs—recruit a friend and buy or rent a tandem bike. Here's the one-hour calorie burnoff for a 150-pounder.

Activity	Calories Burned
Tandeming, 6 mph	240
Tandeming, 12 mph	410
Cross-country skiing	700
Jogging, 5½ mph	740
Jumping rope	750
Running in place	650
Swimming 25 yards/minute	275
Tennis—singles	400
Walking, 3 mph	320

Try this dieter's delight recipe:

One-A-Day Diet Cookies

1 cup whole wheat flour

1 teaspoon low sodium baking powder

1 pinch cinnamon

¼ cup canola or safflower oil

1 egg or ¼ cup tofu

½ cup frozen orange juice concentrate

½ cup puréed carrots (or raw carrot pulp from juiced carrots)

1-2 tablespoon brewer's yeast

2 tablespoons sunflower seeds, toasted

Preheat oven to 350 degrees, In mixing bowl, combine dry ingredients. When well mixed Stir in all other ingredients; mix well. Drop by rounded teaspoonfuls onto ungreased baking sheet. Bake for 15 minutes.

Makes 48 "mini" cookies, 50 calories and 2 grams of fat each.

See foods for healing zones: 2, 6, 7, 8

Also see: Vitamin C, Herbs, Coronary Heart Disease, Water, Juices

DIETER'S NUTRITIONAL SAFETY NET

Losing weight by reducing fat in your diet can put you at a nutritional loss of the eight nutrients listed in the following chart. Here's what to eat for super healing protection.

NUTRIENT	FOUND IN	PROPERTIES
Vitamin A	Eggs, diary foods, red & yellow fruits & vegetables	Antioxidant; protects against heart disease; prevents fatigue; aids in protein synthesis.
Vitamin C	Citrus fruits, parsley, red bell peppers, broccoli	Antioxidant, cholesterol fighter; aids in thyroxin synthesis, which regulates metabolism.
Vitamin E	Whole grains, vegetable oils, nuts & nut oils, wheat germ	Protects against oxidation of cholesterol, which can damage arteries.
Calcium	Dairy foods, leafy greens, cabbage, nuts and seeds, wheat germ	Prevents osteoporosis and muscle fatigue. May be depleted by diet high in fat and animal protein.
Chromium	Brewers and nutritional yeast; wheat germ, corn	Trace mineral which regulates blood sugar and stops sugar cravings.
Magnesium	Rice bran, tofu, nuts and seeds	Constituent of bones and teeth; aids in energy production. Often deficient if diet is high in fat.
Essential fatty acids (EFA)	Vegetable & nut oils, nuts and seeds	Essential fatty acids may be deficient in very low-fat diets. Protects cell membranes; promotes healthy skin, hair, and nails; lowers "bad" cholesterol.
Selenium	Nutritional yeast, soy foods, whole grains	Trace mineral which works synergetically with vitamin E to prevent free radical damage

11 WAYS TO STAY ON A HOLIDAY DIET

Holiday dieting is not easy. One big gingerbread cookie has 200 calories, and cranberry sauce (which no Thanksgiving turkey or turkey substitute is complete without) has more sugar than a jug of Kool-Aid™. In fact, a typical holiday or Thanksgiving menu, with such staples as nuts, cranberry sauce, gravy, stuffing and pie—with seconds—can rack up more than 5,000 calories—two or three days' worth of body fueling rolled into one.

But you don't have to fall off the weight-loss wagon just because it's Hanukkah, the Fourth of July, Christmas, or New Year's. Here are 11 healthy holiday "How Not-To's."

1. When you feel like you could eat your holiday head off, grab a calorie countdown and learn the awful truth. Then grab hunger by the ears. Two acupressure techniques that put the brake on bingeing: Insert your index fingers gently into your ears with palms turned toward face. Place thumbs on the little bump of cartilage at the front of the ear. Massage this bump between thumbs and index fingers for a minute or more. An alternate technique: Find the small depressions in front of your ears. Rub with index fingers, using a circular motion, for a minute or two. Repeat as needed. Meanwhile, memorize these morsel totals:

Food	Calories
3 oz. dark meat turkey	160
3 oz. white meat turkey	135
1 cup plain mashed potatoes	160
2 medium pieces candied sweet potatoes	290
1 cup creamed corn	185
1 cup broccoli with 1 pat butter	80
¼ cup cranberry sauce	102
¼ cup turkey gravy	128
½ cup bread stuffing	251
1 3½″ wedge mincemeat pie	504
1 3½″ wedge pecan pie	431

2. Hanukkah Halvah-and-cracker snacks doing your diet in? Switch to raw zucchini slices, spread with homemade 10-calories-a-

tablespoon Mock Boursin Cheese Spread: Mix 1 pound of uncreamed (farmer's) cottage cheese or soft tofu with one mashed minced clove of garlic. Season to taste with chopped parsley, pepper, and Italian herbs. Chill. Add festive fresh green peas in the pod as a salted-peanut substitute for 75% fewer calories total.

3. Have pickles, not peppermints, at the Fourth of July picnic. The overpoweringly sweet-sour but spicy flavor of this 15-calorie-a-piece vegetable satisfies the craving for sweets. One with each meal and two after dinner is said to suppress a runaway appetite.

4. To eat out and keep calories low, eat ethnic. Typical holiday meal totals? Mexican, 612; Italian, 941; and Chinese 1,247. Worst sodium offenders? American (1,380 grams) and Middle Eastern (3,773). And don't waste calories at parties. Head for the hors d'oeuvres tables, choose two or three large, low-calorie, high-fiber tidbits (raw vegetable sticks, fresh fruit, plain crackers), and slowly savor them to block the urge to binge.

5. Avoid celebration munchies that jangle nerves and stimulate the appetite, including chocolate, cocoa, and avocados. All contain caffeine or caffeine-like stimulants. Instead, reach for yogurt, which contains tyrosine, a safe but stimulating amino acid.

6. Easter brunch followed by an Easter family dinner? Don't binge. Carry a bottle of plain water, and take a slug when you get the urge to overindulge. Water dampens the appetite and flushes out excess sodium that causes bloating. At home, keep frozen herb tea (peppermint, chamomile, or green tea) in ice cube trays. When you get the urge to nibble, suck a cube. It keeps your mouth filled and your hunger fulfilled. To get your RDA for vitamin C at the same time, add 1 teaspoon of powdered vitamin C before freezing. Vitamin C is the dieter's "powdered willpower."

7. Health foods that can add up to hefty holiday calorie counts, too? Watch out for banana chips, 100 calories per ounce; dry roasted almonds, 270 calories an ounce; sesame tahini, 80 calories per tablespoon; chick peas, 250 calories per cup; and sunflower seeds, 80 calories a handful.

8. Avoid the Halloween (or any other holiday) sugar blues. Two ounces of holiday hard candy supply 35 to 40 grams of refined sugar (5 teaspoons). And a small candy bar (or chocolate bunny) supplies 250

calories, 50% from fat. Reach for a peach or a pear, which derives 50% of its calories from complex carbohydrates.

9. Spend a lot of time under the mistletoe or hit the kissing booth, not the strawberry shortcake stand, at that May Day picnic. Scientists say that the average kiss consumes between 6 and 12 calories. At the rate of two kisses a day—one in the morning and one at night—in one-year you could lose 2½ pounds.

10. If you're tipping the scales after the trimming-the-tree buffet or Halloween pigout, repent for a few days with baby foods. With a little spice or herbs to improve seasoning, baby foods aren't half bad. Puréed apricot makes a good fruit mousse substitute. And it's easy to control calories because each jar averages 100 calories.

11. Last but not least? How do you fit a fresh fruit fruit cake or birthday carrot cake into a diet that allows only 1,000 calories a day? Easy. Add a calorie-busting workout. Here's how a good holiday run-around can add up:

	Time	Calories burned
House cleaning	3 hrs.	666
Washing, waxing the kitchen floor	1 hr.	384
Writing and addressing holiday cards	2 hrs.	200
Baking holiday cookies and decorating	1 hr.	150
Cooking Thanksgiving dinner	3 hrs.	486
Going for a work-it-all-off job	1 hr.	600
Raking leaves or shoveling snow	2 hrs.	384
Ice skating or roller blading	1 hr.	360
Ballroom dancing	1 hr.	366*
Playing cards/board games	1 hr.	150

* As many calories as 30 minutes of aerobics

THE SUPER HEALING NUTRITION DIET

DAY ONE

(See recipes for items marked with an asterisk.)

Breakfast

> Fresh fruit cup (grapefruit/kiwi/orange section) with bran sprinkles (oat, wheat, rice, or corn)
>
> 1 scrambled egg or eggless (tofu) scrambled egg
>
> Toasted corn or millet muffin
>
> Herb tea with honey

Snack

> 1 mini oat bran muffin or 2 sesame crackers
>
> 1 cup low-fat dairy or nondairy milk

Lunch

> 1 cup Celery Borscht* or instant reconstituted bean soup
>
> 2 cauliflower croquettes with Two-Root Coulis or tofu mayo

Dinner

> 1 slice Clear-Conscience Cheesecake (O-D) or fresh grapes
>
> 10-Sprigs Parsley Tea or green tea

Snack

> Tropical Fruit Smoothie

DAY TWO

Breakfast

> 1 medium tangerine or ¹/₂ pink or white grapefruit or 1 cup pommelo sections
>
> 2 buckwheat pancakes with 1 tablespoon honey or fruit syrup

Snack

> Green tea, hot or iced and ¹/₄ cup roasted, unsalted nuts and seeds

Lunch

> ¹/₂ cup Avocado guacamole with natural potato or corn chips
> Reduced-fat herb dressing
> 1 whole wheat roll with unsalted butter or Broccoli Butter
> 1 cup skim milk or 1% soy milk
> 1 cup fresh fruit or vegetable of your choice

Dinner

> 1 white or sweet baked potato with tahini or Parsley Pesto
> 1 cup tossed green salad
> Green tea or ginseng spice tea

Snack

> Rice cakes, any flavor, with 1 teaspoon Super Healing Hummus or Tofu
> Mayo

DAY THREE

Breakfast

> 1 cup fresh orange or carrot juice or Breakfast Gimlet
> 1 slice cinnamon toast with 1 ounce farmer (or dry curd) cheese or
> scrambled tofu
> Coffee or grain beverage with skim milk

Snack

> 1 cup Carrot Slurpy (p. 65) or tomato-celery juice with cherry tomatoes

Lunch

> 4 ounces broiled tofu in whole wheat pita bread with sliced red onions,
> lettuce
> Capsicum Citrus Salad or health deli cole slaw
> Berry thick "shake" (1 cup skim milk, 2 tablespoons each strawberries
> and plain yogurt)

Dinner

Broccoli gazpacho with sprouted lentils
1 baked yam with whipped tofu topping
1 cup chicory or dandelion greens with Juicy Fruit Vinaigrette
1 cup popped corn with Super Healing Salt or salt-free seasoning
1 glass alcohol-free sparkling wine

Snack

Cup of instant miso broth

DAY FOUR

Breakfast

1 cup whole wheat cereal with steamed apple or pear slices and toasted walnuts, or Breakfast in a Single Bite (p. 53)
1 cup steamed milk or Health Cappuccino

Lunch

Thermos couscous with broccoli or Brussels sprouts
2 rye crackers
2 Asparagus Dills (p. 20) vegetable crackers
1 medium peach or sugar-free canned peaches
1 cup skim or soy milk
1 cup Blue Ginger Beer or natural ginger (or root) beer

Snack

Green tea and berries or melon in season

Dinner

2 tofu hot dogs with salt-free salsa
Snow peas, spinach, onion salad with yogurt dressing, whole wheat croutons
Sparkling white or purple grape juice

Snack

1 cup dairy-free yogurt

DAY FIVE

Breakfast

$^{1}/_{2}$ cup sliced cherimoya or papaya or dried fruit rings

1 cup hot oat bran cereal with maple sugar or Super Healing Fruit or Fiber Sugar

Midmorning

Carob cocoa with Whipped Tofu Cream

Lunch

Eggless egg salad on whole grain bun or whole wheat croissant

Tossed green salad and sesame oil dressing

1 cup fresh fruit cocktail

1 cup steamed milk or grain "coffee"

Snack

1 cup tropical fruit cocktail (papaya, banana, mango, cherimoya, etc.)

Dinner

Frozen grain burger

1 cup cold steamed broccoli and sprouts in dill vinaigrette

1 cup of natural lemon pudding or yogurt (dairy or dairy free)

Herb tea, your choice

Snack

Tofu-Banana Smoothie

DAY SIX

Breakfast

2 Breakfast in a Single Bite (cookies or mini-muffins or waffles), or

Packaged whole grain fruit and fiber cereal with packaged soy milk

Apple cider or cranapple juice

Lunch

$^{1}/_{4}$ cup Parsley Pesto on 1 cup steamed rice, barley, or millet prepared for thermos night before)

2 plum tomatoes with lemon/pepper

2 sugar-free fig bars or ginger snaps

Mineral water

Snack

Carrot Slurpy with 2 sesame crackers

Dinner

Frozen whole wheat pizza

Lentil/spinach salad with Green Goddess dressing

Alcohol-free beer

Snack

Decaf latté with 1 rice cracker

DAY SEVEN

Breakfast

1 cup super hi protein cereal (amaranth, quinoa, triticale) with half-and-half or skim milk

1 cup skim milk or 1 cup fresh Two-Citrus Crush or

Berry juice, your choice

Snack

2 ounces tofu jerky or sugar-free fruit leather

Lunch

1 cup thermos asparagus gazpacho (prepared the night before) and tofu croutons

2 ounces low-fat natural cheese

1 medium apple

1 cup skim milk

1 cup fresh juice, your choice

Dinner

Vegetarian BLT

Whole Wheat Pasta and Beans

Herb tea

2 oatmeal or peanut butter cookies

Snack

Super Healing Posset or steamed low-fat milk

TEN BASIC SUPER HEALING RECIPES

Butter, margarine, cream, sugar, and salt: Can't live with them, can't live without them unless you know a few healthy alternative tricks. Try the following substitutes. Note: For a shelf full of superhealing salt substitutes, see recipes p. 276, Substitutes (p. 191 and 35) Super Healing Hints (p. 363), and Dairy Substitutes (p. 174).

Half 'n Half Butter #1

Combine 3 parts sesame tahini with 1 part soy sauce. Thin with lemon juice. Use on baked potatoes, over steamed grains and vegetables and pasta, and as a bread spread.

Sweet Super Healing Butter: Combine 3/4 cup tahini (or other nut butter) with 1 part honey, date, or rice syrup.

Super Healing Tofu Mayo (eggless)

2 cups soft tofu, mashed

2 tablespoons olive oil

1 or 2 cloves garlic, crushed

2 tablespoons lemon juice

1 teaspoon mustard

1 teaspoon honey (optional)

Drain tofu and press out excess water.

Combine all ingredients in a blender or food processor. Purée until smooth and creamy. (Add 1 teaspoon water if needed.)

Makes 2 cups.

Healing Half 'n Half*

½ cup dry skim milk

½ cup hot water or warm whey

1 tablespoon almond oil

Combine, liquefy, and refrigerate

Swiss Whip Cream*

Grate Swiss very fine and gradually add tomato juice, 1 drop at a time. Mix until it's the consistency of thick whipped cream.

Super Healing Fruit and Fiber Sugar

2½ cups noninstant rolled oats

2 cups Grape Nuts™-type cereal

½ cup bran (oat, wheat, corn) or wheat germ

½ cup nonfat dry dairy or nondairy milk powder

1 pinch each cinnamon and allspice

2 dried apple rings or 2 dried apricots, finely diced

2 or 3 tablespoons undiluted apple juice concentrate

Preheat oven to low 275 degrees.

Combine all ingredients. Spread on a flat nonstick pan, spreading mixture into a thin layer.

Bake for 45 minutes until mixture is very dry.

Grind to a powder in blender or processor. Store in airtight jar.

Use as a low-calorie high-fiber granulated table sugar substitute.

---

* Also see Dairy Substitutes for more options.

Fast-Fix Nut Sugar

Process 2 cups unsweetened flaked coconut in blender (with or without pinch of cinnamon or tablespoon of bran—oat, wheat, rice, or corn).

Variation: Toast before grinding.

Healing Plus Purées

Did you know that 1 ounce of tomato purée (paste) supplies twice the antioxidant power of one fresh tomato and double the beta-carotene? And what's true for tomatoes holds for any other whole food whose goodness is concentrated by condensing into a purée or paste or sun drying (tomatoes, raisins) into dry powder.

A little dab will do you of any of the following. Use as dips, spreads, and sauce and soup starters.

Vegetable Purée

> *3 cups celery root, trimmed, peeled, and cut into ¹/₂-inch cubes*
>
> *2 medium baking potatoes, peeled and cut into 1-inch cubes*
>
> *2 medium turnips, peeled and cut into ¹/₂-inch cubes*
>
> *4 leeks (white part only), washed well and sliced into 1-inch pieces*
>
> *Freshly ground pepper to taste*

Place celery root, potatoes, turnips, and leeks in large saucepan, cover with cold water, and bring to a boil. Reduce heat, simmer for 30 minutes.

Drain, pass vegetables through a ricer. Add pepper and serve warm.

Makes four servings.

Parsnip-Potato-and-Roasted-Garlic Purée

> *4 large parsnips, peeled and cut into ¹/₂-inch thick rounds*
>
> *2 large baking potatoes, peeled and cut into ¹/₂-inch cubes*
>
> *10 large cloves roasted garlic, peeled*
>
> *¹/₂ cup low-fat milk*
>
> *2 teaspoons salt, plus more to taste*
>
> *Freshly ground pepper to taste.*

Place the parsnips in a large saucepan and cover with water. Place over medium-high heat and bring to a boil. Reduce heat and simmer for 5 minutes. Add the potatoes and cook until parsnips and potatoes are soft, about 15 minutes. Drain well and pass the vegetables through a ricer into a medium-size bowl.

Stir the roasted garlic and the milk into the purée until well combined. Salt and pepper to taste. Divide among 4 plates and serve immediately.

Yield: 6-8 servings.

Sweet-Potato Purée Plus

> *2 large sweet potatoes, pricked several times with a fork*
>
> *2 tart apples*
>
> *1/8 teaspoon ground cardamom*
>
> *Freshly ground pepper to taste*

Preheat oven to 450 degrees. Place sweet potatoes on baking sheet and roast 15 minutes. Add whole apples. Roast until potatoes and apples are soft (25 minutes).

Skin potatoes. Pass apples and potatoes through food mill. Stir in cardamom and pepper to taste.

Serve warm.

Makes four servings.

35 HINTS FOR SUPER HEALING NUTRITION

1. Plenty of peas will sweeten soup. An abundance of onions will do the same for spaghetti sauce.

2. Cinnamon is not forever. To keep fresher longer, refrigerate. The same goes for ginger and cloves. Vanilla beans keep best stored side by side with a humidifying cake that can be moistened as needed. (Tobacco stores sell them.)

3. A perfect brown-not-burned pie crust every time even if you're cooking with wheat flour substitutes? Place a 1½-inch-wide strip of foil around crust; bake as recipe indicates. Remove foil the last 15 minutes of baking.

4. Did you know that cherries are members of the rose family, lemons are related to azaleas, peaches are related to almonds, and tomatoes are botanically classified as orchard fruits? Have a Healthy Mary before your next workout: Combine equal parts of tomato or orange juice and yogurt. Add a twist of lemon or lime. Pour into frosted tumbler.

5. Lost and found. By age 70 you will have lost 40 pounds of body weight in the form of dead skin (16% of body weight is skin). By 75, if you never have a manicure, your fingernails will be 13 feet long.

6. Store-bought jam has 55 calories a glob. Make 60-second Health Spread: Purée soft blueberries with a squirt of lemon juice. Refrigerate, and it's ready to spread in an hour.

7. For cornier fresh corn, line the steaming pan with corn husks before adding water.

8. To keep your nails from splitting, coat them with olive oil. Plain petroleum jelly also works as a protective coating.

9. Five time savers:

♦ For no-stick raisin chopping: freeze raisins, then lightly spray bowl and blades of a food processor with vegetable spray.

♦ For tomatoes that slip out of their skins, freeze and peel. Freezing is also the way to save surplus tomatoes.

♦ Freezing Parmesan and other hard cheeses makes them grate more easily and eliminates small chunks that get stuck in grater holes.

♦ Vegetables taste fresher reheated with a curl of lemon peel (just two minutes does the trick). Mash avocados with a teaspoon of lemon juice to prevent discoloration. Freeze and thaw when needed for dips and spreads.

♦ Bag juiced citrus shells and keep in the freezer to use as serving cups for frozen yogurt, fruit, and pudding, or grate for seasoning other dishes.

10. Need a 10% fat pastry butter? Make your own nutritious prune purée: Purée 4 ounces of pitted prunes with 3 tablespoons water. Use in place of butter in thick-textured cookies, cakes, and brownies. Prunes are rich in fiber, vitamin A, iron, and potassium.

11. Downsize fat and calories and upgrade your health: A standard 12-inch pizza crust has 900 calories and 20+ grams of fat. For a 200-calorie zero-fat crust, make your own using 15% flour and 85% whipped egg white.

12. Dieting? Hold your nose and turn off your appetite. With a clothes pin on your nose, say researchers, you can't tell the difference between chocolate and celery. So pig out on Pascal celery but think Godiva.

13. To reduce light-sensitive vitamin A losses in skim milk, by 60%, buy it in cardboard cartons or yellow or white plastic jugs.

14. Cut your risk of at least six major diseases by taking. the "waist-to-hip" ratio test and doing something about it. An apple-shaped body (with excess fat padded around a midsection atop slim hips and thighs) has a higher risk of developing heart disease, high blood pressure, stroke, diabetes, breast cancer, and endometrial cancer than pear shapes (fat concentrated at the hips, buttocks, and thighs). To calculate your risk, stand with feet together and divide your waist measurement taken at the belly button by that of your hips at their widest point. If that number is above 0.73, it's time to shape up. The good news? Fat cells in the abdomen are the easiest to shrink.

15. To make spices stick to popcorn, lightly coat the kernels with butter-flavored vegetable spray as it cools, and then sprinkle on chili or onion powder or a salt substitute.

16. Did you know that the largest, strongest muscle in the body is the gluteus maximus in the outer hip but that the longest is the sartorius, which extends from the waist to the knee? And that the most calorie-intensive way to work both of them out is to jog or race-walk on sand?

17. Got some overripe peaches? Make additives-free duck sauce. Peel peaches, and purée in processor or blender with a dash of soy sauce, vinegar, or lemon juice to taste. Refrigerate.

18. Nourishing your nails? Get more copper-rich oranges and tangerines into your diet. Copper contributes to smooth skin and normal nail growth. It's also found in almonds, salad greens, and beets.

19. Orange juice allergy? Skin rashes and headaches, according to. Dr. Seymour Diamond, president of the National Migraine Foundation, are tipoffs. The reaction is caused by amines (also found in chocolate, tea, coffee, and red wine). Test it out: Relax for a few minutes and take your pulse. Eat half an orange or drink a glass of juice. Take your pulse 15 minutes later. If it is up more than 10 beats per minute, it indicates an allergy.

20. An elegant, easy way to fix low-fat, oil-free entrees *en papillote* (in a package): Place tofu, tempeh, or similar meat substitute on parch-

ment paper, top with sliced vegetables. season, sprinkle with water, tea, or juice, fold and crimp edges tightly, and steam. Bake in 375-degree oven for 15 minutes.

21. How to have crisp French toast with syrup-catching nooks and crannies built in? Fix it in your waffle maker.

22. Magic act #1—waffle, don't bake, your next batch of bran or corn or multigrain muffins, and use as a foundation for creamed vegetables or yogurty fruits combos.

23. You burn an extra 25 calories if you swing your arms while climbing stairs.

24. To calm a queasy stomach, make a Papaya Pepto: Peel a papaya, remove seed, sweeten if desired; add the juice of one lemon for each 2 cups of fruit; purée.

25. What's a speedy way to remove a speck in your eye? If lifting your lid doesn't do the trick, pop in a flaxseed. As it gently moves beneath your lid, it secretes a jelly-like substance that ousts the invading offender.

26. The air freshener alternative: eucalyptus leaves. The branches are decorative, and longlasting, and all you do is rub the leaves to intensify the aroma. (These are available at floral shops.)

27. Fat chances: Limiting your intake of butter, meat, and pastry helps you lose your fat tooth, says Fred Hutchinson Cancer Research Center, University of Washington. How long does no-gain and no-pain taste-bud retraining take? About six months of eating non- and low-fat yogurt, cheese, salad dressings, and snacks—after which your fatty old favorites, say Center directors, will taste unpleasant.

28. Three freezer tips: Squeeze a dozen lemons, freeze the juice in ice cube trays, and store cubes in freezer bags. Sauté minced onions and freeze in half-cup batches. Cook two or three types of beans and/or two or three types of grains and freeze in 1-cup portions.

29. An I-can't-believe-this-isn't-whipped-cream dessert topping: Whip 2 cups chilled nonfat skim milk with 1 tablespoon rice syrup and $1/4$ teaspoon almond extract to taste until stiff peaks form.

30. Quick-whipped cream #2: Add one sliced banana to the white of one egg. Beat until banana dissolves and cream is stiff.

31. High-tech help for light sleepers: If you need an alternative to ear plugs, get a white-noise machine that uses its own low hum to

"white out" street noise and loud neighbors (available from sleep shops and mail order health product dealers).

32. Like to lighten up your salad dressing? Add 2 tablespoons of sparkling mineral water (plain, lemon, or lime) to 2/3 cup vinaigrette dressing. Adds a subtle tanginess and helps cut calories.

33. Fruit Spritzer Magic Act. Write your name in apple, lemon, or orange juice on a sheet of paper. Let dry until writing vanishes. To make it visible again, hold paper close to a warm toaster or light bulb.

34. Health-whisked soup tip: Smartest way to make cream soup is to stir with a wire whisk. A blender can break down protein particles and cause curdling when the milk and hot liquid combine.

35. Are prescription drugs a must? Safeguard yourself from side-effects. Get a copy of *Consumers Guide to Prescription Medicine* from the Pharmaceutical Manufacturers Association, 1100 15th St. N.W., Washington, DC 20005.

MORE IS LESS
Nutritional Trade-Offs That Let You Eat More and Cut Fat by 30-50%

How to chart a new course if you've got a thumbs-up urge to eat right but a lot of thumbs-down habits? It's not as hard as you think. The trick? Trade-offs that cut fat. Why fat? Because that's the biochemical key to weight loss. While each fat gram contains 9 calories, carbohydrates and proteins contain only 4. But there's another reason. The gastrointestinal tract, brain, liver, and sections of the spinal cord contain receptors that keep track of the carbohydrates you eat, which is critical because carbohydrates are broken down into a quick energy called glucose that prevents complications—nerve and kidney damage and circulatory problems. So when you reduce carbohydrates your body fights back by triggering the appetite. But there are no such receptors for fat. So what you eliminate you don't miss.

In a recent Cornell University study of two groups of women on an 11-week diet, women put on the low-fat regimen automatically consumed fewer calories and shed an average of 5 pounds without any hunger backlash.

What's the max with fat? For men on a 2,500-calories-a-day diet, the actual RDA range is 75 to 95 grams, but a healthier ceiling is 50 to 60 grams. Here are 16 trade-offs that cover your eating in, out, on the road, in the office, at the movies, and during coffee breaks and Happy Hours and allow you to eat more but get one third to one half of the fat, sodium, and sucrose of the original main dish, side dish, or snack.*

16 FAT AND CALORIE TRADE-OFFS

THUMBS DOWN Instead of this:	THUMBS UP Make, choose, order, or brown-bag this:
1 fast-food cinnamon-raisin Danish pastry Fat: 21 grams Calories: 440	2 fast-food fat-free fruit bran muffins Fat: 0 grams Calories: 375–400
1 egg fried in butter, 3 strips bacon, 2 slices white toast with 2 pats butter and 2 teaspoons strawberry jam Fat: 26 grams Calories: 450	2 eggs fried in nonstick, nonfat vegetable spray, 1 English muffin with 1 pat butter or margarine or olive oil, 1 fresh orange Fat: 15 grams Calories: 300
1 cup "natural" granola-style cereal with ⅔ cup whole milk Fat: 23 grams Calories: 325	1.5 cups unsweetened whole grain dry cereal in 1 cup 1% low-fat milk or soy milk with ½ banana Fat: 8 grams Calories: 295
1 blueberry toaster pastry Fat: 6 grams Calories: 220	2 slices whole wheat toast with 2 teaspoons no-sugar-added berry preserves Fat: 3 grams Calories: 200
1 glazed doughnut Fat: 13 grams Calories: 235	1 small blueberry muffin (1.5 ounce) plus 1 sliced kiwi fruit Fat: 6 grams Calories: 175

---

* Did you know, for instance, that spreading mustard, not mayo, on your sandwich 5 days a week leads to a 13-lb. weight loss at year's end?

THUMBS DOWN Instead of this:	THUMBS UP Make, choose, order, or brown-bag this:

1 ounce breakfast croissant
with ham (6 ounces)
    Fat: 17 grams
    Calories: 550
	1 bagel with 2 thin slices low-fat ham
	    Fat: 6 grams
	    Calories: 250

1 standard slice cheesecake
    Fat: 18 grams
    Calories: 200
	1 cup nonfat frozen vanilla yogurt
	and 3 gingersnaps
	    Fat 5 grams
	    Calories: 200

4 cups vegetable-oil-popped popcorn
drizzled with 2 tablespoons butter
flavoring (movie theater)
    Fat: 35 grams
    Calories: 420
	4 cups air-popped popcorn, no butter
	    Fat: 2 grams
	    Calories: 200

1 bag potato chips (3 ounces) with
2 tablespoons creamy dip
    Fat: 38 grams
    Calories: 650
	2 whole wheat pitas (1 ounce)
	with 2 tablespoons mustard dip
	    Fat: 5 grams
	    Calories: 190

1 packaged chocolate-chunk cookie
(0.9 ounce)
    Fat: 6 grams
    Calories: 120
	3 graham crackers
	    Fat: 2 grams
	    Calories: 90

1 ice cream sandwich (2.7 ounces)
    Fat: 7 grams
    Calories: 290
	2 fruit popsicles (twin)
	    Fat: 0
	    Calories: 140

1 cup potato salad with regular
mayonnaise
    Fat: 21 grams
    Calories: 325
	2 ears fresh corn with 1 pat
	butter
	    Fat: 0.5 gram
	    Calories: 280

Salted roasted peanuts (3 ounces)
    Fat: 14 grams
    Calories: 375
	Thompson seedless grapes, 3 clusters
	    Fat: 2 grams
	    Calories: 100

1 cup lettuce with 2 tablespoons
bottled Italian dressing
    Fat: 14 grams
    Calories: 160
	1½ cups lettuce with croutons, shredded
	carrots, tomato, and 1 tablespoon low-fat
	vinaigrette dressing
	    Fat: 7 grams
	    Calories: 150

1 cup potatoes au gratin, made
from a dry mix
    Fat: 10 grams
    Calories: 250
	2½ medium baked potatoes (without
	skin) topped with 1½ tablespoons nonfat
	yogurt and ½ tablespoon chopped
	chives each
	    Fat: 0
	    Calories: 200

1 cup chocolate pudding, made
with whole milk
    Fat: 10 grams
    Calories: 250
	1 cup gelatin dessert, sugar-free
	    Fat: 0
	    Calories: 35

Even better than a store-bought swap is a homemade one. Try this recipe:

Lemon Nuts (The smokehouse-almond alternative)

2 cups whole raw almonds

2 tablespoons olive or canola oil

2 tablespoons fresh squeezed lemon juice

1 tablespoon fresh grated lemon

Sauté almonds in oil in large skillet over medium-low heat for 1 to 2 minutes. Sprinkle with lemon juice and stir until absorbed. Add peel; stir until well blended. Remove nuts from skillet with slotted spoon and drain on paper towels. Store in airtight margarine tub or apothecary/canning jar. Makes 2 cups, 75-95 calories a handful, 8-10 grams unsaturated fat.

Variations: Substitute cashew, pecan, or walnut halves; use lime or ginger juice in place of lemon juice.

TARGET 2,000*
Nutrition-Supportive Exercise

Healing or not, super nutrition doesn't come without calories and it doesn't cover *all* the high-level wellness bases. You still have to get physical once your life is filled with apples, broccoli, and brown rice. Research indicates that the less fit you are, the more likely you are to die from heart disease or cancer. Exercise also helps prevent osteoporosis, diabetes, and high blood pressure, elevates mood, and regulates the appetite, according to the American Holistic Medical Association.

Research also indicates that your metabolic rate rises about 10% after a meal because of the processes involved in digestion of a meal.

---

* Research indicates that expending a minimum of 1,050 calories a week in physical exercise provides peak protection against heart disease by 15% or more. This usually means an hour five or six times a week.

This is called the thermic effect (TE) of food, and the lower the fat content of the food, the greater the effect will be. The even better news is that you can double the TE by doing some light physical exercise within 30 minutes of eating. In fact, you can actually transform your meal into a calorie-burning (rather than a weight-increasing) experience if you combine light activity with a sensible diet.

So what's the 10-grain, 10-speed food and fitness connection? Take a look at your options.

	Cal/hr	Cal/hr	Cal/hr/lb
Aerobic Exercise			
Soccer	666	481	3.7
Table tennis	342	247	1.9
Tennis (singles)	522	377	2.9
Tennis (doubles)	324	234	1.8
Volleyball	396	286	2.2
Walking (2–2.5 mph)	288	208	1.6
Walking (3.5 mph)	432	312	2.4
Water skiing	540	390	3.0
Cycling (10 mph)	486	351	2.7
Jogging	756	546	4.2
Jumping rope	684	494	3.8
Rowing machine	558	403	3.1
Swimming (slow crawl)	630	455	3.5
Weight training	342	247	1.9
Stair climbing (per 12-stair flight)	4.5	3.3	0.025
Fun Stuff			
Badminton	468	338	2.6
Billiards	198	143	1.1
Dancing (ballroom)	288	208	1.6
Fishing (standing)	234	169	1.3
Golf (walking)	411	299	2.3
Hiking (hilly)	648	468	3.6

(continued on next page)

	Cal/hr	Cal/hr	Cal/hr/lb
Horseback riding (trot)	504	364	2.8
Playing piano	198	143	1.1
Scuba diving	684	494	3.8
Sex	240	170	1.3
Skating	468	338	2.6
Racquetball	738	533	4.1
Miscellaneous			
Gardening (dig/hoe)	576	416	3.2
House cleaning	288	208	1.6
Ironing	162	117	0.9
Mopping	306	221	1.7

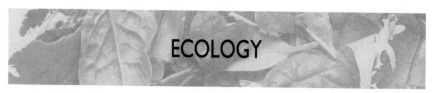

ECOLOGY

Raise your super healing consciousness and extend it to the earth and other people. Here are 26 good ways to be the good green global citizen you were meant to be.

1. Protect yourself and your family from environmental toxins that cling to nonorganic produce with a fruit and vegetable wash formulated to remove 2,000 times more surface dirt than water alone and reduce malathion residue by 50% (ask at your health food store).

2. Spring into spring with an herbal wreath. They're easy to put together: Tie fresh or dried herbs in little bundles and attach them to a straw wreath form so they overlap each other. Make a swag to hang over the doorway or window by using rope as the form. Experiment with colors and fragrances (e.g., wire-edged ribbons for a bright, Victorian feeling).

3. Be a Power of Ten. Buying organic perpetuates planetary as well as personal health and healing. Here are nine good green deeds you do each time you choose organic produce: You contribute to building living soils; promote growth of clean, healthy food; ensure pure water supply; protect clean air; promote wastes recycling; help in reversing global warming; help with preservation of wildlife habitats; encourage diversity; and honor rural life and farming.

4. Be a Power of Ten II: Thinking about writing a letter protesting the wasteful packaging practices of a company you do business with? One person who puts it in writing, say researchers, is the equivalent of 10 who don't or won't.

5. So where can you get the healing best in foods that's coming to you? Try the Americans For Safe Food guide to 75 mail order organic food sources. Write or call Americans For Safe Food, 1875 Connecticut Avenue, NW, Suite 300, Washington, DC 20009-5728; (202) 332-9110. Cost: $1.50.

6. Shop green and clean. *National Green Pages* gives you reliable lists of eco-friendly companies plus mail order products from "businesses with a vision." And to support indigenous peoples striving to make a decent living, write *Co-op America*. 2100 Main St., #403, Washington, DC 20063; (202) 872-5307.

7. Pass it on. Curlpak™, a new packaging material made of paper-thin, fluffy curls of wood from wood scrap blocks previously destined for the landfill, can go directly into a compost pile after unpacking. Two more styrofoam substitutes: shredded computer paper or real popcorn.

8. Don't store your produce in non-biodegradable plastic—invest in reusable ripening bags impregnated with a finely ground zeolite stone, a mineral that absorbs ethylene gas, slows down the ripening process, and keeps foods fresh longer. By mail, $10 plus postage for 20 bags from Vermont Country Store in Manchester Center, VT, (802) 362-2400, or other environmental supply catalogs.

9. Practice pollution control with indoor plants. Bromeliads and orchids remove harmful toxins such as carbon dioxide, methyl alcohol, and ethyl alcohol from the air while you sleep.

10. Travel green. Take a trek that uplifts body, mind, and spirit—learn Stone Age survival skills, live with indigenous craftspeople, take a family vision-quest vacation, tour the world's sacred grounds. For more information call Travel Program Director, Institute of Noetic Sciences, 50 River Rd., Grandview-on-Hudson, NY 10960, (800) 353-2276; Gordon Frost Folk Art Tours, PO Box 2, Benicia, CA 94510; (707) 747-1316; Journeys Together, PO Box 1254, La Mesa, CA 91944, (619) 224-4175; The Educated Traveler, PO Box 220822, Chantilly, VA 22022, (800) 648-5168.

11. Easy on your skin, easy on the earth: Five reasons natural beauty products are a better buy: They reduce waste; don't animal test; use renewable resources; are sustainably harvested, and reinvest a percentage of their profits back into the environment. One good by-mail source to get you started: Environmentally Sound Products, 8845 Orchard Tree Lane, Towson, MD 21286, (800) 886-5432.

12. Do your eco-bit for energy conservation. Use bulb-life extenders. Placed on the base of a light bulb, they dim lights by 30 to 70% and cut energy costs in half. Other smart bulb buys—Power Misers™, Convert-a-Bulb™, and full-spectrum fluorescents (at health food and health pharmacies. See listings p. 379).

13. Join the fight for pesticide reform. (Toxic residue on fruits and vegetables exceeds the safety-for-kids limits by 100%, says the National Academy of Science.) Write the House Health and Environment Subcommittee of the Energy and Commerce Committee. Express your support of a ban on all carcinogenic chemicals in the food supply.

14. Coffee without the chemicals: Did you know coffee is the most chemically treated food crop on the planet? Look for certified organic grinds blended with herbs for one sixth the usual caffeine.

15. Be a super healing minimalist. Set your thermostat at 70 degrees and your end-of-summer electric bill will be 40% lower than it would be at 78 degrees. Reduce your exposure to health-hazardous chemicals (70,000 have entered the environment since 1970)—use one no-risk, biodegradable, does-it-all cleaner/degreaser for everything from soup bowls to toilet bowls. Available at natural health stores, or call Earth Fundamentals 1-800-50-*EARTH*.

16. Sixty percent of all fruits and vegetables carry pesticide residues to market. The four crops likeliest to give you a pesticide over-

dose—apples, celery, peaches, and potatoes. Rx: Visit small-farmer-owned U-pick ranches for peace-of-mind produce.

17. Potpourri lost its punch? Recycle it into the cat litter box.

18. Donate lint from your dryer to the birds for nest lining.

19. Recycle crumpled newspapers for a cost-effective paper towel alternative for washing mirrors and windows.

20. Be a cash-and-carry catalyst for the common good. Three good green funds that specialize in responsible investing: Pax World Fund, 1-800-767-1729; Rightime Social Awareness Fund, 1-800-242-1421; Schiald Progressive Environmental, 1-800-275-2382.

21. Summer in a jar. Here's a hurry-up way to dry your blooms: Mix 10 parts white cornmeal to three parts borax. Bury flowers in mixture and set aside until they set.

22. Green thumber: Buy earth-friendly, low- or nontoxic insecticides such as Adios™, BT, horticultural oils, pyrethrins, or rotenone botanical solution.

23. Beauty is in the eye of the beholder. Put your postage stamp yard or half-plus acre to esthetic good use. Grow a native wildlife garden—designed to attract butterflies and songbirds and to produce edible blooms for your salad bowl. Details and catalogs from Prairie Nursery, PO Box 306, Westfield, WI 53964.

24. Do your banking with eco-friendly checks that advertise a cause you care about—from women's rights to world hunger. Using recycled paper and nontoxic soy ink are two more plusses. For information, call 800-243-2585. See Mail Order Sources.

25. Tie one on and help the environment. One Song Enterprises (800-771-SONG) sells men's neckties recycled from old sidewalls. Or check your environmental products supplier for Deja shoes (casuals and sneaks) made from recycled milk jugs, coffee filters, and polystyrene cups.

26. Eco bytes: Buy some health and healing with every bite, scoop, slice, or cupful. Buy all your household staples from firms that subscribe to nonexploitive workplace practices and tithe to the needy and the environment. For a scoreboard, see the guide "Shopping for a Better World" at health food or book stores.

MAIL ORDER SOURCES

Organic Produce

Americans For Safe Food
1875 Connecticut Ave. NW
Washington, DC 2009-5728
1-202-332-9110

Offers guide to mail order sources

Center for Science
 in the Public Interest
1501 16th St. NW
Washington, DC 10036

List of nationwide dealers

Gold Mine Natural Food Co.
1947 30th St.
San Diego, CA 92102-1105
1-800-475-FOOD

Natural and macrobiotic foods,
cookware, juices, etc.

Natural Lifestyle Supplies
16 Lookout Dr.
Asheville, NC 28804
1-800-752-2775

Natural and macrobiotic foods,
cookware, juices, etc.

Whole Health Direct
1-800-721-1400

Consumer Nutrition Hotline
1-800-366-1655

Organic Herbs, Vegetable Seeds, Flowers (catalogs available)

Peace Seeds
2385 S.E. Thompson
Corvallis, OR 97333

Unusual vegetables, such
as apple green eggplant.
Catalog arranged by
botanical families

Peter Pepper Seeds
c/o H.W. Alfrey
P.O. Box 415
Knoxville, TN 37901

Unusual peppers (peter,
dogtooth, squash) plus
other vegetables.

Salt Spring Seeds
Box 33
Banges, BC,
CANADA VOS IEO

Organic seeds, including 100 varieties of dried beans.

Seed Savers Exchange
3076 North Winn Road
Decorah, IA 52101

Dedicated to preserving heirloom and endangered nonhybrid vegetables and fruits and grains. More than 10,000 vegetable varieties offered by members to members ($1 for membership information brochure).

Seeds of Change
621 Old Sante Fe #10
Santa Fe, NM 87501
505-438-8080

500 varieties of certified-organic seeds

Shepherd's Garden Seeds
6116 Highway 9
Felton, CA 95018
408-335-6910

Unusual vegetables, including mescium mixtures.

Tomato Growers Supply Co.
P.O. Box 2237
Fort Myers, FL 33902

180 tomato varieties; 52 pepper varieties.

Horticultural Enterprises
P.O. Box 810082
Dallas, TX 75381

Pepper specialists; more than 30 varieties of hot and sweet pepper.

Environmentally-Friendly Foods and Household Products

(from rain-forest corn flakes to fountain pens, recycled paper products, non-rechargeable batteries, plastic substitutes, homemade soaps, herbal pesticides, and dried tofu)

Fruit and Vegetable Washes

Mountain Ark
P.O. Box 3170
Fayetteville, AR 72702
1-800-643-8909

Environmentally Sound Products
8845 Orchard Tree Lane
Towson, MD 21286
1-800-886-5432

Earth Fundamentals
66 Witherspoon Street, Suite 250
Princeton, NJ 08542
1-609-443-5090
FAX 1-609-443-5090
Toll Free 1-800-50-EARTH

Aromatherapy Essentials

Oshadhi Essential Oils
Box 824
Rogers, AR 72757
1-501-636-0579

Catalog of oils, floral
waters, natural perfumes.

Cruelty-free Beauty and Home Products

Contact PETA
P.O. Box 42516
Washington, DC 20015
1-301-770-6061 (PETA)

Miscellaneous

Andre Prost
1-800-243-0897

Low-fat coconut milk.

King Arthur Flour
Norwich, VT

Breads, whole grain
flours, seeds, spices,
flavorings, cookware.

Grain and Salt Society
Box DD
Magalea, CA 95954
1-916-872-5800
FAX 916-872-5524

Natural Grey Celtic
sea salt.

Health and Healing Hotlines

Herb Research Foundation
1-800-748-2617

American Botanical Council
1-800-373-7105

Cancer Information Service
1-800-422-6237

American Institute for Cancer Research
1-800-843-8114

Natural Health Hotline
1-900-933-9355
(P.O. Box 70847
Fairbanks, AL 99707)

Health Marketing Systems
(MN, IL, WI, NB, IA, ND, SD & all GNC Stores)
1-800-373-3738

American Diabetes Association Tele-library
800-847-SCAN

EAT SAFE Hotline (Food and Water Inc)
1-800-EAT-SAFE

Health Information Network Medication Information
1-900-990-9700

Physician Referrals:
AM-Board of Medical Specialties
1-800-776-2378

Ask-a-Nurse
(Referral Systems Group)
1-800-535-1111

Peoples Medical Society
1-800-624-8773

PharmaCall
1-900-446-3679

Ask the Pharmacist
1-900-420-0275

Computer-Based Info

National Library of Medicine
1-301-496-6308
(50+ databases)

Or check out the Blackbag Bulletin Board List, a guide to more than 300 computer-accessible health bulletin boards, $5 from Edward Del Grosso, MD, 29A-2 Golfview Drive, Newark, Delaware 19702.

Health Advocacy Groups

Center for Science in the Public Interest
1875 Connecticut Ave. NW, Suite 300
Washington, DC 20009-5728
1-202-332-9110

Food & Water, Inc.
Depot Hill Rd.
RR 1, Box 114
Marshfield, VT 05658-9702

Pure Food Campaign
1130 17th St. NW, Suite 630
Washington, DC 20036
1-202-775-1132

American Academy of Allergy and Immunology
611 East Wells St.
Milwaukee, WI 53202
1-414-272-6071

Alternative Health Practitioners

Aromatherapy:

National Association for Holistic Aromatherapy
PO Box 17622
Boulder, CO 80308-7622
1-303-444-0533

Herbology:

American Botanical Council
PO Box 201660
Austin, TX 78720
1-800-373-7105

Holistic Medicine:

American Holistic Medical Association
4101 Lake Boone Trail, Suite 201
Raleigh, NC 27607
1-919-787-5146

Holistic Dentistry:

Holistic Dental Association
PO Box 5007
Durango, CO 81301
1-303-259-1091

Homeopathy:

National Center for Homeopathy
801 N. Fairfax St., Suite 306
Alexandria, VA 22314
1-803-548-7790

Massage:

American Massage Therapy Association
820 Davis St.
Evanston, IL 60201
1-708-864-0123

Naturopathy:

American Association of Naturopathic Physicians
2366 Eastlake Ave. E, Suite 322
Seattle, WA 98102
1-206-323-7610

If you're looking for a spiritual healer, a good place to start is the National Federation of Spiritual Healers. For a referral, contact PO Box 2022, Mount Pleasant, SC 29465, 1-803-849-1529.

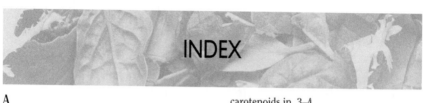

INDEX